THE FOOT
AND ITS DISORDERS

THE FOOT
AND ITS DISORDERS

EDITED BY

LESLIE KLENERMAN
ChM FRCS(Eng) FRCS(Ed)

Consultant Orthopaedic Surgeon,
Northwick Park Hospital, and Clinical Research Centre,
Harrow, Middlesex

FOREWORD BY
SIR HENRY OSMOND-CLARKE
KCVO CBE

Past-President, British Orthopaedic Association,
former Vice President, Royal College of Surgeons of England;
Consultant Orthopaedic Surgeon, The London Hospital and
Robert Jones and Agnes Hunt Orthopaedic Hospital, Oswestry

SECOND EDITION

BLACKWELL SCIENTIFIC PUBLICATIONS
OXFORD   LONDON   EDINBURGH
BOSTON   MELBOURNE

© 1976, 1982 by
Blackwell Scientific Publications
Editorial offices:
Osney Mead, Oxford OX2 0EL
8 John Street, London WC1N 2ES
9 Forrest Road, Edinburgh EH1 2QH
52 Beacon Street, Boston,
   Massachusetts 02108, USA
99 Barry Street, Carlton, Victoria 3053
   Australia

First published 1976
Second edition 1982

Printed in Great Britain
at the Alden Press, Oxford.
Bound by Butler & Tanner Ltd,
Frome and London

DISTRIBUTORS

USA
   Blackwell Mosby Book Distributors
   11830 Westline Industrial Drive
   St Louis, Missouri 63141

Canada
   Blackwell Mosby Book Distributors
   120 Melford Drive, Scarborough
   Ontario M1B 2X4

Australia
   Blackwell Scientific Book
   Distributors
   214 Berkeley Street, Carlton
   Victoria 3053

British Library Cataloguing in
   Publication Data

The Foot and its disorders.—2nd ed.
   1.   Foot—Diseases
   I.   Klenerman, Leslie
   617′.585   RC951

ISBN 0–632–00863–6

Contents

Contributors   vii

Foreword to the First Edition   ix

Preface   xi

1   Evolution of the Foot   1
R.K. GRIFFITHS

2   Functional Anatomy   19
L. KLENERMAN

3   The Mechanics of the Foot   31
W.C. HUTTON, J.R.R. STOTT AND I.A.F. STOKES

4   Examination of the Foot   50
L. KLENERMAN

5   The Foot in Childhood   55
J.A. FIXSEN

6   Hallux Valgus and Associated Conditions   83
M.A. EDGAR

7   Common Causes of Pain in the Region of the Foot   129
L. KLENERMAN, K.I. NISSEN AND H. BAKER

8   The Painful Foot in Systemic Disorders   164
A. ST J. DIXON

9   The Foot in Diabetes   177
E.M. THOMAS

10   Common Neurological Disorders affecting the Foot   193
L. KLENERMAN AND J.A. FIXSEN

11   Fractures of the Foot   203
     D.W. WILSON

12   Radiology of the Foot   305
     P. RENTON

     Radiography of the Foot   378
     W.J. STRIPP

13   The Principles and Complications of Foot Surgery   400
     L. KLENERMAN

14   Surgical Footwear and Appliances   410
     W.H. TUCK

15   Chiropody   430
     P.J. READ

     Index   448

Contributors

H. BAKER MD FRCP
Consultant Dermatologist, The London Hospital and St John's Hospital for Diseases of the Skin, London.

A. ST J. DIXON MD FRCP
Consultant Physician, The Royal National Hospital for Rheumatic Diseases and St Martin's Hospital, Bath.

M.A. EDGAR MB MChir FRCS(Eng)
Consultant Orthopaedic Surgeon, The Middlesex Hospital and Royal National Orthopaedic Hospital, London.

J.A. FIXSEN MChir FRCS(Eng)
Consultant Orthopaedic Surgeon, The Hospital for Sick Children, Great Ormond Street and St Bartholomew's Hospital, Smithfield, London.

R.K. GRIFFITHS MB ChB BSc MFCM
Lecturer, Department of Social Medicine, University of Birmingham.

W.C. HUTTON BSc MSc MIMechE
Principal Lecturer, Department of Mechanical Engineering, The Polytechnic of Central London.

L. KLENERMAN ChM FRCS(Eng) FRCS(Ed)
Consultant Orthopaedic Surgeon, Northwick Park Hospital and Clinical Research Centre, Harrow, Middlesex.

K.I. NISSEN MD FRCS(Eng)
Formerly Consultant Orthopaedic Surgeon, Royal National Orthopaedic Hospital, London.

P.J. READ FChS DipFE
Head of Chelsea School of Chiropody, London.

P. RENTON FRCR
Consultant Radiologist, University College Hospital and Royal National Orthopaedic Hospital, London.

I.A.F. STOKES BA PhD
Bioengineer, Department of Rehabilitation, University of Vermont, Vermont, USA.

J.R.R. STOTT MA MB MRCP
Research Medical Officer, RAF Institute of Aviation Medicine, Farnborough, Hants.

W.J. STRIPP FSR
Superintendent Radiographer, The Royal National Orthopaedic Hospital, London.

E.M. THOMAS MB FRCS(Eng)
Consultant Orthopaedic Surgeon, King's College Hospital, London.

W.H. TUCK MBE FBIST
Appliance Research Unit, Royal National Orthopaedic Hospital, Stanmore, Middlesex.

D.W. WILSON MB BS FRCS
Consultant Orthopaedic Surgeon, Royal Free Hospital, Hampstead, London.

Foreword to the First Edition

In my own practice I have always found it invaluable to have on my bookshelves texts which provide easy reference to major topics such as the shoulder, the knee and so on. Here for the first time is a similar product on the foot and its disorders edited by Leslie Klenerman, supported by a group of experts. The content comprises accounts of the foot, its mechanics, the cause and treatment of disorders, due both to local and systemic causes, and very useful accounts of the help that can be given by adequate footwear and chiropody.

This is an excellent work from which all up-to-date information can be obtained. Its bibliography is extensive and follows each chapter which makes for easy access to the large collection of isolated papers of the past and present.

JANUARY 1976   H. OSMOND-CLARKE

Preface

The second edition of this book has been considerably enlarged in response to criticism, and it is hoped that a number of the obvious deficiencies have now been overcome. There are five new chapters, three are short and two are long. The short chapters deal with clinical examination, neurological disorders as they affect the feet and the principles and complications of foot surgery.

The size of the book has been considerably increased by the addition of two important chapters on fractures of the foot and radiology. I make no apology for the length of these chapters as both subjects are of major importance and form an integral part of the study of the foot.

I would like to thank Mrs Patricia McKillop for her meticulous typing of the manuscript and checking of references.

JANUARY 1982   LESLIE KLENERMAN

1

Evolution of the Foot

R.K. GRIFFITHS

Man is the only primate who walks upright with his feet on the ground. This simple and undeniable fact secures an important place for the foot in studies of man's evolution. We cannot understand the evolution of the foot unless we understand its function and for this reason alone these enquiries are likely to be of interest to the orthopaedic surgeon.

The relationship between structure and function is determined by a complex equation incorporating the effects of natural selection and functional adaptation. This is true whether we are examining fossils or living feet. In both cases there may be the added complication of pathology. Assessment of the importance of these three effects, genetic, functional and pathological, may determine either the kind of therapeutic intervention most likely to succeed in a living foot or the taxonomic status of a fossil one. In the case of evolutionary studies pathology is only important in that it must be excluded, but this is often the case in therapeutic interventions which are designed to make the best of that reserve of functional capacity that remains. Before we can examine the fossil record of the foot we must therefore be aware of the effects of natural selection and functional adaptation and understand how the structure of the modern foot correlates with its function.

ADAPTATION AND NATURAL SELECTION

In the past it has often been assumed that these two processes are the same thing. Lake (1935) barely identifies that there are two things at work when he says, 'A well developed foot judged by evolutionary criteria may stand up to considerable abuse, failing only when the maltreatment becomes excessive; but a badly adjusted foot may fail under the stresses of ordinary locomotion without any misuse what-soever.' The words developed and adjusted are used to cover the relationship between structure and function without any attempt to assess the contribution made by its different parts. Preuschoft (1971) accepts that there are two processes at work but seems to believe that they are indistinguishable. He says, 'Perhaps the reader will not accept the existence of a causal relationship between shape and mechanical stressing . . . or will consider it as not sufficiently proved. But the generally accepted mechanisms of mutation and selection will also lead to forms which are optimally adapted to the stresses to which they are subjected. In all cases

1

a maximum of security against failure will be connected with a minimum of ballast in the form of superfluous bone material.'

The point that Preuschoft fails to make is that the two processes that he clearly identifies do not proceed at the same rate. The mechanism of mutation and natural selection has to take at least one and often many generations to achieve change in shape whereas adaptation can produce major differences within the life of the organism completely independent of any change produced by natural selection in later generations. We have only to look at the asymmetrical arms of the professional tennis player, the comparatively huge thighs of the weightlifter, or the calcium content of the newly-returned astronaut to see that large changes are possible in response to functional demands which are not passed on from one generation to the next, and which often do not persist for the life of the organism.

On the other hand, the process of natural selection has led to a wide variety of species of primates related to man and several races of man, and no matter how we might expose each of these to identical conditions we will always be able to tell them apart.

The central questions to which we must return when we study adaptation are quite simply these: (a) how much of the given structure has been rigidly determined for the lifetime of the organism by its genetic make-up; and (b) how much can be changed by the variety of functional constraints to which it is subject? We are looking at a complex relationship created partly by the previous history of the organism in terms of its evolution; partly by the pattern of environmental constraints to which it has been subject and partly by the capacity of its individual tissues to adapt. When we look at structure we are seeing this complex equation frozen at one instant in time. This is true whether we are looking at living or dead material, although we have the advantage when the organism is alive that we can study the response over a period of time and estimate the rate of change of some of the components of the equation. The fundamental question remains the same, how much can be changed and how much can not. Orthodontics provides a good example of the way this relationship determines the most effective therapeutic strategy. If an individual is born with a small jaw and large teeth the strategy is to attack the genetic element of the relationship by removing some of the teeth and then use the adaptive potential of the remaining tissues which allows the teeth to be moved through the bone in response to externally applied pressures. The second part of the approach will not work without a successful application of the first part.

FUNCTIONAL CORRELATION IN COMPARATIVE ANATOMY

International athletics provides us with an interesting microcosm of a sort of natural selection at work, and it must now be obvious that there are correlations between the shape and the body dimensions of athletes successful in certain events, particularly in field events. The period of success in each athlete's life is normally short and, as is always the case with fellow humans, their morphology is not available for experimental analysis. The more traditional approach has been to use other primates, who resemble man in such things as general metabolism and protein structure, but who demonstrate a wide range of locomotor habit within which we can study functional and morphological correlation.

All locomotor muscles act on lever systems and it is the proportions of these levers that influence behaviour. Engineering lever systems with which we are familiar, such as wheel barrows or pulley blocks normally have a velocity ratio which is greater than one, whereas biological systems rely from a mechanical point of view on much less efficient systems. In assessing biological systems several factors have to be taken into account. The locomotor behaviour of the animal within its habitat is the pre-eminent constraint, and this in turn puts certain demands upon the locomotor equipment of the animal; at the same time the whole system is influenced by the body size and weight of the animal. In a wider evolutionary sense other factors such as the sophistication of the nervous and visual systems also have important roles to play, but matter little when we are concerned only with understanding the structure of the appendicular skeleton.

Change is possible in all the components of the locomotor system both in pathological conditions and in response to functional constraints. It is well known that muscle increases in bulk in response to increased work. There is experimental evidence, at both the histological and biochemical levels, that changes in pattern of nerve stimulation can change muscle fibre types. Exercise does not alter the positions of attachment of muscles and hence their engineering efficiency but within these limits the effects of training are fairly well established and are used both in sport and therapy.

There is no doubt that bone changes in response to the forces acting upon it, but the nature of all the changes remains to be exactly defined. The calcium content appears to vary according to load-bearing but the site of deposition is less clear. It has been suggested that trabecular pattern accords with lines of stress in bone but analysis of the stress situation in three dimensions is complicated. A variety of descriptive and experimental work exist, dating back to Wolfe (1899), and it has been evident since 1936 (Stuhler) that a close structural relationship exists between the two constituents collagen and mineral. White *et al* (1977) showed that in calcified turkey leg tendon there is a gap in the collagen chain of about 33 nm which is eminently suitable for accommodating apatite crystals which, from x-ray and neutron diffraction studies, are thought to be of about the same length. Chatterji *et al* (1972) were able by x-ray diffraction to demonstrate an orientation in the human femur which increased with age after one year and they observed also that the extent of orientation of apatite crystals was greater at the front of the femur than at the back. A number of workers have suggested that the strength of bones in different sites and in different animals can be ascribed to the degree of orientation of the microscopic constituents of the bone (Currey 1979) and the importance of the mineral content in determining the mechanical properties of the bones has also been demonstrated. All of this work suffers from the problem that most of the observations about structure are based upon the study of slices or surfaces of bones, whereas study of mechanical properties is carried out on macroscopic specimens. Neutron diffraction (Bacon *et al* 1979b) allows us to combine microscopic and macroscopic observation because high intensity neutron beams are able to penetrate thick slices of bone (7–8 mm for optimum results). The neutrons are diffracted by the apatite crystals in suitably prepared pieces of bone, so if more of the crystals are orientated in a particular direction, the neutron diffraction pattern is deformed in a way which allows a precise measurement of the degree of the preferred orientation of the apatite crystals. This preferred orientation has been shown to correlate both with the external appearance of bone and other measurements of trabecular pattern in simple situations and in more complicated situations to correlate closely with the pattern of muscle pull on the bone. Where it has been possible to compare the result of experiments with photo-stress models with those obtained by neutron diffraction, it appears that the neutron diffraction technique gives a more detailed picture (Bacon *et al* 1979a). Similarly these results have been shown to correlate with those obtained by Bassett (1965) where the preferred axis of the osteons in samples of bone is described (Bacon *et al* 1980). These results leave little doubt that although the precise mechanisms are not clear, bone can react in such a way as to increase its strength in response to demand. Apparently this strength is achieved in two ways, both by alteration in the direction of the trabeculae and the orientation of the crystalline material but also in terms of the net amount of mineral deposited.

The relative lengths of the lever systems involved in locomotion can have a profound effect on the type of behaviour that is possible for any particular animal. No mechanism has been proposed to suggest that change in length of lever arm is an adaptive response. There is considerable variation within the Primate order and at least some of this appears to correlate with locomotor pattern. There is some evidence that genetic change at the chromosome levels, e.g. in a hybrid (Myers 1979), may change length of lever arms.

If we examine the data contributed by Schultz (1963) we find that a contraction of 1 cm in the calf muscles of the tarsier leads to a rise at the ankle of 8.4 cm whereas the same contraction in a gorilla leads to a rise of only 2.3 cm. For the same rate of contraction the tarsier can thus rise upwards at over three and half times the rate of the gorilla. It is hardly a surprise therefore to find that the method of locomotion of the tarsier is to leap, and it can leap up to 20 times its own length at a time. This is done from a static clinging position. The gorilla, on the other hand, does not leap. Here then is a good example of the velocity ratio adjusted to locomotor habit. However, this piece of engineering has several consequences; the tarsier must exert a force of many times its own body weight with its calf muscles if it is to rise off the ground, whereas the gorilla, with a more mechanically advantageous lever system, requires comparatively less muscle bulk.

The efficiency of the lever system is, of course, also dependent upon the friction at the ankle joint and this in turn depends upon the pressure between the two joint surfaces. There are two components to this pressure, the first being body weight and the second the compressive force of the calf muscle acting across the joint. The actual muscular force required has to be sufficient to overcome not only the body weight multiplied by the mechanical advantage but also the additional friction. For any given lever system there is not therefore a linear relationship between body weight and the muscle required to elevate it. It is hardly surprising that the only primates that move by leaping are relatively small and were a gorilla to be produced with a suitable mutated ankle lever, as compared with a tarsier, it is doubtful if it could adapt its musculature to produce any movement at all. When we are dealing with a muscular system it is not only the length of the actual lever arms involved that is important, but also the length of the muscle itself, which affects the total amount of shortening that the muscle can achieve. This is influenced by the length of the bone proximal to the lever in question. The tarsier has, in addition to its long ankle lever, a relatively long tibia.

The third element that we must consider in analysing functional anatomy is the shape of the joint surface. In the ankle and foot this is of course a complicated matter. Many of the muscles which act across the ankle and foot joints have more than one action, for instance they may flex the toes, extend the ankle and cause inversion or eversion. A number of different techniques have been used to relate muscle action to joint surface, for instance Barnett and Napier (1952) used the technique of geometrical deduction and analysed movement in terms of two axes with different degrees of inclination, one for dorsiflexion and one for plantarflexion. Hicks (1953) described a technique for determining the natural axes of rotation of the various joints of partly dissected, fresh specimens; also showing the position of tendons relative to them on an x-ray which showed the position of the final axis relative to the bones. The difficulty of both of these techniques becomes clear from the study of Newth (1976) which used a modification of Hicks' technique and appeared to show that some muscles, such as tibialis posterior and extensor digitorum longus, have different actions in different species because they pass on different sides of the inversion–eversion axis, and that although their comparative anatomical structure is similar and their primary action the same, their secondary action of either inversion or eversion may be quite different. Conclusions about the functional significance of this are difficult because the power of such secondary actions is very hard to determine. Lewis (1980a, b) shows how the joint surfaces of a number of different primates and other comparable species are modified and has attempted to relate these changes in morphology to changes in locomotor function. Both the study of Lewis and of Newth appeared to provide evidence to suggest adaptation towards an arborial environment which are different from those required for a terrestrial environment. Jenkins (1974) has demonstrated however that where small mammals are concerned there may be little difference in the functional constraints of a forest floor environment from that of an arborial one. In both cases the foot is presented with a very bumpy terrain consisting of many elements oriented in three dimensions. This means that in evolutionary terms it is very difficult to place precise interpretations on progression of changes through animals of different sizes.

All these studies seem to suggest that man's evolution, or at least the details of the evolutionary pathway, are probably considerably more complex than the early and popular notion (as put forward by Keith 1929) that man became upright in the trees (as a brachiator akin to the gibbon).

Whatever interpretation is placed on individual findings the important principle appears to be that the anatomy of joint surfaces and joint axes and the length of lever arms and the position in which muscles are attached are likely to be genetically determined, whereas the power of muscles and the internal organization of the bone is likely to be determined by functional criteria during the life of the animal. This means that there has been no mechanism proposed (other than natural selection*) that can alter the properties of lever systems and joint axes, whereas muscular dimensions and bone strength can adapt to changes in function. The implication from the point of view of therapeutic intervention would seem to be that surgical alteration of lever lengths or joint dynamics, should it be desired, would be effective only when changes are not demanded of the other bones and muscles that are beyond their adaptive capacity. From the evolutionary point of view lever lengths, joint surfaces and muscle attachments are the characteristics most likely to produce information of taxonomic significance.

FUNCTIONAL CORRELATION IN THE HUMAN FOOT

In the past comparative anatomy provided one of the main methods by which form and function were investigated. Early work was based on the simple collation of descriptive material, but there has been a trend over the last 20 years towards increasing quantitation. The availability of more and more powerful computers has meant that an increasing number of workers are using quantitative methods and multivariate analysis as an aid to description, hypothesis generation and experimental analysis. An alternative approach is to use comparative material as test data on which structural or functional hypotheses can be tried. The work of Preuschoft (1969, 1970a, b, 1971) provides numerous examples where theoretically derived shapes and stress analyses are compared with a variety of existing primate specimens whose degree of approximation to the theoretically derived shape tests the validity of the method used to produce it.

As anatomy has advanced into a more rigorous and quantitative science it has been enriched by techniques from other disciplines such as physics and engineering. Russell Jones (1941), in his extensive study, made use of test bed methods to investigate the contribution of different muscle, bone and ligamentous units to the function of the foot. Some of his conclusions have since been re-examined electromyographically by Basmajian (1969) and others, who found Jones to be substantially correct in his conclusion that the muscles do not play a major part in support of the arches. This contrasts with the view of Keith (1929) who believed that muscles were responsible for arch support. Keith had based his opinion on his views of phylogeny; in either case a useful hypothesis was formed that led, when it

* But see Hooper (1977) for evidence that artificial selection is effective.

was tested, to a better understanding. However, there was a considerable interval before methods existed to test Keith's theory and there is always a danger that if ideas are put forward with force, in the absence of a suitable test, then they may gain currency simply by repetition.

It is possible that the same criticism could be applied to the suggestion that the internal architecture of the foot bones represents a half-dome. This idea is based upon observations of the supposed trabecular pattern and has been put forward by several workers (McKenzie 1955; Wood-Jones 1944). Such a theory is based upon assumptions about the way in which bone reacts to weight-bearing, which may themselves be oversimplifications. The same criticism can be applied to the theory as a whole, in that Hicks (1955) has shown that under some circumstances the foot can bear the load either as an arch or as a beam.

Neutron diffraction provides a means for analysing the spongy bone of the foot and quantifying some of the suggestions about its structure that can be traced back to Meyer (1873). Preuschoft (1970b) believed that these pictures of trabecular pattern are in error but the neutron diffraction studies seem to suggest that the picture is more complicated than can easily be determined by simple inspection of x-ray or cross-section material. Fig. 1.1 shows two diagrammatic cross-sections through the foot with the plantar aponeurosis in the relaxed position and then tensed by the windlass mechanism described by Hicks (1953, 1954). Fig. 1.2 shows a similar section through the calcaneum enlarged and with the results of neutron diffraction studies at four sites imposed upon it. The polar diagrams displayed at each site show the ratio between the number of apatite crystals pointing in a particular direction and that which would be expected if the material were a powder or, in other words, if the crystals were equally oriented in all directions. The dotted circle shows the picture that would be obtained if the material was a powder, so that in the simplest situation shown, namely at site C, the orientation in the preferred direction is something like twice that which would be expected from a powder in the main direction of orientation and about half of that in the least

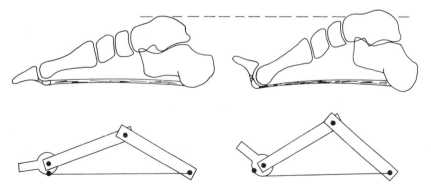

Fig. 1.1 Showing the windlass action of the plantar aponeurosis. By kind permission of Mr J.H. Hicks MCh Orth, FRCS, from *Biomechanical studies of the musculo-skeletal system* (1962). Courtesy of Charles C. Thomas, Springfield, Illinois.

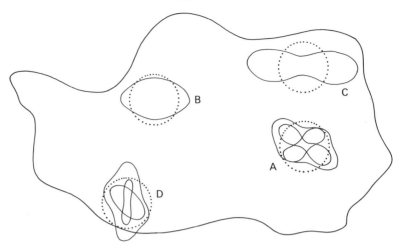

Fig. 1.2 Orientation of apatite crystals in midline saggital sections of calcaneum. At each site the dotted circle is scaled to show the expected value if the crystals had been randomly organized. The polar diagrams represent smooth curves drawn from measurements taken at 10° angles of rotation. The inner diagrams are calculated distributions which, when summated, produce the overall pattern seen in the outer shape.

direction of orientation. This can be compared with site B where the preferred orientation is much less pronounced and the picture more closely approximates to the dotted circle. At sites A and D the polar diagram is skewed in two directions indicating that there are two main axes of orientation of the apatite crystals, the inner elements of the polar diagram showing the orientation of crystals in these two predominant axes while the outer pattern shows the effect of summating the two. These pictures thus given an accurate quantitation to the trabecular pattern through a section of calcaneum just under a centimetre thick in the mid-line. The relationship between the trabecular pattern, as shown by the crystalline orientations, the joint surfaces and the tension in the plantar aponeurosis becomes very clear when these diagrams are examined. At site C, the simplest situation, the crystalline elements are oriented very strongly in the direction which is the resultant force between the Achilles tendon and the joint surfaces in the foot which from that site are, in fact, almost in line with each other. At site B the same predominant orientation along the length of the foot is seen. At a greater distance from the insertion of the Achilles tendon underneath the talar joint the force pattern is clearly much less simple and the consequent orientation more closely resembles a powder. The apatites are distributed almost evenly in most directions with a slight predominant orientation along the length of the foot tending therefore, to support, in part, the notion of a dome, but really operating in order to resist the resultant force, the main force of the foot generated by the leverage of the Achilles tendon. At position A the situation is more complicated, this particular site falling midway between the influence of the plantar aponeurosis and the

Achilles tendon. The predominant orientation, in other words, the longer of the two main directions in the polar diagram points at the talocalcaneal joint the other direction of preferred orientation points at the insertion of the plantar aponeurosis and is presumably a reflection of the impact of this tendon on the posterior part of the calcaneum. Although the existence of some trabecular fibres pointing in this direction is fairly visible from inspection of either cut specimens or x-rays, it has not been remarked upon to any extent by those who have made claims for the dome like structure of the trabecular patterns. The functional significance of this part of the trabecular structure which is revealed by neutron diffraction is, of course, clear. At position D we see a similarly complicated trabecular pattern at a part of the calcaneum which is beyond the insertion of the plantar aponeurosis, where the bone appears to be organized in order to resist forces which point at the two joint surfaces of the talocalcaneal junction and the function of the calcaneum with the rest of the foot.

Neutron diffraction studies unfortunately require the use of European nuclear facilities to which access is relatively restricted and it has not yet been possible to analyse any other bones in the foot. When Hicks (1953, 1954) investigated the foot he showed that the bones of each ray of the foot functioned as a set of independent arches, i.e. structures which are loaded in compression when the plantar windlass aponeurosis was under tension. He also showed that the effect of the windlass mechanism was independent of muscle contraction, which fits in with the observations of Russell Jones and Basmajian, namely that the muscles play little part in raising the arches of the foot. Hicks was also able to show that in the situation where the aponeurosis is not under tension the bones of the foot are loaded as a beam and are thus under bending strain rather than compression. It is not possible to say how much of the time the foot is loaded in each of these two modes in normal or pathological situations. When neutron diffraction studies of the remaining foot bones are available they may provide further information about this by indicating the ratio of apatite crystals pointing in directions which would resist beam forces and those which would resist arch forces. On the basis of the results seen for the calcaneum it would appear that the majority of apatite is organized to resist the kind of forces we would expect when the foot is loaded as an arch and perhaps only those crystals seen pointing at the talocalcaneal joint from position D could be construed as being required for a foot loaded as a beam.

THE FOSSIL RECORD OF THE HUMAN FOOT

There have always been two reasons for looking at the fossil record; the most obvious is to throw light on the possible evolution of man, a subject which is, of course, intrinsically interesting and often highly controversial. The second reason is to view the fossil record as a chronicle of the increasing perfection of certain characteristics which are important to locomotor function in man. In the past this strand of thinking was used to justify the study of evolution of the foot in the hope that it would reveal imperfections in the adaptive process and that these so called 'weak links' in the foot might be a clue to pathology (Lake 1935). The nature of the adaptive process is such that this is probably a naive assumption, for if we cannot account for a particular aspect of the structure then the weak link is probably in our understanding and not in the structure itself. In the last 15 years the study of fossils and the study of biomechanics has tended to go hand in hand, each throwing light on the other.

The fossil record has never been easy to interpret. Each new fossil bone represents some frozen instant of a geological epoch, and is often only part of an animal selected by a random process from a population, whose numbers and characteristics we do not know, which lived in an area whose boundaries can only be guessed at and whose habitat may not be fully defined. We are looking at minutiae in detail when we study fossils and it is hardly surprising that each new find has tended to add doubt and confusion rather than clarity to the picture.

There has been deep controversy in the last few years over a number of aspects of human evolution and we have seen findings and claims and counterclaims rebounding around the major journals (Leakey 1973; Wood 1973; Oxnard 1975; Pilbeam 1977; Johannson 1979; Day 1980; Leakey 1980; Johannson 1980; Lisowski *et al* 1972, 1974, 1976). These controversies are only understandable if we know something of the problems which are faced by those who seek to interpret fossils and something of the techniques which are used.

Our understanding of the fossil record requires first of all that we organize it into some sort of chronological order. Techniques for dating fossil material are now fairly sophisticated in ideal conditions, although there are problems if the geology of the region (such as the area of the South African fossils) is very confused. Modern techniques exploit the differences between living material and rock by observing the rates at which they become similar. Two examples illustrate the point: when an animal dies minerals in the surrounding rocks will diffuse into its bones, fluorine is one that is easily analysed; on the other hand the organic content of the fossil becomes fixed at death, in other words the manufacture of those compounds that are only found in living material ceases. All living material contains traces of naturally occurring radioisotopes and these will continue to decay at their normal rate. Their content in the fossil can be estimated and from this, knowing the half-life of their rate of decay, we can extrapolate back in time to the point where their concentration equals their natural occurrence. This is the time at which the fossil died. The accuracy of all these methods depends upon the half-life of the material concerned, as a rough guide they are accurate to within the period of their half-life, over a period of ten times that period. If both the fossil and the surrounding rocks are dated, it should be possible to avoid errors due to earth movement and deliberate forgery such as the Piltdown saga. In very old fossils we have to rely on dating rock strata using the decay of potassium isotopes into argon. Having established the date of the material we come to the problem of taxonomy, and here a whole new class of problems appear. It has never been easy to say exactly what constitutes a separate species, the accepted operational definition is that two types of animal that do not interbreed form two species. This works in most cases when we are dealing with living animals, but is not of great help when we are trying to distinguish two fossils that may be many thousands of years apart in age and hundreds of miles apart in geography. The problem has never been solved to everyone's satisfaction in any single case. In the same context it is not much easier to say whether particular specimens should be assigned to different genera, or to separate species within one genus. We have very poor estimates of the natural variability in the populations from which the fossils were drawn and hence modern statistical methods, which depend upon assessment of the variance of normally distributed characters, are unreliable.

Most fossils have been studied from the point of view of determining their relationship to man rather than examining the degree to which they might be fitted to their presumed habitat. As such they are often not studied as evolutionary problems, rather, man is used as a sort of target and the degree of likeness is estimated. If trends are found which appear man-like in some aspect then the fossil is assigned to a hominoid genus. There are dangers in this as Day has said in reply to a question by the author (Day 1973), '. . . I am also saying that bipedalism has been used as a taxonomic feature and may well be used as a taxonomic feature in the future but at present I am not entirely sure what I mean by it, and I am not entirely sure what other people mean by it and until this has been agreed, not only on an anatomical and biometric basis but also on a truly biomechanical basis, it would be unwise to regard bipedality as a unique feature by which you separate man from others.' Nevertheless Oxnard (1981) was able to say '. . . but because there has never yet been hailed a new find that was not a human ancestor, and because there has never yet been announced a new find that was not bipedal, we may be prefer to be extremely circumspect until the fossils are widely available for study by the entire range of methods and investigators of the present day. My doubts about some of these things would be somewhat allayed if only some fossils would be recognized that are *not* the ancestors of man at these times and in these places. Richard Leakey with the wide range of material that has been discovered by his group at East Turkana, may be providing the first evidence that we have become objective enough to recognize that not everything that we discover is a human ancestor.'

Over the last few years a considerable number of new specimens have been discovered, for instance 14 have been described from Laetoli (White 1977) and additional specimens have also been recovered. There is also a remarkable collection of hominid specimens from Haddar in the Afar triangle of Ethiopia. These are highly fragmented and represent a minimum of 35 and a maximum of more than 65 individuals, some of them, for instance the famous Lucy, remarkably complete for fossils (40% of the skeleton). Others represent quite large groups of individuals, for instance more than 200 specimens representing an absolute minimum of 13 individuals in one group. These figures give some impression of the degree of fragmentation that is common with a lot of fossil material. Many of these specimens consist only of small parts of the skull, teeth and jaws and there are no post-cranial remains. Even where post-cranial bones do exist the whole foot is an unusual occurrence. The specimen found in Olduvai Gorge, known as hominid 8, is still the most complete foot that has been discovered, consisting of the complete tarsus with the metatarsals attached, that are complete apart from the heads and the styloid of the fifth metatarsal. There is also very little of the calcaneum. Certain bones, noticeably the talus, are now represented in a considerable number of specimens and Lisowski *et al* (1976) were able to study measurements from the tali of 21 individual fossil primates from Africa; a considerable series by most fossil standards. However, when we consider the distances which separate these specimens (see Fig. 1.3) and the time which separates them, several million years in some cases, it is clear that the apparent richness of the material is only relative.

Fundamentally there are three methods of study available which might be described as recognition, metrication, and modelling. Each of these techniques has

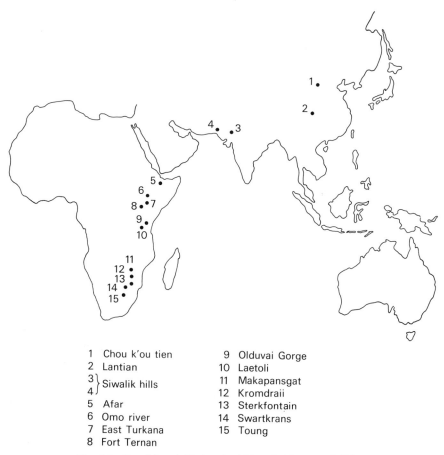

1	Chou k'ou tien	9	Olduvai Gorge
2	Lantian	10	Laetoli
3 } Siwalik hills		11	Makapansgat
4		12	Kromdraii
5	Afar	13	Sterkfontain
6	Omo river	14	Swartkrans
7	East Turkana	15	Toung
8	Fort Ternan		

Fig. 1.3 Fossil hominid sites in Africa, Pakistan and China.

its own advantages and disadvantages but when all three produce the same answer there seems to be reasonable grounds for optimism about the findings.

The most easily understood modelling technique is that of photoelastic stress analysis. Any birefringent translucent material tends to change its refractive index under strain. The resultant changes can be viewed as an interference pattern if the material is transilluminated with plane-polarized monochromatic light. The concentration of strain in the material shows itself as a concentration of interference fringes. This method is attractive because of the apparent ease of interpretation of the findings. Nevertheless it does require very complete specimens from which to construct the models and this of course limits its application to the study of fossils.

Simple recognition is the oldest technique available and because beauty lies in the eye of the beholder sometimes it is the most prone to error. Recognition of course also depends upon reconstruction which in turn may be prone to error if the reconstructor has in mind a preconceived notion as to the end product of his task.

Metrication whether in the form of single measurements or indices from particular specimens or multiple measurements has always been portrayed as a way of avoiding the subjective elements in the former techniques. There is, of course, a subjective element in deciding what to measure and how to measure it. The more sophisticated techniques of multivariate analysis suffer from the further disadvantage that their results are not easily understood and the algebra on which they are based is incomprehensible to the average reader. In geometrical terms the rationale of multivariate statistics is fairly easy to comprehend and is analagous with rotating a specimen in one's hands in order to examine it from a number of view points. In the case of multivariate analysis the object being rotated is a multi-dimensional matrix of data and the hands that are manipulating it are computer programmes which can cope with the algebraic representation of the multi-dimensional space involved. These methods are well documented elsewhere (Oxnard 1973, 1975) but are not without problems in their interpretation and as Day (1973) points out they often fall into the trap of using the very characters that they are studying as a basis of classification and circular arguments may be the result. The inter-relation of these various techniques is well exemplified in the numerous studies on the talus of the Olduvai hominid 8 (OH8) foot and other similar fossil tali.

The OH8 foot was first described by Day and Napier (1964). They concluded that the principal affinities of the foot were with Homo sapiens noting that 'this is particularly apparent in the anatomy of the metatarsal bones'. Their conclusions were based upon their study of the original specimens and the reconstruction of the entire foot. Preuschoft (1971) using elastic modelling studies analysed the forces involved in prehension and in walking and suggested that the latter required strong resistance to bending moments, particularly in the proximal part of the metatarsal, whereas the forces involved in prehension tend to be compressive in this region. Metatarsals of walking feet thus tend to be elliptical in a sagittal plane at their proximal ends and this feature is present in hominid 8, particularly in the fifth metatarsal. However placing undue emphasis on the preponderant robusticity of the fourth and fifth metatarsal as an indicator of advanced bipedal capability requires caution, as Lewis (1980) points out, illustrating a specimen of gorilla (British Museum 1978–1226) which shows just the same feature with a particularly strong and buttressed fifth metatarsal. Lisowski (1967) studying predominantly the talus of the OH8 foot showed that it fell within the range of sub-human primates including the African apes and proconsul and was markedly different from *Homo sapiens*. Day and Wood (1968), studying their reconstruction of the OH8 foot and other tali in a multivariate statistical study, decided that the fossil was intermediate in form between that of bipedal man and the African apes. This study was then subject to trenchant methodological criticisms from Oxnard (1972) who went on to reinterpret their data in a more complete multivariate analysis and showed that the OH8 talus was uniquely different from both the African apes on the one hand and modern man on the other but was, in fact, close to the talus of another fossil—proconsul. Lisowski and Oxnard (1974) carried out a further study on a large number of tali and Wood (1974) reappraised his own multivariate study and cautiously inclined towards the view that OH8 should be attributed to the genus Australopithecus. Oxnard (1975, 1976) in further studies incorporating still more fossil tali and other extant species to the data matrix concluded that the OH8 foot does not represent part of the main line of human ancestry, and Wood (1977) moved further towards this view. Lewis (1980) in a series of three very detailed studies of the joints of the evolving foot is clearly less impressed with multivariate statistical analysis and demonstrates by the traditional techniques of dissection, comparison and recognition that, 'the OH8 foot retained to a considerable extent the essential morphology seen in extant apes and its closest affinities are clearly with the African apes. Its main distinction is seen in the remodelling of the medialcuniform with the consequent dimunition in divergence of the hallax. There can be little doubt that this is a specialization associated with bipedal locomotion, but clearly the gait must have lacked the finely tuned functional qualities found in the modern man . . .'

Lewis's (1980a, b, c) very comprehensive review charts a possible course of evolution for the primate and the human foot which includes a possible marsupial origin for the early primates. In a series of detailed studies of the individual joints of the ankle and foot, Lewis describes the various specializations required for different aspects of arborial and terrestrial life for animals of different sizes and weights. The conclusion that the OH8 foot does not form part of the main strand of human ancestry is thus based upon comparative anatomical, biochemical and biometric studies. Perhaps the final twist in the argument comes from Oxnard (1981) who suggests that there is an error in the original reconstruction of the OH8 foot described by Day and Napier. Oxnard (working from casts) has produced a new reconstruction of which he is able to say, 'now at last there is no anomaly in all of the results. All of the morphometric studies of the talus, whether those of Oxnard and colleagues or whether those of Day and Wood as reinterpreted by Oxnard, suggest non-human functional affinities for that bone. The rearticulation of the whole foot conforms in also suggesting non-human affinities for the entire foot. The apparent human features originally believed to be displayed by the rearticulated foot are spurious, being due to a series of misalignments.' Perhaps the final irony is that at the very moment that we are able to determine that the OH8 foot is not part of the main stream of human evolution, Mary Leakey discovers bipedal footprints (now seen on television) in volcanic ash nearly four million years old (Reader 1981). Not only are these footprints much older than the OH8 foot they are also much larger. Whose footprints has Mary Leakey found?

At the moment there is no clear answer to this question and controversy rages. In 1975 at Koobi Fora in Northern Kenya two discoveries were made of fossils KNM–ER 3733 and KNM–ER 406 which established unequivocally that two species of fossil hominds both existed about one and a half million years ago. KNM–ER 3733 is quite clearly from the genus known as *Homo erectus* where KNM–ER 406 is quite clearly an Australopithecus (Leakey & Walker 1976). The discovery of KNM–ER 1470 dated at around two million years further tends to confirm that more than one kind of probably upright hominid existed at least that long ago. The question that now has to be determined is how far back do these various species go? Do they have a common point and a single identifiable ancestor? Did that ancestor make the footprints? Johannson (1979) clearly believes that they do have a common ancestor and that he has found it in the Haddar region of the Afar triangle of Ethiopia and the specimen now known as 'Lucy' is a member of the tribe. He calls the species *Australopithecus afarensis*. 'Lucy' is too small to have made the footprints so Johannson assumes that there must have been pronounced sexual dimorphism, the males being 60% larger than the females. Mary Leakey, Day and Olsen in one paper (1980) and Richard Leakey and Walker (1980) in another, do not agree with Johannson's conclusions.

Whatever interpretation is put on them, the discoveries of Haddar represent very large amounts of material very often consisting of several bones from the same individual. This now affords the possibility of interpolating several bones from the same individual into multivariate analyses of similar bones. This ought to enhance the taxonomic power of the analysis by an order of magnitude.

The fossil record further back in time is less helpful. Pilbeam *et al* (1977) have found enough fossils to propose that the genus Ramapithecus is the common ancestor to the later forms but their conclusions are based upon skull, jaw and tooth fragments. From 90 hominid specimens representing more than 60 individuals in four species there are only fragments of a cuneiform, a metatarsal, a calcaneum and a talus; hardly enough for a footprint.

Further studies will take a considerable time and we can only speculate about the answers. At the moment it is not surprising that it is Johannson, who discovered 'Lucy', who is making the greatest claims on her behalf. He has the benefit of owning the specimens, but it is part of the ritual of hominid paleontology that every new find is hailed as the missing link by its finder. Sceptics might find it surprising that the discoverers of these missing links have always been able to announce their findings while still in the field. This contrasts with forensic pathologists who always refuse to say anything until they have managed to get the specimens back to the laboratory, yet there are obviously many parallels in their work. It was this excess of confidence among so many anthropologists which led Lord Zuckerman (1966) to initiate studies based upon measurement rather than 'expert' recognition. Ashton, Oxnard, Lisowski and their co-workers (including this author) have followed in his footsteps.

Despite these caveats there does seem a real possibility that an animal with the general form of *Homo erectus*, with a brain of the order of 800 cm^3, may have existed not for a few hundred years, but for several million years. This may have co-existed for some time in the company of at least one other extinct ape/man who may also have been bipedal to a degree. The footprints at Laetoli will certainly keep the foot near the centre of the stage in studies of evolution and seem to have pushed the origins of bipedality back to a point at least $3\frac{1}{2}$ million years ago. Just as we saw with the studies of the OH8 foot that over 15 years the various methods of enquiry gradually converged on a concensus, it appears that another consensus may be around the corner. Biochemists (e.g. Goodman, 1973) have examined proteins common to man and other animals and translated their amino acid sequences into gene codons. From these they have been able to estimate the length of evolutionary time required to produce the necessary changes in the DNA molecule. They have, of course, had to assume that these changes in the genetic material take place at a constant rate and that they do not oscillate or regress; nevertheless estimates based on these methods repeatedly suggest that man diverged from the great apes some $3\frac{1}{2}$ to 5 million, or even 7 million, years ago.

In a few more years we may be asking not how did man come to evolve but why did the other upright, or semi-upright, apes die out, and we may be looking much further into antiquity for the origins of man. The ultimate survival of a species does not depend usually on the ability of single tissues or systems to adapt to change but rather on the ability of the gene package of the whole animal to survive. It may be, therefore, that the ultimate perfection of the human foot was not crucial to man's survival (Wood-Jones (1944) briefly proposes the opposite view) but rather that this development was inevitable because bipedality was becoming the order of the day in the Primates of the time. It seems most probable that it was the most intelligent of the ape/men that survived. Whether an advancing brain caused man to walk upright or whether the brain developed because he kept his feet on the ground remains to be discovered.

REFERENCES

Bacon G.E., Bacon P.J. & Griffiths R.K. (1979a) Stress distribution in the scapula studied by neutron diffraction. *Proceedings of the Royal Society, London, Series B* **204,** 355–62.
Bacon G.E., Bacon P.J. & Griffiths R.K. (1979b) The orientation of apatite crystals in bone. *Journal of applied Crystallography* **12,** 99–103.
Bacon G.E., Bacon P.J. & Griffiths R.K. (1980) Orientation of apatite crystals in relation to muscle attachment in the mandible. *Journal of Biomechanics* **13,** 725–9.

BARNETT C.H. & NAPIER J.R. (1952) The axis of rotation at the ankle joint in man, its influence on the form of the talus and the mobility of the fibula. *Journal of Anatomy* **86**, 1–9.

BASMAJIAN J.V. & MacCONAIL M.A. (1969) *Muscles and Movement*. Williams & Wilkins, Baltimore.

BASSETT C.A. (1965) Electrical effects in bone. *Scientific American* **213** (4), 18–25.

CHATTERJI S., WALL J.C. & JEFFREY J.W. (1972) Changes in the degree of orientation of bone materials with age in the human femur. *Experientia* **28**, 156–7.

CURREY J.D. (1979) Mechanical properties of bone tissues with greatly differing functions. *Journal of Biomechanics* **12**, 313–19.

DAY M.H. (1973) In *Concepts of human evolution*. Symposium of the Zoological Society of London **33**, 49–50.

DAY M.H. & NAPIER J.R. (1964) Hominid fossils from Bed 1 Olduvai Gorge, Tanganyika: Fossil foot bones. *Nature* **201**, 967–70.

DAY M.H., LEAKEY M.D. & OLSON T.R. (1980) On the status of *Australopithecus afarensis*. *Science* **207**, 1102–3.

GOODMAN M. (1973) In *Concepts of Human Evolution*. Symposium of the Zoological Society of London **33**, 339–75.

HICKS J.H. (1953) The mechanics of the foot. I. The joints. *Journal of Anatomy* **87**, 345–57.

HICKS J.H. (1954) The mechanics of the foot. II. The plantar aponeurosis and the arch. *Journal of Anatomy* **88**, 25–30.

HICKS J.H. (1955) The foot as a support. *Acta Anatomica* **25**, 34–45.

HOOPER A.C.B. (1977) A further study of the effects of selection for relative bone length. *Journal of Anatomy* **124** (2), 495.

JENKINS F.A. (1974) In *Primate Locomotion*. Academic Press, New York.

JOHANNSON D.C. & WHITE T.D. (1979) A systematic assessment of African hominids. *Science* **203**, 321–30.

JONES R. (1941) The human foot. An experimental study of its mechanics and the role of its muscles and ligaments in the support of the arch. *American Journal of Anatomy* **68**, 1–39.

KEITH SIR ARTHUR (1929) The history of the human foot and its bearing on orthopaedic practice. *Journal of Bone and Joint Surgery* **II**, 10–32.

LAKE N. (1935) *The foot*. Tindall & Cox, London.

LEAKEY R.E.F. (1973) Evidence for an Advanced Plio-Pleistocene Hominid from East Rudolf Kenya. *Nature* **242**, 447–50.

LEAKEY R.E.F. (1976b) New hominid fossils from Koobi Fora formation in Northern Kenya. *Nature* **261**, 574–6.

LEAKEY R.E.F. & WALKER A.C. (1976a) Australopithecus, Homo erectus and the single species hypothesis. *Nature* **261**, 572–4.

LEAKEY R.E.F. & WALKER A.C. (1980) On the status of *Australopithecus afarensis*. *Science* **207**, 1103.

LEWIS O.J. (1980a) The joints of the evolving foot. Part I the ankle joint. *Journal of Anatomy* **130** (3), 527–43.

LEWIS O.J. (1980b) The joints of the evolving foot. Part II the intrinsic joints. *Journal of Anatomy* **130** (4), 833–57.

LEWIS O.J. (1980c) The joints of the evolving foot. Part III the fossil evidence. *Journal of Anatomy* **131** (2), 275–98.

LISOWSKI F.P., ALBRECHT G.H. & OXNARD C.E. (1974) The form of the Talus in some Higher Primates: a multivariate study. *American Journal of Physical Anthropology* **41**, 191–216.

LISOWSKI F.P., ALBRECHT G.H. & OXNARD C.E. (1976) African Fossil Tali: further multivariate morphometric studies. *American Journal of Physical Anthropology* **45**, 5–18.

MEYER G.H. (1873) *Die Static und Mechanic des Nerschlichen Knochengevastes*, Leipzig.

MYERS R.H. & SHAFER D.A. (1979) Hybrid Ape off-spring of a mating of Gibbon and Siamang. *Science* **205**, 308–10.

McKENZIE J. (1955) The foot as a half dome. *British Medical Journal* **3**, 1068–70.

NEWTH S.J. & GRIFFITHS R.K. (1976) Functional adaptation in the Primate ankle. *Journal of Anatomy* **122** (1), 199.

OXNARD C.E. (1972) Some African Fossil Foot Bones: A Note on the Interpolation of Fossils into a Matrix of Extant Species. *American Journal of Physical Anthropology* **37**, 3–12.

OXNARD C.E. (1973) *Form and Pattern in Human Evolution.* University of Chicago Press, Chicago.

OXNARD C.E. (1975) *Uniqueness and Diversity in Human Evolution.* University of Chicago Press, Chicago.

OXNARD C.E. (1975) The place of the Australopithecives in human evolution: grounds for doubt. *Nature* **258**, 389–95.

OXNARD C.E. (1981) Convention and Controversy in human evolution. *Homo* **30**, 225–46.

PILBEAM D., MEYER C.E., BADGLEY C., ROSE M.D., PICKFORD M.H.L., BEHRENSMEYER A.K. & IBRAHIM SHAH S.H. (1977) New hominoid primates from the Siwaliks of Pakistan and their bearing on hominoid evolution. *Nature* **270**, 689–95.

PREUSCHOFT H. (1969) Statische Untersuchangen am fur der Primates I. *Zeitschrift fur anatomie Entwickle-Gesch* **129**, 285–345.

PREUSCHOFT H. (1970a) Statische Untersuchangen am fur der Primates II. *Zeitschrift fur anatomie Entwickle-Gesch* **131**, 156–92.

PREUSCHOFT H. (1970b) In Bourne G.H. (ed.), The Chimpanzee. *Larger* **3**, 221–94.

PREUSCHOFT H. (1971) Body posture and mode of locomotion in early pleistocene hominids. *Folia Primat* **14**, 209–40.

READER J. (1981) *Missing links.* Collins, London.

SCHULTZ A.H. (1963) Symposium on the Primates. *Zoological Society of London.*

STUHLER R. (1936) Die Lagerung der anorganischen kristallite im Knochen. *Naturwissenschafter* **24**, 523.

WHITE S.W.W., HULMES D.S.J., MILLER A. & TIMMINS P.A. (1977) Collagen—mineral axial relationship in calcified turkey leg tendon by x-ray and neutron diffraction. *Nature (Lond.)* **266**, 421–5.

WHITE T.D. (1977) New Fossil Hominids from Laetolil, Tanzania. *American Journal of Physical Anthropology* **46**, 197–230.

WOLFE J. (1899) Die Lehre von der functionellen Knochengestalf. *Virchows Archiv; A: Pathological anatomy and histology* **155**, 256.

WOOD B.A. (1974) Locomotor Affinities of Hominid Tali from Kenya. *Nature* **246**, 45–6.

WOOD B.A. & HENDERSON A. (1977) The functional anatomy of the Olduvai (OH8) foot. *Journal of Anatomy* **124**(1), 252.

WOOD-JONES F.W. (1944) *Structure and function as seen in the human foot.* Ballière, Tindall & Cox, London.

ZUCKERMAN S. (1966) Myths and methods in anatomy. *Journal of the Royal College of Surgeons of Edinburgh* **11**, 87–114.

2

Functional Anatomy

L. KLENERMAN

Although the basic gross anatomy which is taught to students does not change, advances in technical expertise have provided new methods of investigation. These have produced a better understanding of functional anatomy. For example, electromyography has given rise to a much more accurate knowledge of muscular action and the techniques of the engineer have enabled the load-bearing aspects of the foot to be studied in detail (see Chapter 3).

The foot has two main functions, support and propulsion. It combines stability with flexibility and its propulsive action is that of a flexible lever. Compared to the hand, the cortical area of the brain devoted to the foot and its digits is very small (Jones 1949), furthermore the ordinary shoe-wearing individual does not undertake any skilled movements with his toes. Nevertheless it is possible to develop great neuromuscular control of the feet, as is shown by the grace of the ballet dancer and the skill of the occasional armless individuals who can paint and undertake most activities with their feet normally performed with the hands (Fig. 2.1).

It is assumed that the reader knows the gross anatomy of the foot; the purpose of this chapter is to correlate some aspects of this knowledge with function in relation to clinical work and to stimulate further reading and thought.

BONE STRUCTURE

The anatomy of the foot in most people's memory is usually dominated by descriptions of medial, lateral and transverse arches. This latter arch can readily be discounted, as in a normal foot the metatarsal heads can be seen to lie in the same horizontal plane (Acton 1960). The concept of medial and lateral longitudinal arches is static and based on the obvious similarity between the arch shape of the foot and the arch as seen in buildings.

This concept cannot simply be transferred to the weight-bearing foot, which is moving and subject to changing forces. An arch is fixed at each end and bent upward to resist and to conduct into its supports loads, which tend to flatten it. Because the arch is curved, the upper edge has a greater circumference than the lower, so that each of its blocks must be cut in wedge shapes that press firmly against the whole surface of neighbouring blocks and conduct loads uniformly.

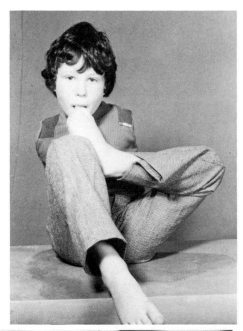

Fig. 2.1 This boy with no arms is completely independent. He can write and feed himself without difficulty.

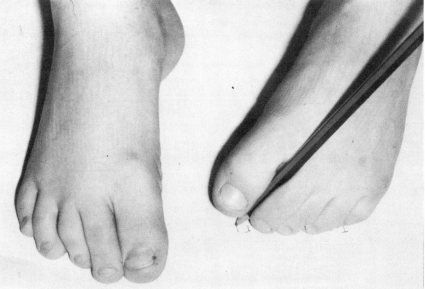

The segments cannot slide over each other and the joints cannot take tension.

This cannot be applied to the foot, which is a multi-segmented beam in compression on its dorsal surface and in tension on its lower surface. This allows for flexibility and movement, and indeed, if one ignores the os calcis of the plantigrade foot, there is great similarity between the feet of digitgrade animals and man. Hicks (1961) has shown that apparent flattening or raising of the medial longitudinal arch is due to flexion and extension occurring in the first ray at the tarso-metatarsal junction.

Changes in the form of the external appearance of the normal foot on static weight-bearing are due to alterations and displacements of soft tissues (Carlsöö & Wetzenstein 1968). One cannot speak of any true changes in the form of the foot skeleton during this type of weight bearing. In terms of support, the intrinsic muscles, tibialis anterior and peroneus longus have been shown to be inactive on static weight-bearing (Basmajian & Stecko 1963) and this is strong evidence that the ligaments and plantar aponeurosis must play a predominant role in the support of the static foot skeleton. Even when loads up to 200 pounds have been applied to the legs there has been no evidence of muscular activity. With 400 pounds the muscles do come into play but then only a few, such as tibialis anterior and posterior are found to be active. The ligaments of the foot are histologically identical to the plantar fascia. Plantar fascia has thus been studied extensively from the biomechanical aspect (Wright & Rennals 1964) because its length and accessibility permit it to be tested more easily than specimens of ligaments. It has been shown that the degree of stretching is not proportional to the load, but does decrease considerably with increased load.

In other words, plantar fascia has a progressively increasing modulus of elasticity and as increasing load is applied the specimen becomes stiffer or more able to resist deformation. This pattern of behaviour is thought to result from the mixture of collagen and elastic fibres found in the ligaments.

Accessory bones in the foot

Abnormal ossicles may be found in the foot and, if not recognized, make the interpretation of radiographs difficult, as they may be mistaken for evidence of trauma. Accessory bones may be due to additional centres of ossification or be present as sesamoid bones, which occur in tendons where an acute angulation occurs or where the tendon is subjected to pressure. These bony variations may be found either bilaterally or unilaterally, but the latter situation is more common in the foot. Basmajian (1971) lists the following common examples:

1   The os trigonium or separate posterior tubercle of the talus.
2   The tibiale externum or separate navicular tuberosity.
3   A bipartite medial cuneiform in the upper and lower halves.
4   A sesamoid within the tendon of peroneus longus where it changes direction to pass beneath the cuboid into the sole of the foot.
5   A sesamoid bone in the tibialis posterior tendon.
6   The tuberosity of the base of the fifth metatarsal existing as a separate bone (os vesalianium).

Congenital tarsal fusions may occur between almost any two bones and probably arise as an absence of joint cavitation (O'Rahilly 1953). Peroneal spastic flat foot is generally due to talocalcaneal or calcaneonavicular fusion. The abnormal junctions may be either bony or cartilaginous.

JOINTS OF THE ANKLE AND FOOT

The ankle joint has two axes of movement (Barnett & Napier 1952). One exists when the joint is in the flexion two-thirds of its range and the other when it is in the extension one-third. The foot thus moves in the ankle like a poorly mounted wheel and swerves slightly from side to side as dorsi- and plantarflexion takes place (Wyller 1963). Most people are aware of the relatively greater instability of their ankles in the plantarflexed as compared with the dorsiflexed position.

Normally the swerve is compensated by the action of the subtalar and talonavicular joints, i.e. peritalar joint (see below). Inman (1976) suggests that the talus is a frustrum (or section) of a cone. A section cut at 90° to the axis of the cone is circular when projected on to a transverse plane of the cone and corresponds to the fibular facet. A section cut obliquely is elliptical and corresponds to the tibial facet. The fibular facet being further from the apex of the cone produces greater dimensions. The subtalar joint, like the ankle, is for practical purposes a hinge in its function but its axis is at an angle of 42° to the ground and 16° to the sagittal plane (Fig. 2.2). A hinge joining two segments at an angle becomes what is called by

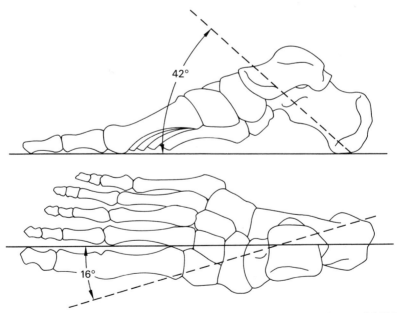

Fig. 2.2 The axis of the subtalar joint (from Manter 1941) (By kind permission of G.K. Rose FRCS and the Editor of *Journal of Bone and Joint Surgery*).

engineers a torque converter. Rotation of one segment about its long axis causes similar rotation in the other segment (Rose 1962).

The only tarsal joints with mobility amounting to more than slight gliding are the subtalar, talonavicular and calcaneocuboid joints. As pointed out by Shephard (1961; Fig. 2.3) in a very clear description, the functional combinations are:

1   The talonavicular and subtalar joints together allow movement of the remainder of the foot about the stationary talus and is referred to as the 'peritalar joint'.

2   The talonavicular and calcaneocuboid joints are the midtarsal joint, and allow rotation between the fore and hind parts of the foot.

The peritalar joint is much more mobile than the midtarsal.

There is sometimes confusion about the movements that may take place in the foot. Inversion and eversion (rotation of the foot about its long axis), adduction and abduction (rotation about a vertical axis) are sometimes considered, incorrectly, as isolated movements. They cannot occur independently. The complex movements of inversion and eversion refer to changes in position and form of the whole foot when the foot is off the ground (Warwick & Williams 1973). A further source of confusion is that inversion and eversion are often loosely used when supination and pronation are meant (Shephard 1951). Furthermore inversion is usually associated with plantarflexion of the ankle joint and eversion with dorsiflexion.

The terms pronation and supination of the foot are used only when the foot is

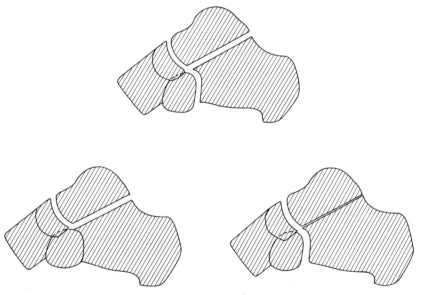

Fig. 2.3 Functional joints of the tarsus. (Top) the only joints with a material range of movement are the subtalar, talonavicular and calcaneocuboid; (bottom) the two functional combinations of these joints are the peritalar joint (left) and the mid-tarsal joint (right). (By kind permission of E. Shephard FRCS and the Editor of *Journal of Bone and Joint Surgery*).

bearing weight. Pronation is, by analogy with the hand, a downward rotation of the medial border and great toe towards the ground and supination is the reverse of this, being the movement to bring the lateral border into more direct plantigrade contact (Warwick & Williams 1973). The twist imparted to the foot by pronation and, to some extent, undone in supination, has been compared to a twisted plate able to untwist in a resiliant manner (MacConaill 1945).

A small amount of flexion-extension type of movement occurs in relation to each ray of the foot. This is not entirely independent for each individual ray as the interconnections through the lengths of each segment causes them to follow each other to some extent (Hicks 1953). An understanding of the working of the joints of the foot is of practical importance for orthopaedic surgeons in relation to both problems of orthopaedics and trauma. For example, it seems likely that club feet are a congenital dislocation of the talocalcaneonavicular joint ('peritalar' joint). Furthermore, traumatic dislocations of the talus can be classified in relation to the midtarsal and peritalar joints, or total dislocation of the talus may occur (Kenwright & Taylor 1970). It is of interest that occasionally where congenital bony fusions of the tarsus occur which preclude normal subtalar and midtarsal movement, abnormal ankle joints may be found. These have been described as of the 'ball and socket' type (Lamb 1958), and allow abnormal mobility at the ankle to compensate for stiffness of the foot (Fig. 2.4).

THE TOES

It is of some importance to recall the common variations of the lengths of the toes that may occur (i.e. digital formula). The big toe is usually the longest digit (69% of

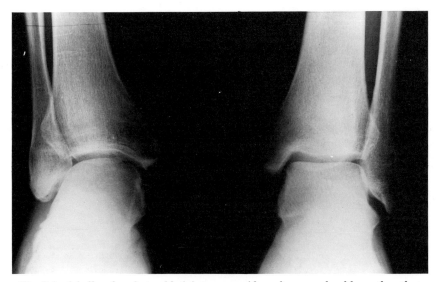

Fig. 2.4 A ball and socket ankle joint on one side and a normal ankle on the other.

subjects), great and second toes equal in length 7%, and the second toe is longest in 5% (Lake 1952). The lengths of the metatarsals do not coincide with the digital formula and it is the second metatarsal that is typically the longest. Toe length is significant in the assessment of patients for surgical procedures that shorten the great toe, as in Keller's operation. If the second toe is thereby left very long, prophylactic shortening is necessary to prevent the development of a hammer toe deformity.

In a nonprehensile foot, such as the human, the range of movement of the toes lies in dorsiflexion rather than plantarflexion. In this respect the toes differ from the fingers, whose working range lies between the neutral and the flexed position. The articular cartilage of the metatarsal heads is continued further dorsally than it is on the metacarpal heads. Dorsiflexion occurs twice during the stance phase of walking. Active dorsiflexion starts just before heel contact and continues until after the ball of the foot has been in contact with the ground. Passive dorsiflexion occurs after the heel leaves the floor before push-off, as the toes are forced dorsally by the weight of the body (Bøjsen-Moller & Lamoreaux 1979).

The function of the toes is two-fold; prehensile and ambulatory (Lambrinudi 1932). In modern man the prehensile function is secondary and the toes function mainly in the straight position. They thus effectively extend the area of weight-bearing forwards and thereby help reduce the load on the metatarsal heads. The share of the body weight taken by the pads of the toes varies, depending upon the position of the foot in the gait cycle. In the later part of foot contact the toes play a predominant part, carrying about one third of the load at 50% of the cycle (see Chapter 3). In walking the lumbricals flex the metatarsophalangeal joints and the interossei draw the metatarsal heads together and thus prevent the foot from spreading. Both groups also extend the interphalangeal joints and prevent the toes curling up and clawing. The interossei of the foot differ from those in the hand in that the second instead of the third ray is the axis about which abduction and adduction take place in the foot. The little toe in particular is often held in contempt by surgeons. Jones (1949) pointed out that it has some importance in weight-bearing and should not be removed without good reason. Even relatively functionless toes seem to be of some use in the maintenance of balance as in the situation after filleting procedures, such as Fowler's or Kates' and Kessel's operations (see Chapter 5). After amputation of all toes it is essential to provide shoes of normal length with two blocks, to enable the patient to walk normally (Flint & Sweetnam 1960) as balance is disturbed by shortening the lever action of the foot.

GAIT CYCLE

A single walking cycle on a horizontal surface consists of 60% stand phase and 40% swing phase (Fig. 2.5). A 'gait cycle' is the period from the time one of the feet strikes the ground until the same foot makes contact with the ground again. There

SPECIAL KINESIOLOGY

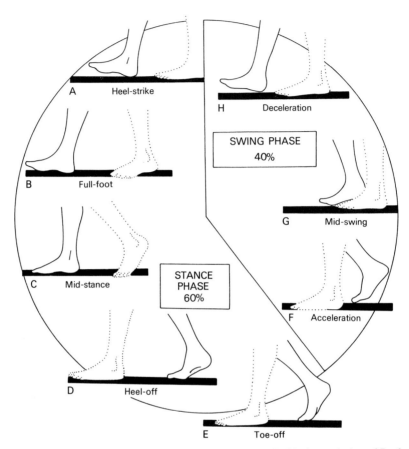

Fig. 2.5 A single walking cycle on a horizontal surface. (By kind permission of Professor John V. Basmajian and *Anatomical Record*.)

is a time at the beginning and the end of each cycle when both feet are on the ground. The speed of walking governs the time each leg will remain in contact with the ground. At the point of 'mid-stance' the body weight is entirely over the foot (MacConail & Basmajian 1969). The distribution of weight through the foot during various parts of the gait cycle will be discussed in Chapter 3.

PULSES

It is essential to take stock of the circulation whenever one examines the feet. The dorsalis pedis pulse is normally palpable on the dorsum of the foot midway between the medial and lateral malleoli. It is a continuation of the anterior tibial artery which changes its name as it crosses the ankle joint. However, in 3.5% (18.76) of 536 limbs Grant (1952) found the dorsalis pedis artery was a continuation of the perforating branch of the peroneal artery. The posterior tibial pulse is normally felt midway between the medial malleolus and the point of the heel where the artery ends beneath the flexor retinaculum by dividing into the medial and lateral plantar vessels. Absence of the posterior tibial vessel is an occasional finding with compensatory enlargement of the peroneal artery.

In a series of men 40 years of age or younger known to be free of peripheral vascular disease the incidence of absence of dorsalis pedis pulses was 4.5%. In this same group there was only an incidence of 0.5% of absent posterior tibial pulses. The absence of a dorsalis pedis pulse does not necessarily carry the implication of peripheral vascular disease whereas in contrast in the case of the absent posterior tibial pulse, this is much more likely (Stephens 1952).

THE SKIN

Skin thickness ranges from 0.5 mm (as in the eyelid) to 4.5 mm in the sole of the foot. The thickness of the plantar skin is due to the thick epidermis with a wide layer of keratin on its superficial surface. This is the state from birth, but with intermittent pressure and friction the thickness increases (Fig. 2.6). Between the plantar aponeurosis and the skin there are numerous fibrous bands that bind the two together. The sole pad develops during the early months of intrauterine life and is

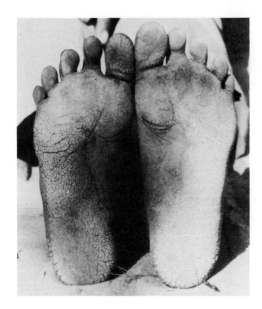

Fig. 2.6 The feet of an adult African who has never worn shoes. (By kind permission of Professor L. Solomon, University of the Witwatersrand, Johannesburg.)

responsible for the smooth convex contours and the flat footed appearance of the feet in the embryo and young child. Later the sole pad is confined mainly to areas of the greatest weight-bearing and is consequently best developed at the heel, along the fibular border of the sole and across the plantar aspects of the metatarsal heads to join the pad of the great toe (Jones 1946). Dissection reveals that the ball of the foot contains a connective tissue framework with transverse, vertical and sagittal fibres, all connecting the skin with the proximal phalanges of the toes. Dorsiflexion of the toes tightens the framework and thereby restricts passive movements of the skin, enabling shear forces to be transferred to the skin.

As might be expected from a consideration of the excellent results that follow a Syme's amputation, the tissues of the heel can bear the body weight for an unusually large proportion of the stance phase of the walking cycle without ill effects (Barnett 1956). The pressures borne by plantar skin are greater than is necessary to produce ischaemia, necrosis and ulceration (Hay & Walker 1973) but as one is constantly varying position, trophic changes do not occur unless fixed deformity is present. In severe neural leprosy with sensory as well as motor paralysis below the knee, the patient can always walk provided that contractures have been prevented and sores dealt with. This may equally apply to some patients with complete sciatic paralysis (Seddon 1972).

In contrast to the sole, the skin covering the dorsum of the foot is thin and has very little subcutaneous fat. Therefore the skin on the dorsum of the foot cannot tolerate much trauma. In order to minimize surgical trauma, flaps should be kept as thick as possible and care should be taken in retraction. The skin over the extensor digitorum brevis has the poorest supply of all (Pyka & Coventry 1961) as few cutaneous arteries run through the substance of the belly of this muscle. The only supply to this area of skin is from a few thin and long arteries. Incisions on the soles of the feet heal well, as is the case with incisions elsewhere in skin subjected to pressure (K.I. Nissen, pers. comm.), such as in the buttock and palm.

The value of the highly specialized skin on the sole of the foot is most appreciated when it is lost following an injury. It is possible to produce a satisfactory covering with split skin grafts if a pad of free fat remains. However, when there is no cushion of subcutaneous tissue a flap is required. All distant flaps (from abdomen, thigh etc) are inherently defective because they do not contain fibrous elements which bind the skin to the underlying tissues in the normal sole and reduce shearing stresses. Useful local flaps may be fashioned from the skin on the lateral aspect of the ankle, which is nourished by the terminal branches of the peroneal artery and some elements of the sural nerve or skin based on the inner aspects of the heel supplied by the medial calcanean artery and nerve (Maisels 1961).

REFERENCES

Acton R.K. (1967) Surgical anatomy of the foot. *Journal of Bone and Joint Surgery* **49A,** 555–67.

BARNETT C.H. (1956) The phases of human gait. *The Lancet* ii, 617–21.

BARNETT C.H. & NAPIER J.R. (1952) The axis of rotation at the ankle joint in man. Its influence upon the form of the talus and mobility of the fibula. *Journal of Anatomy (Lond.)* 86, 1–9.

BASMAJIAN J.V. (1967) *Muscles Alive*, 2nd edition, p. 241–2. Williams and Wilkins, Baltimore.

BASMAJIAN J.V. (1971) *Grant's Method of Anatomy*, 8th edition. Williams and Wilkins, Baltimore.

BASMAJIAN J.V. & STECKO G. (1963) The role of muscles in arch support of the foot. *Journal of Bone and Joint Surgery* 31B, 1184–90.

BØJSEN-MOLLER F. & LAMOREAUX L. (1979) Significance of free dorsiflexion of the toes in walking. *Acta Orthopaedica Scandinavica* 50, 471–9.

CARLSÖÖ S.L. & WETZENSTEIN H. (1968) Change of form of the foot and the foot skeleton upon momentary weight-bearing. *Acta Orthopaedica Scandinavica* 39, 413–23.

FLINT M.M. & SWEETNAM R. (1960) Amputation of all toes. *Journal of Bone and Joint Surgery* 42B, 90–6.

GRANT J.C.B. (1952) *A Method of Anatomy*, p. 441. Ballière, Tindall & Cox, London.

HAY M.C. & WALKER G.F. (1973) Plantar pressures in healthy children and in children with myelomeningocele. *Journal of Bone and Joint Surgery* 55B, 828–33.

HICKS J.H. (1953) The mechanics of the foot. I. The joints. *Journal of Anatomy* 87, 345–57.

HICKS J.H. (1954) The mechanics of the foot. II. *Journal of Anatomy* 88, 25–30.

HICKS J.H. (1961) The three weight-bearing mechanisms of the foot. In Evans F.G. (ed.) *Biomechanical Studies of the Musculo-Skeletal System*, p. 161–91. Thomas, Springfield, Illinois.

INMAN V.T. (1976) *The Joints of the Ankle*, p. 29. Williams & Wilkins, Baltimore.

JONES F.W. (1946) *Buchanan's manual of anatomy*, 7th edition, Baillière, Tindall & Cassell, London.

JONES F.W. (1949) *Structure and Function as Seen in the Foot*, 2nd edition. Baillière, Tindall & Cassell, London.

KENWRIGHT J. & TAYLOR R.G. (1970) Major injuries of the talus. *Journal of Bone and Joint Surgery* 52B, 36–48.

LAKE N.C. (1952) *The Foot*, p. 126. Baillière, Tindall & Cassell, London.

LAMB D. (1958) The ball and socket ankle joint—a congenital abnormality. *Journal of Bone and Joint Surgery* 40B, 240–43.

LAMBRINUDI C. (1932) Use and abuse of toes. *Postgraduate Medical Journal* 8, 459–63.

LAMBRINUDI C. (1938) The feet of the industrial worker. Functional aspect: Action of foot muscles. *The Lancet* ii, 1480–82.

MACCONAILL M.A. (1945) The postural mechanism of the human foot. *Proceedings of Royal Irish Academy, L, Section B*, 14, 265–78.

MACCONAILL M.A. & BASMAJIAN J.V. (1969) *Muscles and movements: a basis for human kinesiology*, p. 74. Williams & Wilkins, Baltimore.

MAISELS D.O. (1961) Repairs of the heel. *British Journal of Plastic Surgery* 14, 117–25.

MANN R. & INMAN V.T. (1964) Phasic activity of intrinsic muscles of the foot. *Journal of Bone and Joint Surgery* 46A, 469–81.

MANTER J.T. (1941) Movement of the subtalar and transverse tarsal joints. *Anatomical Record* 80, 397–409.

McKENZIE J. (1955) The foot as a half dome. *British Medical Journal* 1, 1068–70.

O'RAHILLY R. (1953) A survey of carpal and tarsal anomalies. *Journal of Bone and Joint Surgery* 35A, 626–39.

PYKA R.A. & COVENTRY M.B. (1961) Avascular necrosis of skin after operations on feet. *Journal of Bone and Joint Surgery* 43A, 955–60.

ROSE G.K. (1958) Correction of the pronated foot. *Journal of Bone and Joint Surgery* 40B, 674–83.

SEDDON H. (1972) *Surgical Disorders of the Peripheral Nerves*, p. 223. Churchill Livingstone, Edinburgh.

SHEPHARD E. (1951) Tarsal movements. *Journal of Bone and Joint Surgery* **33B,** 258–63.
STEPHENS G.L. (1952) Palpable dorsalis pedis and posterior tibial pulses. *Archives of Surgery* **84,** 662–4.
WARWICK R. & WILLIAMS P.L. (1973) (eds.) *Grays Anatomy,* 35th edition, p. 464. Longman, Edinburgh.
WRIGHT D.G., DESAI S.M. & HENDERSON W.H. (1964) Action of subtalar and ankle joint complex during stance phase of walking. *Journal of Bone and Joint Surgery* **46A,** 361–82.
WRIGHT D.G. & RENNELS D.C. (1964) A study of the elastic properties of plantar fascia. *Journal of Bone and Joint Surgery* **46A,** 482–92.
WYLLER T. (1963) The axis of the ankle joint and its importance in subtalar arthrodesis. *Acta Orthopaedica Scandinavica* **33,** 320–8.

3

The Mechanics of the Foot

W.C. HUTTON, J.R.R. STOTT & I.A.F. STOKES

The function of the foot is essentially mechanical. As the final linkage in the lever system of the leg, it has to transmit the forces of stance and locomotion to the ground in a way that is related to the terrain. Given the appropriate neuromuscular control and aided by suitable footwear, the human foot is remarkable in the way it has adapted to function successfully on such diverse terrain as rock faces, football fields, snow slopes and ice rinks.

On an evolutionary time scale these changes in function have been suddenly imposed on a structure that has only recently become adapted to upright stance and locomotion. It would not be surprising if analysis of the mechanics of the foot were to suggest the incompleteness of this evolutionary process, and that some of the disorders of the foot are the result of asking it to function in a way for which it is not yet adapted. For example, from an engineer's point of view, the first metatarsal would seem designed to carry a large proportion of the load on the forefoot, but measured loads on the first metatarsal are often surprisingly small in comparison with those on the slender second and third metatarsals, and it is these bones, rather than the first metatarsal, which are particularly liable to fatigue fracture. It seems as though the first metatarsal has not yet lost the structure it needed as an opposable digit, nor yet fully gained the mechanical function its size deserves.

The wearing of shoes, while allowing a whole new range of activities, may also influence normal foot function and lead to unusual stresses on the foot. This can be particularly true when shoes are designed to meet the demands of fashion rather than function. It is recognized that hallux valgus is associated with the wearing of shoes, but it is still not clear what new stresses on the foot and which designs of shoe are most liable to lead to the disorder. Part of the difficulty in obtaining more precise information is that of making relevant measurements. A well-fitting shoe does not leave much space for measuring devices, and footwear specially adapted for the purpose takes no account of the wearing-in process that makes a shoe conform to its owner's foot.

A number of diseases that affect the foot alter the way in which it functions. It is useful to study the mechanical consequences of such conditions in order to follow the progress of the disease and to assess the value of therapeutic efforts. Equipment for this purpose, hitherto largely confined to the research environment, is beginning to find a more routine clinical use.

This chapter begins by outlining the methods available to study the function of the foot and then considers the mechanics of the foot in walking and standing. Running imposes higher loads on the foot than walking (Stott *et al* 1973), but there is a lack of detailed information about the mechanics of running, in particular the magnitude of the stresses within the foot. A qualitative description of running and jumping has been given by Dyson (1967) and James and Brubaker (1973).

METHODS OF STUDY

There are two complementary elements in the study of the mechanics of the foot. The first is termed kinematics, and deals with the relative movements of the lower limb elements during various activities. The second element, kinetics, is concerned with the analysis of forces exerted on the foot for the purpose of weight-bearing and locomotion. It is only when considered together and in relation to the detailed anatomy of the foot, that an understanding of the mechanics of the foot, as yet far from complete, begins to emerge.

Kinematics of gait

Eadweard Muybridge (1887) pioneered the use of cinephotography in the study of human movement, and the extensive records that he obtained continue to be of use to both artists and scientists.

Present photographic techniques label significant anatomical points either with reflecting markers fixed to the skin, or, in highly motivated volunteers, by means of stainless steel pins screwed into bone (Levens *et al* 1948). The subject is then photographed walking, either using the techniques of stroboscopic photography (Murray *et al* 1964) which generates multiple exposures on a single frame from which measurements can be made directly, or using cinephotography together with a projection system capable of measuring the displacement of any marked point on the subject between successive frames (Sutherland & Hagy 1972). The process of obtaining quantitative date from photographic records is very time consuming. Techniques are now available which enable a number of anatomical points, marked with miniature infra-red light emitting diodes, to be tracked automatically by means of a television camera linked to the signal analysis facilities of a computer.

Angular movements at certain joints may be studied more conveniently by means of goniometers. Wright *et al* (1964) describe their use in measuring movements of the subtalar and ankle joints. The goniometer is fixed across the joint in such a way that its axis of rotation is aligned with that of the joint. Its output can be calibrated in terms of the angular displacement of the joint. Analysis of movement at other joints within the foot during walking have received relatively little attention compared with the study of gait as a whole. These movements, though small, are significant in maintaining the structural stability of the foot.

Kinetics of the foot

Direct measurement of forces acting within the foot is not currently possible though some of these forces can be estimated from a detailed knowledge of the anatomy of the foot and from measurement of the forces between the foot and the ground (Stokes *et al* 1979a). A number of methods are available for the measurement of external forces on the foot.

Force plates

A force plate consists of a load-sensitive surface set into a walkway which measures the changing forces imposed on it during the period of foot contact. If the record of force is analysed in conjunction with kinematic data, the forces acting at other points in the leg can be calculated. For example, by considering the lower limb as three levers, the femur, the tibia, and the foot, hinged to move in the sagittal plane, Elftman (1939) has calculated the angular forces acting at the ankle, the knee and the hip, and has determined the transfer of energy that occurs between the lower limb elements and the trunk. In a similar manner it is possible to deduce the cycle of loading on the hip joint during walking (Paul 1967).

One of the first force plates was developed by Manter (1938) to study the dynamics of quadrupedal walking. This consisted of a light platform, supported on springs. The displacement of the loaded platform was magnified by a lever system and recorded by cinephotography. As advances were made in electronics, more sophisticated techniques were developed. A group at the University of California (1947) and Cunningham and Brown (1952) both described a force plate which used strain gauges as the transducing elements. The design developed by them was improved by Harper *et al* (1961). Rydell (1966) in a study of the forces acting on the femoral head prosthesis, used a force plate system which consisted of two identical plates, five metres long, placed side by side, one for each foot. The plates were suspended from load cells which enabled them to measure the vertical and horizontal components of force on each foot during walking.

A typical force plate in current use consists of a rigid rectangular plate about 50 cm by 30 cm set into the floor of a walkway and supported near each corner by load cells. Vertical, longitudinal and transverse forces and also torques can be measured separately. It is also possible to derive the centre of load, the point on the force plate at which the force exerted between the foot and the ground can be considered to act (Fig. 3.4).

An essential feature that has to be considered in the design of a force plate is the frequency response of the system. This is a measure of how fast and with what accuracy the system will respond to abrupt changes in load. To transduce accurately the forces imposed on it, a load-measuring system must have a lowest natural frequency which is substantially higher than any of the applied frequencies (Marsden & Montgomery 1972).

Pressure transducers

The use of pressure transducers provides a convenient method of studying the forces on selected areas of the foot. One particular advantage they have over other methods is that they can be worn inside shoes and thus enable studies on the mechanical effect of footwear and therapeutic insoles. There are however a number of problems associated with interpretation of the records generated by transducers.

The sole of the foot is irregular in contour and varies in compliance from the relatively unyielding region under the metatarsal heads to the softer areas under the midfoot. As a result, the force transmitted across the region of foot contact changes quite markedly with small changes in position. It is important to know how a transducer, which may have a fairly large pressure sensing area, summates forces that are varying from point to point across its surface. In addition, it is often difficult to be sure that by its presence between two relatively incompliant surfaces, the transducer is not altering the pressure it attempts to measure. A further difficulty that is inherent in sampling only a few points under the sole of the foot is the problem of inferring the pressure elsewhere on the foot. Unless a very large number of small transducers are used, there is no possibility of integrating pressure values over a specific area to derive the total force transmitted.

Schwartz and Heath (1949) used pressure transducers to obtain recordings from 503 subjects. They showed wide variations in foot function between individuals, but published no quantitative analysis of their results. Bauman and Brand (1963) measured the pressure between the foot and the shoe by means of a capacitance-type pressure transducer 1 mm thick. The method was designed to evaluate footwear for patients with leprosy in whom excessive pressures under certain metatarsal heads was demonstrated. Holden and Muncey (1953) described the modification of a shoe to hold a capacitance pressure transducer in the heel and also the use of a transducer 3 mm thick for pressure recordings at other sites between the foot and the shoe. Collis and Jayson (1972) used pressure transducers 2 mm thick to study the pressures under the heel and the metatarsal heads in both normal subjects and patients with rheumatoid arthritis. They found the highest pressures in normal feet under the second and third metatarsal heads and showed that patients with rheumatoid arthritis could alter their gait to reduce the pressure under a painful joint. Inactivity of the toes was found to be reflected in higher pressures under the corresponding metatarsal heads.

Force distribution measurement

Beely (1882), a general practitioner from Berlin, made one of the first recorded attempts to determine the load pattern under the foot. He stood on a linen bag filled with rapidly setting plaster of Paris. From the negative casts produced, he made positive casts of the foot from which he was able to study changes in contour of the sole of the foot in various stance postures and when carrying loads.

The kinetograph described by Morton (1935) enabled a more quantitative approach. The apparatus consisted of a long baseboard covered with a rubber mat, the top surface of which was corrugated. The mat was covered with an inked fabric and a layer of paper. As the subject walked on the apparatus, the corrugations were deformed, and the width of the ink impression gave a measure of the maximum pressure exerted during walking. Elftman (1934) reported on a similar type of apparatus, but by means of cinephotography he was able to produce a permanent record of the changes in pressure distribution with time. Barnett (1954) studied the phases of human gait by means of a device which consisted of 1 cm square section perpex rods standing on end on a thick slab of sponge rubber: 650 rods were arranged to form a block having an upper surface 16×40 inches. The downward displacement of each rod was recorded photographically as the subject stepped on to the block.

These methods rely for their accuracy on measuring the deformation of rubber under load. As a material rubber is not ideal for measuring rapidly changing loads on account of its viscoelastic properties. Deformation is dependent not only on the magnitude of the load but also the length of time for which it is applied. A further problem associated with measuring systems that yield significantly under load is that peaks of load become more uniformly distributed than when walking on a rigid surface.

An improvement on the type of system used by Barnett was developed by Arcan and Brull (1976). They used an array of metal plungers pressing onto a photoelastic coating on glass. When illuminated with polarized light, photoelastic materials exhibit dark fringes, the pattern of which indicate the stress in the material. This apparatus is more rigid and has a faster response to changing forces compared with the methods using rubber materials.

An apparatus to give a dynamic visual display of force distributions was developed by Chodera and Lord (1979). It consisted of a plastic foil placed on a glass plate illuminated through its edge, on which a subject can walk or stand, thus pressing the plastic foil into contact with the glass. The contact areas between the glass and the plastic foil reflect light downwards and the intensity of reflected light varies with the applied pressure. The image produced by the foot was recorded using a television camera and displayed using a contour plot or a colour scale to indicate pressure levels (Betts 1979). Clinical application of this system is described by Betts *et al* 1980.

A modification of the force plate principle undertaken by the authors to record force distribution has been to subdivide a force plate into twelve independent strips each recording against a base of time the vertical component of load. The strips can be orientated either transverse or longitudinal to the direction of walking and their output used to generate the longitudinal and transverse load profiles. A further development has been the construction of a force plate subdivided into 128 squares, each 15 mm × 15 mm recording vertical load (Fig. 3.1). Data is collected and analysed by computer (Dhanendran *et al* 1978).

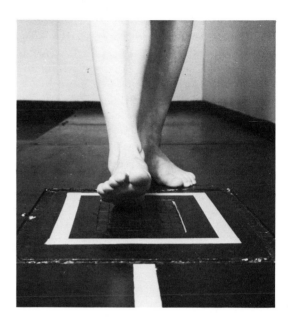

Fig. 3.1 A subject on the walkway stepping on to the subdivided force plate. The vertical load on each of the 128 square areas is recorded, processed and displayed by a computer.

THE FOOT IN WALKING

During normal walking at about 112 steps/minute the foot spends about 60% of time in contact with the ground (stance phase) and the remaining 40% swinging through to take up its new position ahead of the supporting foot (swing phase) (Murray *et al* 1964). It follows that both feet are in contact with the ground simultaneously for 10% of the walking cycle immediately after the heel meets the ground (heel-strike). These values change only slightly with changes in walking rate; at 150 steps per minute the stance phase is reduced to 57% of the walking cycle. For this reason, in the description that follows, the timing of events is referred to in terms of percentage of the walking cycle, the cycle of events for one foot starting at heel-strike, and ending when the same foot meets the ground again two steps later (Fig. 3.2.)

The centre of gravity of the body moves up and down as we walk. The amplitude of this vertical oscillation is about 5 cm. At the same time, the forward velocity of the trunk is being alternately increased and decreased, so that when the forefoot first reaches the ground at 5% of the cycle, the trunk is at its lowest point and its forward velocity is at a maximum. Similarly, when at 30% of the cycle the opposite foot is in the middle of its swing phase, the trunk is at its highest and its forward velocity is at a minimum. In addition, the centre of gravity of the body moves laterally about 3 cm to each side of the midline in order to bring itself more nearly over the supporting foot; the maximum deviation to one side occurs at 20% of the cycle after heel-strike on that side.

These displacements and changes in velocity are approximately sinusoidal. They represent a compromise between mechanical efficiency and anatomical constraints. The displacements of the trunk and the changes in horizontal velocity are the result of forces exerted by the muscles of the leg and their total effect can be seen in the reaction forces as measured by a force plate (Fig. 3.2).

The stance phase of walking has been extensively studied (Barnett 1956; Harper et al 1961; Murray et al 1964; Drillis 1958). At heel-strike, there is 3–4° of transverse rotation of the pelvis to bring the acetabulum forward, and the knee is extended in order to lengthen the forward reach of the leg. The ankle joint is sufficiently dorsiflexed to project the heel forward for initial contact. Subsequent quick plantarflexion allows early contact of the entire foot with the floor (Fig. 3.2). The early phase of foot contact is associated with deceleration of the body-mass both vertically and in the forward direction. This is achieved, first by activity of the tibialis anterior and the long extensor muscles, which retard the forefoot as it comes to the ground, and then by allowing about 20° of knee flexion against the restraining action of the quadriceps. The vertical force recorded by force plate at this time (15% of the walking cycle) usually exceeds body weight by 10–20%. At the same time, the record of the component of force in the direction of walking, after a transient backward force as the heel registers with the ground, shows a maximum retarding force. Up to this time in the cycle, no activity can be recorded in the intrinsic muscles of the foot, but from this point until the end of the stance phase, the intrinsic muscles together with the tibialis posterior and the peroneal muscles all show moderate activity (Mann & Inman 1964). Their effect is to brace the foot in preparation for the transfer of load on to the forefoot and for the subsequent push-off phase.

An aspect of the dynamics of gait important for the stability of the foot during walking is the sequence of rotation movements occurring about the long axis of the leg and the associated torque as recorded by the force plate. Fig. 3.2 shows the axial rotations occurring in the leg during the walking cycle (Levens et al 1948). It can be seen that the femur adds rotational movement to that of the pelvis and that the tibia contributes still more rotation. Thus the thigh and leg do not absorb rotation imposed by the trunk, but rather increase it, and this rotation makes an important contribution to the function of the foot.

When the foot is in contact with the ground the ankle and subtalar joints act together somewhat like a universal joint to convert rotation in the long axis of the tibia into a rotation about an anteroposterior axis in the foot (Wright et al 1964). More precisely, internal rotation of the tibia is converted into pronation of the foot and external rotation of the tibia into supination.

The degree of pronation of the foot has an important bearing on the mobility of the midtarsal joint. This joint is formed by two pairs of articulating surfaces, the talonavicular and the calcaneocuboid, the former a condyloid joint, the latter a saddle joint. When the foot is pronated the principal axes of these joints are more nearly in line and there is some flexion–extension mobility at the midtarsal joint. When the foot is supinated, the movement of the talus on the calcaneum at the subtalar joint throws the axes of the talonavicular and calcaneocuboid joints out of line and the midtarsal joint is effectively locked (Elftman 1960). It appears

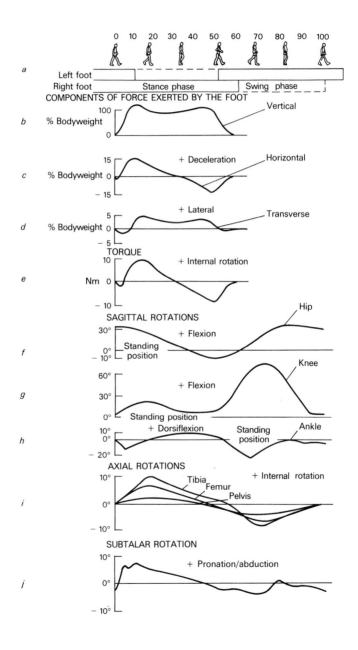

therefore that rotatory movements in the tibia during the stance phase of walking serve to control the rigidity of the foot at the midtarsal joint.

At heel strike the tibia is undergoing internal rotation. From the time of full foot contact with the ground until 15% of the cycle, the foot is pronating and consequently while the heel is the principal load-sustaining part of the foot, the forefoot is relatively mobile. From this point in the cycle, until after the foot leaves the ground, external rotation is occurring in the tibia and hence supination in the foot. Thus, at a time when the load is being transferred to the forefoot, supination of the foot converts it into a rigid lever in preparation for the push-off phase.

The torques recorded by the force plate represent the extent to which the tissues of the foot resist the rotational forces imposed upon them by the tibia. The magnitude and sequence of these forces show wide variation from one individual to another. The most usual pattern is that the foot exerts an internal rotation torque of 2–5 Nm (Newton metres) early in the stance phase at 12% of the cycle, followed by external rotation torque reaching 3–10 Nm towards the end of the stance phase, at 45% of the cycle.

The vertical forces in excess of body weight during the heel phase impart an upward acceleration to the trunk. Between 25% and 30% of the cycle, as the other leg is swinging through, the force plate records a vertical load of about 75% of body weight. From this point onwards, the vertical load increases to reach a second maximum at 45% of the cycle, when it exceeds body weight by about 25%. At the same time an increasing horizontal component of force produces forward acceleration of the trunk. The second peak of load is the result of muscular activity in soleus and gastrocnemius. Their contraction is initially isometric and prevents dorsiflexion of the ankle beyond about 10°, so that as the supporting leg passes the vertical position, the heel lifts from the ground and the foot pivots about the metatarsal heads. When active plantarflexion occurs there is almost simultaneous flexion at the knee so that this period of calf muscle activity also helps to accelerate the leg forwards and upwards to begin its swing phase.

Because the line of the metatarsal heads is not transverse to the direction of walking, but inclines laterally and backwards by about 30°, as the foot tips forward on the metatarsal heads the lateral metatarsal heads tend to leave the ground and

---

Fig. 3.2 A summary of the forces and joint movements throughout the walking cycle. (a) The relative timing of stance and swing phases for each foot. Graphs (b) to (e) show typical forces during the stance phase as recorded by a force plate; (b) the vertical component of force, (c) the anteroposterior component, (d) the transverse component and (e) the torque about a vertical axis. (Redrawn from Rehman *et al* (1948) by permission of *Archives of Physical Medicine*.) Graphs (f) to (h) show the relative angular movements in the sagittal plane at the hip, knee and ankle. (Redrawn from Murray *et al* (1964) by permission of the *Journal of Bone and Joint Surgery*.) Graph (i) shows the rotation occurring about the vertical axis of the pelvis and about the long axis of the femur and the tibia. (Redrawn from Levens *et al* (1948) by permission of *Journal of Bone and Joint Surgery*). Graph (j) shows the movement at the subtalar joint about its axis, which in the standing position lies on a line passing forwards, upwards and medially through the head of the talus. (Redrawn from Wright *et al* 1964 by permission of *Journal of Bone and Joint Surgery*).

the centre of load moves medially. Several mechanisms act to diminish this effect and maintain load on the lateral metatarsal heads. The first is that external rotation of the tibia continues to produce supination of the foot. Also backward and lateral inclination of the ankle joint axis (about 20°) adds a small component of supination to the predominant movement of plantarflexion. Finally, limited flexion–extension movement at the tarsometatarsal joints allows some readjustment of the metatarsal heads.

The dorsiflexion of the toes that occurs in the second half of the stance phase as the heel leaves the ground has the effect of increasing tension in the plantar aponeurosis. This has been termed the windlass effect (Hicks 1953), though the importance of this mechanism in bracing the longitudinal arch of the foot has probably been over estimated. The toes assume an important role at this stage of the walking cycle. There is increased activity in the long and short toe flexors (Mann & Inman 1964) and the load transmitted through the toes can reach 50% of body weight.

Fig. 3.3 shows the longitudinal and transverse load distribution patterns at 5% intervals of the walking cycle during the period of foot contact of a normal subject. The forefoot is in contact with the ground from 5% of the cycle after heel-strike. There follows a smooth transfer of load from the heel to the forefoot and by 30% of the cycle the heel is leaving the ground. At no time does the midfoot carry significant amounts of load. During the later part of foot contact the toes play a prominent part carrying about one third of the total load.

From these diagrams the position of load at successive instants in the walking cycle can be calculated. Fig. 3.4 plots its movement during the period of foot contact. This may prove to be a useful and concise way of expressing force distribution data.

THE FOOT IN STANDING

A number of conflicting theories have been put forward about the way in which the foot distributes the body weight when standing. Morton (1935) suggested that the load is shared equally between the heel and the forefoot, and that the first metatarsal segment carries one third and the remaining metatarsals one sixth of the forefoot load. Jones (1944) considered that, in addition to the heel and forefoot, the lateral border of the foot makes an important contribution to load-bearing. Burger (1952) found a weight distribution ratio between heel and forefoot of 5:3 and a more equal division of load between the metatarsals than was suggested by Morton. Dickson and Diveley (1953) state that the load on the foot is concentrated on three areas, the heel and the heads of the first and fifth metatarsals. Jones (1941) agreed with Morton on the 1:1 weight distribution between heel and forefoot. On the basis of cadaver studies, however, he considered the lateral four metatarsals to act as a unit relatively independently of the first metatarsal. In studies on 100 medical students, he found a wide scatter in the ratio of load between the first and the lateral four metatarsals with a mean ratio of 1:2.5.

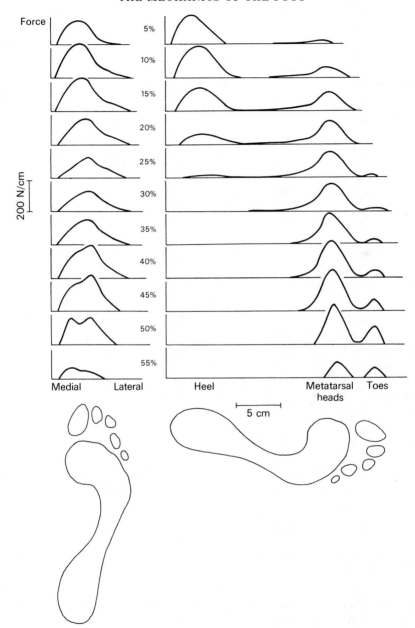

Fig. 3.3 The distribution of load on a normal foot during walking. These graphs are drawn from recordings made with the subdivided force plate used by the authors. The subdivided force plate makes it possible to draw longitudinal and transverse profiles of the distribution, which are shown in the figure at 5% intervals of the walking cycle. The smooth outline of load on the forefoot, the absence of significant load carried by the mid-foot, the moderately high load imposed on the toes and the load being imposed on the medial rather than lateral side of the foot, are typical features of the normal pattern.

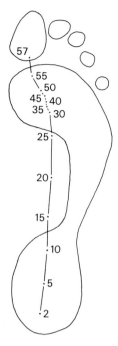

Fig. 3.4 The pathway of the centre
of load, the point through which the
load on the foot can be considered to
act, during the stance phase of
walking. Each point was derived by
finding the centre of load of the
longitudinal and corresponding
transverse distribution patterns at
successive instants, expressed in the
diagram as percentages of the
walking cycle for a normal foot.

Our own investigations using the subdivided force plate described above show
that on a firm flat surface the weight of the body is carried almost entirely by the
heel and the forefoot, and, as in walking, the normal midfoot carries very little
load. The way in which the body weight is shared between heel and forefoot was
found to be quite widely variable, and a variety of comfortable stances could be
achieved with the heel carrying between one and three times the load on the
forefoot. Calculation of the centre of load on the foot shows it to be 1·5–5 cm in
front of the ankle joint. As is well known the upright posture requires continuous
activity in the soleus muscle.

The role of the toes in stance has received little attention. We have found that
in upright stance the toes carry 5–10% of the fore-foot load, but as more weight is
transferred to the front of the foot, the toes bear an increasing proportion of this
load. They are particularly active in restoring balance. Following a gentle but
unexpected push from behind, typically 25% of the increased load imposed on the
forefoot may be taken by the toes. The effect of this is to move the centre of load on
the front part of the foot forward by about 1·5 cm and thus increase the effective
lever length of the foot. We have also found wide variation in the load distribution
across the forefoot. There is no suggestion of a transverse arch producing greater
loading on the medial and lateral borders of the forefoot; the opposite tends to be
the case with the highest loads falling on the central metatarsals. The pattern can,
however, be rapidly altered in order to maintain balance (Fig. 3.5).

During standing the longitudinal arch of the normal foot has been shown to be

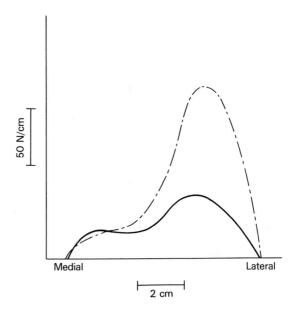

Fig. 3.5 An illustration of the change of load distribution across the right forefoot during standing (continuous trace) which resulted from a gentle but unexpected push to the right (dashed trace). Equilibrium is restored by increasing the total load on this foot, and also by supination of the foot to increase the load on the lateral side. Load shifting of this kind is used continuously in standing in order to maintain balance.

well maintained (Carlsöö & Wetzenstein 1968). X-ray studies revealed no signifi-cant change in the form of the skeletal structure of the foot between non-weight bearing and sustaining the full body weight. Jones (1941) in his study of the role of muscles in supporting longitudinal arch of the foot, points out that in standing the stress on the arch is proportional to the load carried by the forefoot and is independent of the load imposed on the heel. He demonstrates that the line of action and the muscle bulk of peroneus longus and tibialis posterior (muscles thought to be important in arch support) are inadequate to maintain the arch against the stresses upon it. Furthermore, electromyographic studies (Basmajian and Bentzon 1954, Basmajian and Stecko 1963) have shown that these muscles, and also flexor hallucis longus, abductor hallucis and the intrinsic muscles, are inactive in stance in the normal foot. They do, however, show activity during stance in subjects with pronated feet (Gray 1969).

The resemblance between the longitudinal sections through one of the three medial metatarsals and a masonry arch is unfortunate in that it has led to the supposition that there are mechanical similarities, and to the search for structures which tie together the bases of the longitudinal arch of the foot. The major determinant of the longitudinal stiffness of the foot is the alignment of the talonavicular and calcaneocuboid components of the midtarsal joint.

Maintaining the axes of each component out of alignment not only prevents movement at the midtarsal joint but effectively produces a longitudinal fold at midtarsal level between the three medial metatarsals originating on the navicular and the two lateral metatarsals based on the cuboid. This has the effect of stiffening the bony structure of the forefoot as a whole, much as a thin strip of card is stiffened by a right angle fold along its length.

Collapse of the longitudinal arch is a frequent end result of traumatic damage to the midtarsal joint and it has long been known that the same result is produced by cutting the calcaneonavicular (spring) ligament. This ligament by its strong fibrous tie between the plantar aspects of the two components of the midtarsal joint, limits the extent to which their axes can be brought into line, and thus plays an important part in maintaining the longitudinal rigidity of the foot.

LOAD DISTRIBUTION IN THE DISEASED FOOT

Hallux valgus

The development of hallux valgus is associated with a progressive shift of load from the medial to the lateral side of the foot and also a reduction in load carried by the hallux and, to a lesser extent, by the remaining toes. The changes are shown in Fig. 3.6 which also shows the increased load on the midfoot, a frequent associated finding. Pressure measurements inside fashion shoes during walking have shown striking increases in pressure under the hallux and first metatarsal head in certain types of shoe when compared with walking barefoot. These findings may be relevant to the causative role of shoes in hallux valgus. Studies to determine the effect of corrective procedures (Stokes *et al* 1976) show that far from restoring a more normal load pattern, the abnormalities of load distribution are more marked after either Keller's operation or first metatarsal wedge-type osteotomy. This worsening of load distribution is however minimized in patients undergoing osteotomy as this type of operation results in a large reduction in metatarsal angle. Reduction in load carried through the first metatarsal is compensated for by increased load under the lateral metatarsals and may result in post operative lateral metatarsalgia.

Diabetes mellitus

Diminished load on the toes is an early finding in developing diabetic neuropathy of the feet. Changes occur in the distribution of load on the metatarsal heads. At sites of neuropathic ulcers particularly high loads are found (I.A.F. Stokes *et al* 1975). Fig. 3.7 illustrates these changes in the foot of a 52-year-old diabetic with neuropathic ulceration under the fifth metatarsal head. The record also shows an area anterior to the heel at 10–40% of the walking cycle which is suggestive of damage to the midtarsal joint perhaps as a result of the development of a Charcot joint.

Rheumatoid arthritis

Loss of load carried by the toes is also an early feature of rheumatoid arthritis

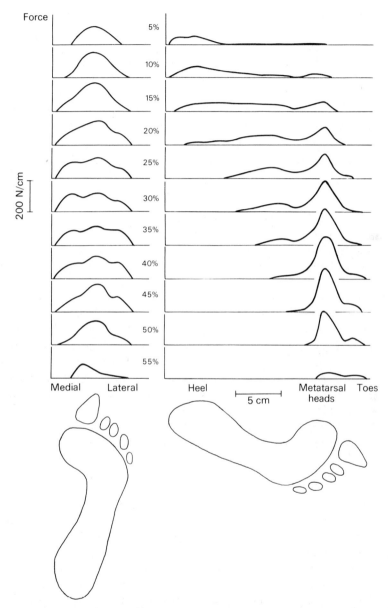

Fig. 3.6 Transverse and longitudinal load distribution patterns at 5% intervals of the walking cycle of a 50-year-old woman with hallux valgus. The reduction in load carried by the toes has led to a corresponding increase of load on the metatarsal heads. There is also a shift of fore-foot load away from the medial side of the foot. This patient shows an increased load under the midfoot characteristic of weakness of the longitudinal arch.

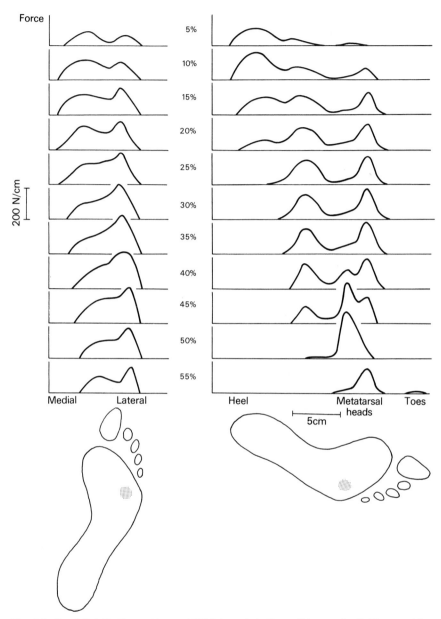

Fig. 3.7 Load distribution patterns at 5% intervals in the walking cycle of a 52-year-old man with diabetic neuropathy and ulceration under the fifth metatarsal head. The toes make a negligible contribution to load-bearing. Considerable load falls on the midfoot with an additional peak of load under the midtarsal region occurring at 10–45% of the cycle. Another sharp peak of load appearing at 30–50% of the cycle can be seen in both longitudinal and transverse recordings, to correspond with the site of the ulcer.

involving the feet. Changes become more marked with increasing radiological evidence of the disease. In severe involvement of the foot the load under the first metatarsal may be decreased (Sharma *et al* 1979).

CONCLUSIONS

Research into the biomechanics of the foot is beginning to yield results relevant to the normal foot and to a number of foot disorders. From the point of view of the clinician, a quantitative test of foot function is needed to complement the radiographic investigation of structural disorders. Many of the systems used for research purposes are expensive to implement, and rely on computers to collect, analyse and present the results. The reduction in cost of computing systems over recent years however makes increasingly feasible the development of such systems for routine clinical use. A large number of patients will certainly benefit from a better understanding of their disordered foot function and of the consequences of therapeutic intervention.

REFERENCES

ARCAN M. & BRULL M.A. (1976) A fundamental characteristic of the human body and foot, the foot-ground pressure pattern. *Biomechanics* **9**, 453–7.

BARNETT C.H. (1954) A plastic pedograph. *Lancet* **ii**, 273.

BARNETT C.H. (1956) The phases of human gait. *Lancet* **ii**, 617–21.

BASMAJIAN J.V. & BENTZON J.W. (1954) An electromyographic study of certain muscles of the leg and foot in the standing position. *Surgery, Gynaecology and Obstetrics* **98**, 662–6.

BASMAJIAN J.V. & STECKO G. (1963) The role of muscles in arch support of the foot. *Journal of Bone and Joint Surgery* **45A**, 1184–90.

BAUMAN J.H. & BRAND P.W. (1963) Measurement of pressure between foot and shoe. *Lancet* **i**, 629–32.

BEELY F. (1882) Zur Mechanik des Stehens. *Langenbecks Archiv. für Chirurgie* **27**, 457–71.

BETTS R.P. (1979) A simple grey scale to colour converter. *Journal of Medical Engineering and Technology* **3**, 31–7.

BETTS R.P., FRANKS C.I., DUCKWORTH T. & BURKE J. (1980) Static and dynamic foot pressure measurements in clinical orthopaedics. *Medical and Biological Engineering and Computing* **18**, 674–84.

BURGER E.S. (1952) The measurement of the static forces at the weight bearing points of the feet with reference to critical heel heights and 'split heel' factors. *Chiropody Record* **35**, 1–17.

CARLSÖÖ S. & WETZENSTEIN H. (1968) Change of form of the foot and the foot skeleton upon momentary weight-bearing. *Acta Orthopaedica Scandinavica* **39**, 413–28.

CHODERA J. & LORD M. (1979) In Kenedi P. *et al* (eds.) *Pedobarograph foot pressure measurements and their application in disability*, p. 173. Macmillan Press, London.

COLLIS W.J.M.F. & JAYSON M.I.V. (1972) Measurement of pedal pressures. *Annals of the Rheumatic Disease* **31**, 215–17.

CUNNINGHAM D.M. & BROWN G.W. (1952) Two devices for measuring the forces acting on the human body during walking. *Proceedings of the Society for Experimental Stress Analysis* **9**, 75–90.

DHANENDRAN M., HUTTON W.C. & PAKER Y. (1978) The distribution of forces under the human foot—an on line measuring system. *Measurement and Control* **11**, 261–64.

DICKSON F.D. & DIVELEY R.L. (1953) *Functional Disorders of the Foot*, 3rd edition. Lippincott, Philadelphia.

DRILLIS R. (1958) Objective recording and biomechanics of human gait. *Annals of the New York Academy of Sciences* **74**, 86–109.

DYSON G.H.G. (1967) *The Mechanics of Athletics*, 4th edition. University of London Press, London.

ELFTMAN H. (1934) A cinematic study of the distribution of pressure in the human foot. *The Anatomical Record* **59**, 481–7.

ELFTMAN H. (1939) Forces and energy changes in the leg during walking. *American Journal of Physiology* **125**, 339–56.

ELFTMAN H. (1960) The transverse tarsal joint and its control.*Clinical Orthopaedics* **16**, 41–5.

GRAY E.R. (1969) The role of leg muscles in variations of the arches in normal and flat feet. *Physical Therapy* **49**, 1084–8.

HARPER F.C., WARLOW W.J. & CLARKE B.L. (1961) The Forces Applied to the Floor by the Foot in Walking. *National Building Studies Research Paper 32*. HMSO, London.

HICKS J.H. (1953) The mechanics of the foot. II. The plantar aponeurosis and the arch. *Journal of Anatomy* **88**, 25–30.

HOLDEN T.S. & MUNCEY R.W. (1953) Pressures on the human foot during walking. *Australian Journal of Applied Science* **4**, 405.

JAMES S.L. & BRUBAKER C.E. (1973) Biomechanics of running. *Orthopaedic Clinics of North America* **4**, 605–15.

JONES F.W. (1944) *Structure and Function as seen in the Foot*. Baillière, Tindall & Cox: London.

JONES R.L. (1941) The human foot. An experimental study of its mechanics and the role of its muscles and ligaments in the support of the arch. *American Journal of Anatomy* **68**, 1–39.

LEVENS A.S., INMAN V.T. & BLOSSER J.A. (1948) Transverse rotation of the segments of the lower extremity in locomotion. *Journal of Bone and Joint Surgery* **30A**, 859–72.

MANN R. & INMAN V.T. (1964) Phasic activity of intrinsic muscles of the foot. *Journal of Bone and Joint Surgery* **46A**, 469–81.

MANTER J.T. (1938) The dynamics of quadrupedal walking. *Journal of Experimental Biology* **15**, 522–40.

MARSDEN J.P. & MONTGOMERY S.R. (1972) An analysis of the dynamic characteristics of a force plate. *Measurement and Control* **5**, 102–6.

MORTON D.J. (1935) The foot in stance. In *The Human Foot*, p. 105. Columbia University Press, New York.

MURRAY M.P., DROUGHT A.B. & KORY R.E. (1964) Walking patterns in normal men. *Journal of Bone and Joint Surgery* **46A**, 335–60.

MUYBRIDGE, EADWEARD (1979) *Muybridge's complete human and animal locomotion all 731 plates from the 1887 Animal locomotion* Dover, New York.

PAUL J.P. (1967) Forces transmitted in the joints of the human body. *Proceedings of the Institute of Mechanical Engineers* **181** (30), 8.

REHMAN I., PATEK P.R. & GREGSON M. (1948) Some of the forces exerted in the normal human gait. *Archives of Physical Medicine* **30**, 698–702.

RYDELL N.W. (1966) Forces acting on the femoral head prosthesis. *Acta Orthopaedica Scandinavica* (suppl.) **88**.

SCHWARTZ R.P. & HEATH A.L. (1949) The oscillographic recording and quantitative definition of functional disabilities of human locomotion. *Archives of Physical Medicine* **30**, 568–78.

SCHWARTZ R.P., HEATH A.L., MORGAN D.W. & TOWNS R.C. (1964) A quantitative analysis of recorded variables in the walking pattern of 'normal' adults. *Journal of Bone and Joint Surgery* **46A**, 324–34.

SHARMA M., DHANENDRAN M., HUTTON W.C. & CORBETT M. (1979) Changes in load bearing under the rheumatoid foot. *Annals of Rheumatic Disease* **38,** 349–552.

SUTHERLAND D.H. & HAGY J.L. (1972) Measurement of gait movements from motion picture film. *Journal of Bone and Joint Surgery* **54A,** 787–97.

STOKES I.A.F., STOTT J.R.R. & HUTTON W.C. (1974) Force distributions under the foot—a dynamic measuring system. *Biomedical Engineering* **9,** 140–3.

STOKES I.A.F., FARIS I.B. & HUTTON W.C. (1975) The neuropathic ulcer with loads on the foot in diabetic patients. *Acta Orthopaedica Scandinavica* **46,** 839–47.

STOKES I.A.F., HUTTON W.C. & STOTT J.R.R. (1979a) Forces acting on the metatarsals during normal walking. *Journal of Anatomy* **129**(3), 579–90.

STOKES I.A.F., HUTTON W.C., STOTT J.R.R. & LOWE L.W. (1979b) Forces under the hallux valgus foot before and after surgery. *Clinical Orthopaedics and Related Research* **142,** 64–72.

STOTT J.R.R., HUTTON W.C. & STOKES I.A.F. (1973) Forces under the foot. *Journal of Bone and Joint Surgery* **55B,** 335–44.

UNIVERSITY OF CALIFORNIA (1947) *Fundamental Studies of Human Locomotion and Other Information Relating to the Design of Artificial Limbs.* Prosthetic Devices Research Project, University of California, Berkeley.

WRIGHT D.G., DESAI S.M. & HENDERSON W.H. (1964) Actions of the subtalar and ankle joint complex during the stance phase of walking. *Journal of Bone and Joint Surgery* **46A,** 361–82.

4

Examination of the Foot

L. KLENERMAN

In this short chapter it is intended to provide a background for a clinical approach to the foot. Details of specific physical signs are described in the appropriate sections of the book.

The examination, as always, must follow a careful history, which should include enquiries about general health and past history of illnesses and operations. This time is well spent and should enable one to obtain an assessment of the patient as a whole and the likely response to treatment. In the case of the large number of normal children who are brought by anxious parents for reassurance about their children's feet, it is important to find out about the mother's state of health during pregnancy, the nature of the delivery, birth weight and the milestones in the development of walking, such as when the child first sat up unassisted and when walking started. One may thus avoid overlooking the occasional child with cerebral palsy or muscular dystrophy.

When examining a foot it is important to remember that this is just part of the whole patient. This is of particular importance where there is an underlying generalized disease, such as diabetes or rheumatoid arthritis. It is always necessary to look at the spine in a patient with deformed feet for evidence of an underlying neurological abnormality, such as a pigmented and hairy naevus in the skin of the midline of the back, indicative of spinal dysraphism. This applies particularly to the child and adolescent.

In the examination of the foot of the newborn and toddler one is looking for evidence of mobility and flexibility. The foot of the normal newborn infant should be able to be dorsiflexed easily, so that the dorsum comes into contact with the shin (Fig. 4.1). Pathology such as talipes equinovarus or vertical talus is associated with a rigid foot. When the child first walks the feet are often widely separated for stability. There is little evidence of a medial longitudinal arch because of the presence of additional fat and the frequent association of knock-knee. Intoeing is common, and a variety of asymmetrical variations of this may occur until a proper walking pattern has been established.

Patients should first be asked to walk in shoes to obtain an impression of the gait. Walking in shoes may, however, mask an underlying deformity. The shoes must be studied for areas of wear and patterns of distortion. They also give an indication of the usual type of footwear customarily worn by the patient. With the patient barefoot and the lower limbs exposed, one should rapidly run through a

50

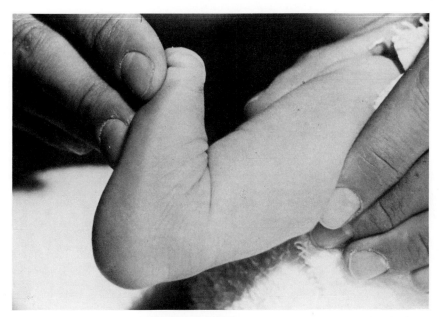

Fig. 4.1 The normal foot in the neonate should be mobile and dorsiflex so that the dorsum can be brought into contact with the shin.

routine list of points to be noted as he stands and then walks. Do the heels reach the ground? Is the heel neutral, valgus or varus? (Figs. 4.2, 4.3). Is there a heel–toe gait? Is the foot fully plantigrade? Does the great toe function? This is a point of particular relevance in the management of hallux valgus.

With the patient recumbent, the sole can be inspected for callosities, warts or evidence of prolapse of the metatarsal heads. The sole of the foot is like a contour

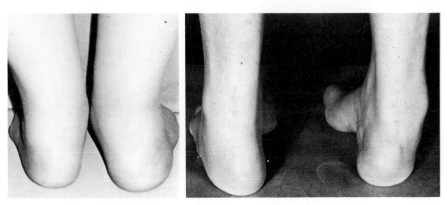

Fig. 4.2 (*Left*) It is uncommon for one heel only to be in valgus.

Fig. 4.3 (*Right*) Cavus feet with varus heels.

map and provides an accurate reflection of the mode of weight-bearing. Occasional nodules due to Dupuytren's contracture or rheumatoid arthritis may be found. The toes may have hammer or mallet toe deformities with corns on the dorsal surfaces of the proximal interphalangeal joints or their tips. The cleft between the digits must be inspected for fungus infection or soft corns, both of which are particularly common between the little and fourth toes.

The circulation must be assessed. The temperature gradient from proximal to distal is felt; marked coldness is easily detected. Very dry feet may result from the autosympathectomy of diabetes. The skin texture, presence of hair and state of the nails are all pointers to the quality of the blood supply to the foot. A shining skin, absence of hair and brittle nails all denote ischaemia. The pedal pulses should be palpated and the perforating peroneal artery sought if the dorsalis pedis is absent. If there is any doubt about the vascular state of the limb, the pressure index should be recorded using a Doppler probe (the ratio of the systolic pressure at the ankle and the antecubital fossa should be approximately one). In patients where this is not the case, the opinion of a surgeon interested in vascular disorders may be needed. Varicosities and skin pigmentation indicative of venous stasis have

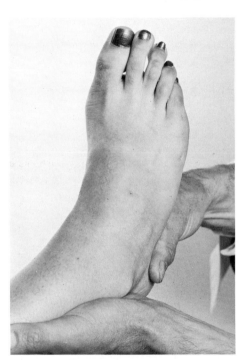 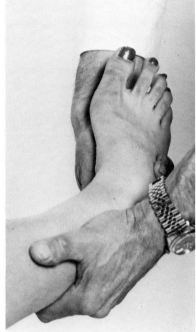

Fig. 4.4 (*Left*) Examination of the subtalar joint. The leg is supported in its lowest third by one hand and the calcaneum is rocked from side to side by the other.

Fig. 4.5 (*Right*) Examination of the midtarsal joint. The subtalar joint is held firm while the forefoot is twisted.

relevance as indicators of potentially slow clearance of swelling of the leg and foot after surgery.

Ankle, subtalar, midtarsal and toe joints are tested for their range of movement. Both sides must always be compared. The range of normal movements depends on the age and physique of the patient and the degree of generalized joint laxity. It is helpful to assess the joint range passively and actively. The range of ankle dorsiflexion should be used for evidence of calf muscle contracture. Dorsiflexion to more than a right angle should be possible without the need to flex the knee. One may easily be misled in the infant and it is sometimes helpful to take a lateral radiograph with the foot in maximum dorsiflexion to make sure of the position of the calcaneum.

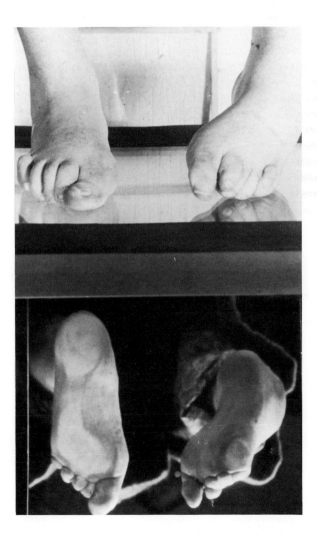

Fig. 4.6 This type of standard photograph taken with the patient on a translucent stand with a mirror beneath it is a useful record of the shape of the foot and the weightbearing surface.

Ideally the movements between the talus and calcaneum should be measured in a plane that is at right angles to the axis of rotation of the subtalar joint with the patient prone and knee flexed to 135° (Inman 1976). Inversion and eversion is usually only about 10° in each direction, although it often appears to be more when projected along the axis of the whole foot. To test subtalar movement, the calf is supported in its lowest third with one hand and with the other the heel is gripped from below (Fig. 4.4). For midtarsal movement the heel is held firmly while the forefoot is moved (Fig. 4.5). Movements of the toes must be noted. Restricted dorsiflexion at the metatarsophalangeal joint of the great toe is particularly significant, as it may be responsible for symptoms. The patient should always be asked to stand on tip-toe. In the normal foot the heel inverts and the longitudinal arch rises.

The clinical examination will need to be supplemented by appropriate radiographs and the details of these will be described in the chapter on radiology. A pre-operative photograph showing the state of the deformity is an invaluable record. Photographs taken with the patient standing on a translucent platform so that the appearance of the sole can be seen in a mirror are particularly valuable for recording changes in weight-bearing (Fig. 4.6). Specific blood investigations for rheumatoid arthritis or gout may also be necessary.

REFERENCES

INMAN V.T. (1976) *The Joints of the Ankle*, p. 29. Williams & Wilkins, Baltimore, USA.

5

The Foot in Childhood

J.A. FIXSEN

Anxiety about the condition of children's feet is extremely common. Children referred to orthopaedic clinics with foot problems or parental anxiety about the condition of a child's feet exceed all other children's referrals. Unless there is a clear understanding of the natural history and development of the foot in childhood it is impossible to give advice about these feet. This problem is exemplified by the question of so-called flat feet.

PES PLANOVALGUS (FLAT FOOT)

There is no clear cut definition of pes planovalgus or flat foot. Clinically, if the medial longitudinal arch of the foot touches the ground, or is closer to the ground than the observer feels it should be, then the foot is described as flat (Fig. 5.1). This is a vague and unreliable method of measurement but more complex methods requiring lateral radiographs or special mats which record the area of the sole in contact with the ground on weight-bearing are not widely used.

It is important to consider the formation of the medial longitudinal arch and its development in childhood. The medial longitudinal arch is dependent on the configuration of the bones, joints and the joint capsules of which it is composed. Under normal relaxed standing conditions it has been shown by electromyographic studies that muscle function is not important (Basmajian & Stecko 1963). The time honoured use of exercises in the treatment of flat feet, therefore, has become of doubtful value.

During the first few years of life there are considerable changes in the normal appearance of the child's foot. At birth the commonest position is mild calcaneovalgus and the foot looks flat, but unlike the true calcaneovalgus foot (Fig. 5.2) there is a full range of plantarflexion. At the end of the first year, when the child commonly starts to stand, the foot almost invariably looks flat because of the large quantity of fatty tissue in the sole, and there is a prominent pad of fat in front of the heel on the medial side filling in the medial arch. Between the first and second years, when walking becomes established, the child walks on a wide base, commonly with the legs turned out and the feet everted so they appear flat. The later the child walks the more obvious this apparent flat foot and the greater the parental anxiety. In the second and third years the feet tend to come together and

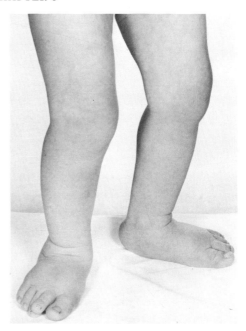

Fig. 5.1 Flat everted feet in a child
of $2\frac{1}{2}$ years who was a late walker.

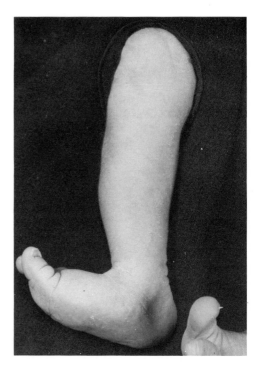

Fig. 5.2 Talipes calcaneovalgus in
a child aged 1 week. At this stage
there was no plantarflexion. Simple
passive stretching rapidly restored a
full range of plantarflexion.

the medial arch becomes established. If this sequence of events is not clearly understood, a large number of children will be treated unnecessarily for a condition which is part of normal development. Morley (1957) in a study of the natural history of knock-knee and flat foot in children, showed that under the age of 18 months 97% of children have flat feet, measured by a weight-bearing sole method. By the age of 10 years only 4% had flat feet. During this period 1% had been treated, usually with shoe wedges, with no effect on the prognosis. Vice versa, any treatment in a condition which spontaneously regresses in over 90% of cases will be considered highly successful unless the natural history of the disorder is taken into account.

Another trap for the unwary is the apparent flat foot (Fig. 5.3). In these children the position of the lower limb as a whole is the cause of the flat foot and not the foot itself. The common conditions which produce apparent flat feet are genu valgum, intoeing due to tibial torsion, femoral anteversion and femoral retroversion. These are almost always so-called normal variants in the growing child (Walker 1972) and correct spontaneously in the majority of children without specific treatment. The problem of flat foot, therefore, becomes one of distinguishing between the common wide variations of normal development and significant abnormality.

The true pes planovalgus also provides us with a therapeutic dilemma. In some races up to 35% of the population will have such feet and it has a marked familial

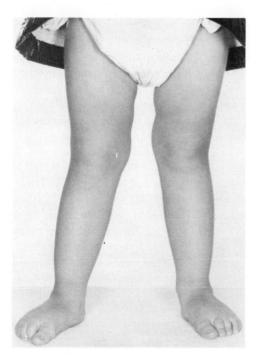

Fig. 5.3 Apparent flat feet in a girl aged 20 months with mild genu valgum.

tendency. Does the condition require treatment and does treatment provide any benefit? There is a notable lack of reliable scientific evidence on both these points.

For the past ten years it has been the policy in the orthopaedic clinics at The Hospital for Sick Children, Great Ormond Street, to divide planovalgus feet into two main categories. The first, and by far the largest, group are those in which the feet are asymptomatic, mobile and there is no evidence of underlying neuromuscular or skeletal abnormality. The second, much smaller group, consists of those which have one or more of the following features: definite symptoms, stiffness or excessive mobility, demonstrable neuromuscular or skeletal abnormality. The first type requires no treatment but the position must be carefully explained to often anxious parents that their children's feet are basically normal and that modifications to the shoes, heel-cups (Helfet 1956) or insoles will not alter the shape of the foot although they may help excessive shoe-wear. Undoubtedly not all orthopaedic surgeons will agree with this view (Rose 1962) but in the absence of clear cut evidence that these feet benefit from treatment or that they suffer from no treatment, we have continued with this policy.

The second type should be examined carefully and if possible a definite diagnosis made. For example, a painful flat foot may be due to an accessory ossicle on the navicular bone or a simple strain of the tibialis posterior tendon after unusual exercise. It may be due to infection in the subtalar joint, tuberculosis and juvenile rheumatoid arthritis may present in this way.

Stiffness of the foot is often associated with pain and may also be associated with one of the forms of tarsal coalition which frequently have a family history (Wynne-Davies 1973). Hypermobility of the foot is commonly associated with generalized joint laxity, which is seen at its most severe in neuromuscular disorders such as benign congenital hypotonia (Walton 1956) and connective tissue disorders such as Ehlers–Danlos syndrome, Marfan's syndrome and osteogenesis imperfecta. An underlying neurological disorder should always be looked for carefully in children presenting with flat feet. At regular intervals a child will present in the orthopaedic clinic with flat feet and turn out to be an undiagnosed case of cerebral palsy, muscular dystrophy or spinal dysraphism. It is most important that the underlying condition is diagnosed and assessed before embarking on treatment for the flat feet.

What types of treatment are available for the second category of patients? Clearly if the condition is due to infection this should be rigorously treated. If the condition is due to a skeletal anomaly this will commonly respond to a period in a below-knee walking plaster or an iron and T-strap. Sometimes excision of a calcaneonavicular bar is effective if the patient is under fourteen years of age (Mitchell & Gibson 1967). Cain and Hyman (1978) report good results with a closing wedge osteotomy of the os calcis in the treatment of peroneal spastic flat foot as suggested by Dwyer (1976). Excessive shoe-wear can be helped by a wedge on the inner side of the sole and heel, by a valgus insole, a Helfet heel cup or Schwarz insole. A more rigid method of controlling a markedly valgus foot is by an outside iron and inside T-strap or double iron. Extra-articular subtalar arthrodesis (Grice

1952—see also Chapter 10) is a very effective method of stabilizing the subtalar joint in the growing foot. Alternatively, Dillwyn Evans (1975) advises in opening wedge osteotomy of the anterior part of the os calcis inserting a tibial bone graft to lengthen the lateral border of the foot. This procedure is not advised in cerebral palsy or spina bifida. Medial osteotomy of the os calcis can correct the valgus of the heel and improve foot function in mobile flat feet (Koutsogiannis 1971).

Triple arthrodesis can be used successfully at maturity. Procedures which simply fuse part of the medial arch seem bound to failure (Seymour 1967). Crego and Ford (1952) in an end result study of various procedures for correcting flat feet in children came to the conclusion that one should only operate for disabling pain failing to respond to conservative treatment; that one exchanges loss of pain for loss of mobility and that talonavicular and naviculocuneiform fusion must be combined with subtalar fusion.

CONGENITAL VERTICAL TALUS OR CONGENITAL CONVEX PES VALGUS

Congenital vertical talus is a rare disorder. It occurred in one of 131 patients (0.76%) attending a special clinic for congenital foot deformities of the newborn (Osmond Clarke 1956). It may occur as an isolated entity or, more commonly, associated with neuromuscular disorders such as meningomyelocele or connective tissue disorders such as arthrogryposis. It has been described in autosomal anomalies, e.g. trisomy 13–15 and trisomy 18 and is often seen in 'whistling face' syndrome (Freeman–Sheldon syndrome, craniocarpotarsal dystrophy). In the so-called paralytic type, i.e. those associated with anomalies of the neuraxis such as meningomyelocele, Drennan and Sharrard (1971) have suggested a neuromuscular imbalance between a weak tibialis posterior and strong evertors of the foot as the cause of the deformity. The appearance of the foot is similar in both the paralytic and non-paralytic types. The heel is elevated. The calcaneum is in equinus and valgus. The forefoot is in fixed calcaneus and eversion. The sole of the foot is convex with the head of the talus forming the lowest point on the medial side (Fig. 5.4, 5.5).

The condition must be distinguished from talipes calcaneovalgus, severe idiopathic flat foot, the flat foot of cerebral palsy and the rocker-bottomed foot of spuriously corrected talipes equinovarus (Lloyd-Roberts & Spence 1958). On the lateral radiograph the calcaneum is in equinus and becomes beaked anteriorly. The talus inclines to the vertical and becomes waisted or hour-glass shaped. The forefoot is in calcaneus and the navicular is dislocated dorsally on to the neck of the talus (Fig. 5.6). Before the age of three, when the ossific centre of the navicular appears, its position can be inferred by the position of the ossified medial cunieform and first metatarsal. A lateral radiograph in full plantarflexion is important (Eyre-Brook 1967) as severe idiopathic flat foot may give the same appearance in a lateral radiograph in neutral, but in full plantarflexion the dorsal dislocation of

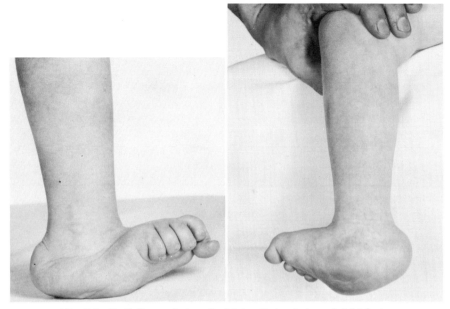

Fig. 5.4 (*Left*) Congenital vertical talus. Lateral view of right foot.

Fig. 5.5 (*Right*) Congenital vertical talus. Medial view of right foot.

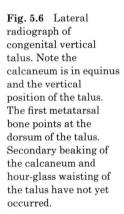

Fig. 5.6 Lateral
radiograph of
congenital vertical
talus. Note the
calcaneum is in equinus
and the vertical
position of the talus.
The first metatarsal
bone points at the
dorsum of the talus.
Secondary beaking of
the calcaneum and
hour-glass waisting of
the talus have not yet
occurred.

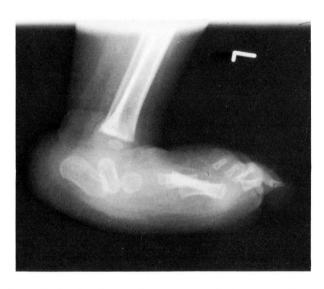

navicular is reduced in idiopathic flat foot but not in true congenital vertical talus.
If conservative treatment is to have any chance of success it should be started as
soon as possible after birth. Silk and Wainwright (1967) recommended repeated
manipulation and plasters to reduce the forefoot into full plantarflexion followed

by elongation of the tendo-Achilles and posterior capsulotomy of the ankle joint to correct the hindfoot equinus. The majority of cases require surgical correction. A number of procedures have been advocated (Eyre-Brook 1967; Harrold 1967; Herndon & Heyman 1963; Colton 1973; Duckworth & Smith 1974). They all involve open reduction of the talonavicular dislocation, correction of the hindfoot equinus and stabilization of the talus in its correct position.

Osmond-Clarke (1956) transferred the peroneus brevis to the neck of the talus. Harrold advocated Kirschner wire fixation. Eyre-Brook excised a wedge of the navicular and inserted it under the neck of the talus. Colton advised removal of the whole navicular and transfer of the tibialis anterior tendon to the neck of the talus to hold it in position. Fitton and Nevelos (1979) believe that excision of the navicular is not necessary if a full peritalar release is performed between the ages of three to six months. They advise complete calcaneocuboid division, lengthening of all the dorsiflexors, the peronei and the tendo-Achilles. The talus is held reduced by a Kirschner wire.

Duckworth and Smith, in a review of a number of procedures, (1974) recommend in the paralytic type transfer of the tibialis anterior to the neck of the talus and the peroneus brevis to the tibialis posterior. Clearly with such a variety of methods available, all of which can give reasonable results, the important point is to fully correct the deformity early in life and to stabilize the corrected foot by whichever method seems most appropriate. The author personally prefers transfer of the tibialis anterior to the neck of the talus with or without excision of the navicular, as necessary.

CONGENITAL METATARSUS ADDUCTUS AND VARUS

Metatatsus adductus often combined with some varus is a common deformity (Fig. 5.7). It is frequently mistaken for talipes equinovarus (Bankart 1921), but the heel is normal or sometimes valgus (Fig. 5.8). Mild forms are common and the condition seems to be increasing in frequency, possibly associated with the acceptance of the prone lying position as the recommended position for nursing newborn babies and infants.

The deformity is best seen from the sole of the foot, when the heel is seen to be in neutral but the forefoot is adducted towards the midline (the so-called hook or skew foot). Radiography shows the metatarsals are adducted relative to the midtarsus and the talocalcaneal angles are normal or even increased on the anteroposterior view (Fig. 5.9).

Treatment

The majority of cases in which the forefoot can be passively corrected beyond the neutral position and the dorsiflexors and evertors are working normally will correct spontaneously without specific treatment. In order to maintain the range of

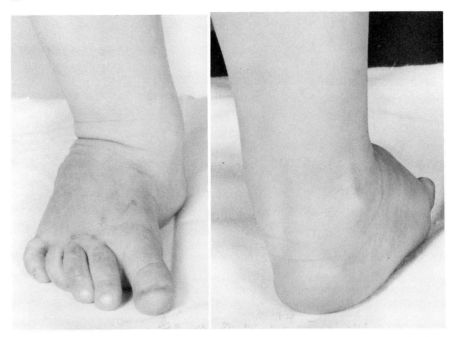

Fig. 5.7 (*Left*) Metatarsus varus in a child aged 15 months. Anterior view to show forefoot deformity.

Fig. 5.8 (*Right*) Metatarsus varus. Posterior view of same child as in Fig. 5.7. Note that the heel is normal.

passive movement the mother can be shown how to stretch the forefoot into the corrected position. It is most important that the hindfoot is held in neutral otherwise there is a tendency to produce a secondary valgus deformity of the hindfoot. Denis Browne hobble boots or reversed boots have been used, but again it is difficult to control the heel sufficiently to prevent the production of a valgus heel.

If the forefoot deformity cannot be passively corrected or fails to respond to maternal stretching then serial manipulations and plasters can be used. Ponseti and Becker (1966) in a careful review suggested that approximately one patient in nine requires definitive treatment. The plasters are not easy to apply. The hindfoot should be held in equinus and inversion while the forefoot is plastered in eversion and abduction. The plasters should extend to the groin and immobilize the knee at 90°. They are changed every 2–3 weeks and correction is usually obtained in 8–10 weeks. Rushforth (1978) reported the natural history of 130 feet followed up for an average of seven years, in which no treatment was given. In his series 86% of feet corrected spontaneously, 10% showed mild persistent deformity which was completely asymptomatic and 4% had stiff, deformed feet. He was unable to predict which feet would fail to correct spontaneously until the patient was 3 years old. It therefore seems reasonable to advise simple observation until the age of three,

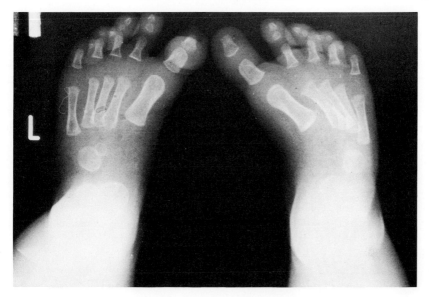

Fig. 5.9 Radiograph of congenital metatarsus adductus and varus. The metatarsals are adducted relative to the tarsus.

unless the condition is causing excessive anxiety, in which case conservative treatment with plasters can be used. At the age of three in persistent cases, release of the abductor hallucis and plastering will usually correct the foot. Recently Browne and Paton (1979) have described an anomaly of the tibialis posterior tendon insertion, as the main bulk of the tendon did not attach to the navicular tuberosity. This should be noted at operation and the tendon re-attached to the navicular tuberosity if necessary. If the release of the abductor hallucis is insufficient then the more extensive procedure of tarso-metatarsal capsulotomy described by Heyman *et al* (1958) can be used. Finally, in very late cases multiple metatarsal osteotomies may be indicated (Berman & Gartland 1971).

There is a rare form of this condition in which the foot is S-shaped or serpentine. In this type the forefoot adductovarus deformity is fixed and the hindfoot is in fixed valgus. Kite (1967) found only 12 out of 2818 cases (0.43%). The condition is often familial and is very difficult to treat. Lloyd-Roberts and Clark (1973) pointed out that this condition, which is notoriously difficult to correct is associated, at least in some cases, with a ball and socket type ankle joint. This feature should be taken into account when considering methods of treating this refractory condition.

CONGENITAL TALIPES EQUINOVARUS (CLUBFOOT)

In this condition there is a fixed structural deformity of both the forefoot and hindfoot at birth (Fig. 5.10). The hindfoot is in equinus and varus, unlike metatarsus adductus or varus where it is normal or valgus. The heel frequently appears small or tucked up under the medial malleolus (Fig. 5.11). The forefoot is also in equinus and varus. There is associated wasting of the calf muscles which can be marked in severe cases and persists despite full correction of the foot deformity.

The deformity occurs in 1–2 per 1000 live births in this country. It is two to three times as common in males as females and is frequently bilateral. There is a strong familial incidence which is 20–30 times that in the normal population (Wynne-Davies 1964). The aetiology remains unknown despite a vast literature and numerous theories. Hippocrates advised treatment by manipulation and bandaging from birth, but the condition remains one of the most difficult to treat successfully.

It is important to examine the child fully as the deformity is frequently associated with other abnormalities or forms part of a specific syndrome. This may not alter the primary treatment but may have a considerable bearing on the prognosis.

A wide range of neurological disorders such as meningomyelocele, spinal dysraphism, sacral agenesis, cerebral palsy, poliomyelitis and sciatic nerve palsy should be considered. Tibial deficiency and congenital constriction rings may

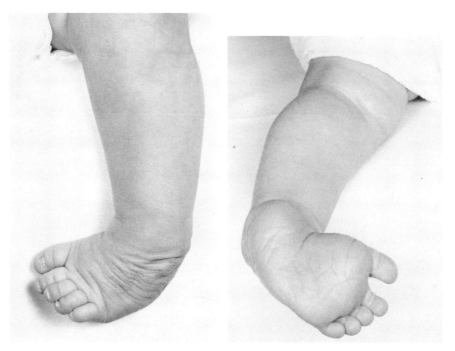

Fig. 5.10   (*Left*) Talipes equinovarus in a child aged 4 months. Anterior view.

Fig. 5.11   (*Right*) Talipes equinovarus in the same child as Fig. 5.10. Posterior view.

produce very severe forms of the deformity. Generalized disorders such as arthrogryposis multiplex congenita, diastrophic dwarfism and trisomy 13–15 should be borne in mind.

Treatment

It is generally agreed that treatment should start as soon as possible after birth. The basis of early treatment is repeated gentle manipulations, maintaining the correction obtained by splintage using adhesive strapping (Figs. 5.12, 5.13), plaster of Paris or metal splints. Forcible manipulation should not be used as this can cause damage to the growing foot and permanent iatrogenic deformity. The method of manipulation and splintage depends upon the preference of the surgeon and the ability of the child's parents to bring the patient at frequent intervals for

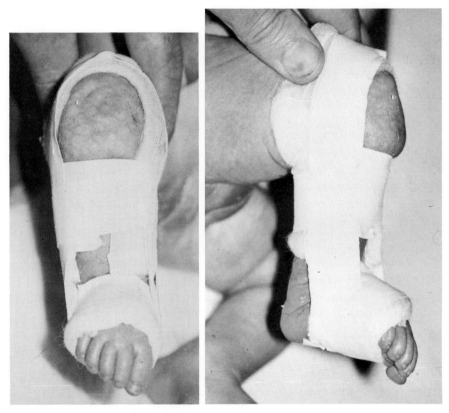

Fig. 5.12   (*Left*) Adhesive strapping applied for correction of talipes equinovarus. Anterior view.

Fig. 5.13   (*Right*) Adhesive strapping applied for correction of talipes equinovarus. Lateral view.

treatment. The author prefers the method of repeated gentle stretching of the foot several times a day by the mother, supervised 2–3 times a week by the physiotherapist. The correction obtained is maintained by adhesive strapping which is changed at frequent intervals but allows the foot to be manipulated with the strapping on. This method requires more frequent visits than the other methods, but probably gives the best results. Alternatively, serial manipulations and plasters by the surgeon once or twice a week can be very effective, particularly if the patient cannot attend sufficiently often for the strapping method to be used, or the mother cannot cope with the repeated stretching procedure. The Denis Browne splint has not proved as successful as its originator hoped (Fripp & Shaw 1967).

The next problem is how long to continue with this type of conservative treatment and how to recognize its success or failure. In the past the use of radiographic as well as clinical assessment has often been neglected. However, clinical assessment can be fallible and in the author's opinion, radiographs at the age of 2–3 months can be very helpful in confirming whether the talocalcaneal angles and the relation of the forefoot to the hindfoot has been accurately restored. The normal and abnormal appearances have been described by Davies and Hatt (1955) (Fig. 5.14).

In the normal foot, in the anteroposterior view, a line drawn through the long axis of the talus should pass down the first ray and that through the long axis of the calcaneum passes down the fourth ray. In the lateral view, a line through the long axis of the talus points downwards along the long axis of the first ray and that through the calcaneum points upwards and bisects the first line at about 30°. In the uncorrected foot (Fig. 5.15) both lines point downwards in calcaneus and bisect at a much more acute angle. In the anteroposterior view, the line through the talus points further laterally, as does that through the calcaneum, which often lies outside the fifth ray altogether.

Two important forms of spurious correction must be recognized following conservative treatment. First the so-called rocker-bottomed foot, in which the forefoot equinus is well corrected but the hind foot remains in equinus. Major degrees of this deformity should be obvious clinically; minor degrees can easily be missed but show up well on a lateral x-ray. Second, the midfoot horizontal breech or 'bean-shaped' foot in which the equinus deformity is corrected but the lateral rotation of the hindfoot persists. This is well shown in the anteroposterior x-ray and in the lateral x-ray where the fibula is displaced posteriorly and the talus appears flat-topped (Swann *et al* 1969; Fig. 5.16). If a further lateral x-ray with the foot in 20–30° medial rotation is taken, then the relation of the fibula is restored and the dome of the talus reappears (Fig. 5.17).

How long should one persist with conservative treatment? This is a contentious subject but if no progress is being made with the foot, if excessive force is being exerted to attain further correction or spurious correction is developing, then conservative treatment should be abandoned in favour of operative methods. In practice the decision is usually made by the end of the first three months of life. If

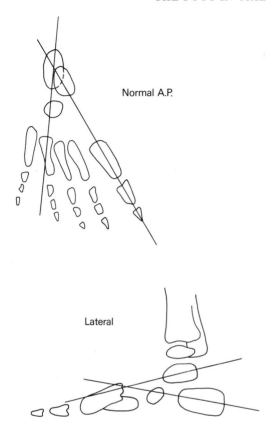

Normal A.P.

Lateral

Fig. 5.14 Outline tracing from the radiographs of a normal foot in a child of 6 months. Anteroposterior and lateral views.

the foot is not fully corrected clinically and radiologically at 12–14 weeks, or even earlier (Main *et al* 1977), then surgery is indicated. If the foot is fully corrected at this time then manipulations can be discontinued but some form of splintage is generally considered necessary to maintain the correction. Denis Browne type hobble boots are very suitable for this (Fig. 5.18). There is no clear cut indication as to how long they should be continued. It seems reasonable to continue with them until the child is standing and walking and active dorsiflexion and eversion of the foot is well established. Many surgeons feel that splintage at night should be continued until the age of three or four years, but there is no definite evidence that this is necessary. Some parents have difficulty in retaining the heels properly in these splints, and the incorporation of a heel strap in the boot is a good solution to this problem.

Once it is clear that surgery is necessary there are two main schools of thought on the approach to surgical correction of the deformity. Clark (1968) considers the basic problem to be one of medial tether and medial dislocation of the navicular on the talus. He, therefore, recommends a radical medial release combined with release of the structures behind the heel to obtain complete correction of the foot.

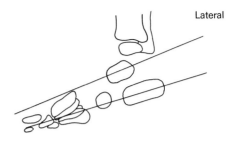

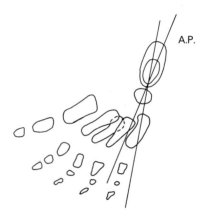

Fig. 5.15 Outline tracing from the
radiographs of a child with
uncorrected talipes equinovarus at
the age of 6 months.

Turco (1979) reported the results in 240 feet treated by a one-stage postero-medial
release in which he uses Kirschner wires. He does not advise this extensive
operation before the age of one year and warns of the dangers of over-correction.
The problem of this type of procedure seems to be the recurrence of the deformity
due to excessive scarring on the medial side, loss of correction if internal fixation is
not used, or over-correction producing a valgus and often stiff foot.

The alternative approach, advocated by Attenborough (1966), relies on a full
soft tissue release behind the heel correcting the hindfoot deformity by elongating
the tendo-Achilles, the tibialis posterior and any other tendons which are tight and
preventing full correction of the hindfoot. A posterior capsulotomy of the ankle
joint is also necessary to correct the position of the talus and calcaneum. In
practice, one often finds that a combination of two approaches is necessary. If the
forefoot is fully corrected by conservative means but the hindfoot remains in
equinus and varus, then simple posterior soft tissue release will suffice. If, however,
there is some persistent forefoot varus as well as hindfoot deformity, some
extension of the dissection on to the medial side of the foot after full hindfoot
correction is necessary. Often releasing the abductor hallucis and the long plantar
ligaments from the calcaneum, as in a Steindler stripping operation, will fully

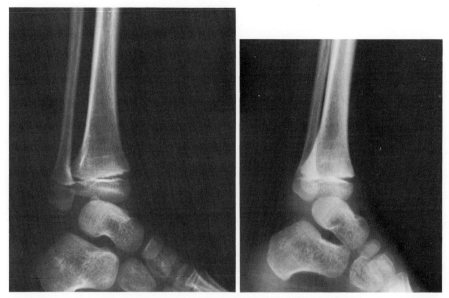

Fig. 5.16   (*Left*) Lateral radiograph of an uncorrected talipes equinovarus to show posterior displacement of the fibula and apparent flat-topped talus.

Fig. 5.17   (*Right*) Radiograph of the same foot as in Fig. 5.16 taken in 20° internal rotation, showing the fibula in its normal relation to the tibia and reappearance of the dome of the talus.

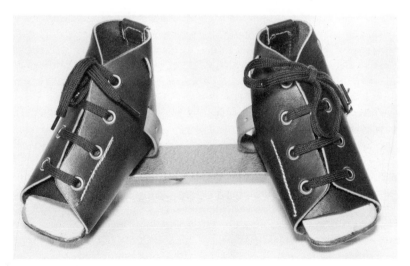

Fig. 5.18   The Denis Browne type hobble boots and bar. Used as a holding splint. Note the heel straps.

correct the foot. In the really rigid deformity a full medial release as described by Clark (1968) and Turco (1971) may be necessary.

The important point is that the foot should be fully corrected at operation and lie easily in the fully corrected position. The position is maintained in a plaster of Paris splint for 6–8 weeks. The plaster is simply to retain the foot in the corrected position and not used to obtain further correction. Once the plaster is removed, hobble boots should again be used to maintain the corrected position at least until walking and active dorsiflexion and eversion of the foot is established. The older the child the more difficult is becomes to obtain full correction.

Until the age of three or four years soft tissue release can still give good results, but bony deformity becomes increasingly important and operations such as calcaneal osteotomy (Dwyer 1963) for the varus heel or medial release combined with calcaneocuboid fusion (Dillwyn Evans 1961) for the 'bean-shaped' foot become necessary. If active dorsiflexion and eversion fail to develop, transfer of either the tibialis anterior tendon (Garceau & Palmer 1967) or tibialis posterior tendon (Singer 1958) to the lateral side of the foot have been advocated. Both these operations require careful evaluation and full correction of any fixed deformity before they are used, as there is a considerable danger of failure either to control the deformity or of overcorrection into valgus. If the foot is still deformed at or near maturity, triple arthrodesis can be used. This procedure was introduced in 1923 by Ryerson. It involves fusion of the subtalar, talonavicular and calcaneocuboid joints excising the required amount of bone from each joint to correct the foot deformity. The ankle mortice must be stable if triple arthrodesis is to be successful. If it is not stable then varus or valgus deformity can recur in the foot by tilting of the talus within the ankle mortice. Triple arthrodesis can produce a stable plantigrade foot of good shape which allows weight to be borne on the correct parts of the sole of the foot and normal footwear to be worn. However, this is achieved at the expense of loss of flexibility of the hind and midfoot. This can produce difficulty in walking over rough ground and increases the strain on the ankle joint, which may show degenerative changes with time. As such it represents a failure of earlier treatment to correct the foot and maintain correction at a stage when a mobile plantigrade foot can be obtained (see Nissen (1957) for further operative details). The question of whether deformity relapses due to failure to gain full correction previously, or recurs following complete correction remains a hotly debated one. It only emphasizes the empirical nature of our treatment and our lack of knowledge of the basic aetiology of this condition.

Although reported series are difficult to compare because of differing standards and modes of evaluation, recent results (Blockey & Smith 1966; Fripp & Shaw 1967) show little apparent improvement over those obtained in 1930 (Brockman 1930). Laaveg and Ponseti (1980) in a long term follow-up of a closely controlled group of feet in which there was no evidence of any other congenital anomaly or underlying condition, made the important point that a mobile but not anatomically perfect foot is functionally more acceptable to the patient than a perfect anatomical correction which is stiff.

CONGENITAL TALIPES CALCANEOVALGUS

This abnormality is a relatively common finding in otherwise normal newborn infants (Fig. 5.2). At birth the foot can usually be dorsiflexed so that the dorsum touches the anterior aspect of the leg and plantarflexed approximately 45°. In this condition plantarflexion is limited or non-existent. There is a considerable excess of first-born children with this anomaly. It is often associated with oligohydramnios and the so-called 'moulded baby' syndrome (Lloyd-Roberts & Pilcher 1965). Five percent of cases are associated with congenital dislocation of the hip and this should always be looked for.

Provided there is no underlying neuromuscular or skeletal anomaly and there is clinical evidence of active invertors and plantarflexors, the condition usually responds rapidly to simple stretching. The mother is shown how to passively stretch the foot into maximum plantarflexion. This should be repeated several times daily at a convenient time and frequency, e.g. each time the baby is fed. The foot is usually fully corrected by the end of the first or second month. It is advisable to follow up the child until walking is established to ensure that no deformity persists. Some orthopaedic surgeons (Gianestras 1973) pursue a much more aggressive policy of treatment with serial plasters followed by modifications to the shoes. However, in the author's own experience, that has not been necessary except in cases with underlying neuromuscular or skeletal problems.

PES CAVUS

In this condition (Figs. 5.19, 5.20) the medial and, sometimes in more severely affected cases, the lateral longitudinal arch is abnormally high. There is a fixed equinus deformity of the forefoot relative to the hindfoot. The toes are commonly clawed and the heel frequently goes into varus and calcaneus. Radiologically a standing lateral radiograph should be taken to demonstrate the deformity. The patient usually presents with shoe-wear problems due to the high arch, clawing of the toes or varus of the heel. Pain and callosities over the metatarsal heads which are prominent are rare in young children but common in adolescents and adults.

Alternatively the patient may present with a clumsy gait and a history of repeated falls which are usually due to an underlying neurological abnormality rather than the cavus deformity itself. Brewerton et al (1963) in a study of the aetiology of pes cavus showed that if a neurological abnormality was carefully looked for it was present in 66% of cases. The commonest neurological condition associated with pes cavus in their series was peroneal muscular atrophy. Other conditions which should be looked for are anterior poliomyelitis, spinal dysraphism, meningomyelocele, muscular dystrophy, Friedreich's ataxia and cerebral palsy. A family history is very common even when no definite neurological abnormality can be detected. It is, therefore, useful to examine the feet of the parents and siblings. Accurate diagnosis of the underlying neurological condition

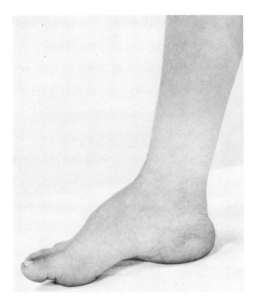

Fig. 5.19   Pes cavus. Medial view.
Note the high medial longitudinal
arch and early clawing of the big toe.

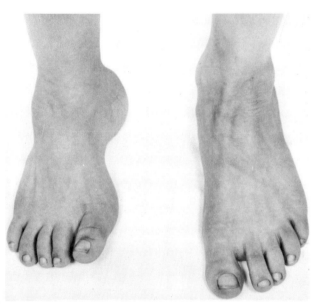

Fig. 5.20   Pes cavus. (Right) Anterior view. Note again the early clawing of the big toe and
the heel is in varus.

is important both for the general and orthopaedic management of the patient.
Expert neurological advice and investigations such as electromyography, nerve
conduction studies, muscle biopsy and myelography may be necessary.

True congenital pes cavus or pes arcuatus is rare. The condition is present at birth but is often not noticed until shoe-wear becomes a problem. In this condition both medial and lateral longitudinal arches are elevated and the toes are not clawed. There is no evidence of an underlying neurological abnormality.

Orthopaedic treatment in mild cases consists of advice regarding shoe-wear and the fitting of an arch support with a metatarsal pad behind the metatarsal heads to spread the load-bearing area more evenly. During the growing period the height of the arch can be reduced by Steindler's procedure in which the plantar fascia is divided through a medial or lateral incision. The intrinsic muscles of the sole of the foot and the long plantar ligament are released by stripping them from the calcaneum. Clawing of the toes may be corrected before the deformity becomes fixed by transfer of the toe flexors to the toe extensors at the level of the proximal interphalangeal joint. The clawing of the big toe is corrected by the so-called Robert Jones tendon transfer, in which the extensor hallucis longus is transferred to the neck of the first metatarsal and the interphalangeal joint of the big toe is stabilized by tenodesis or fusion. Taylor (1951) reported satisfactory results from these procedures. If the varus of the heel is a problem this can be corrected by a calcaneal osteotomy excising a wedge of bone from the lateral side of the calcaneum (Dwyer 1959). If at maturity there is a fixed cavus deformity of sufficient severity, it may be corrected by dorsal wedge osteotomy of the apex of the arch in the midtarsal region. This is frequently combined with the Steindler plantar release in order to flatten the arch satisfactorily. Other methods of reducing the cavus are the tarsal V-osteotomy described by Japas in 1968 and the tarsometatarsal truncated wedge arthrodesis (Jahss 1980). If persistent equinus and varus of the heel is also present then a triple arthrodesis is necessary. Finally, if there is significant calcaneus of the heel the two-stage arthrodesis described by Elmslie (Cholmeley 1953) should be employed.

In this operation, at the first stage, the plantar fascia is stripped as in the Steindler procedure. A dorsally based wedge is excised in the midtarsal region to correct the cavus relative to the hindfoot. Six weeks later, at the second stage, the calcaneus of the hindfoot is corrected by excising a posteriorly based wedge from the subtalar joint. In the procedure as originally described, half the tendo-Achilles was used as tenodesis by attaching it to the back of the tibia with the hindfoot in slight plantarflexion. It is doubtful if this is of more than temporary value. In poliomyelitis cases the flexor hallucis longus, flexor digitorum longus, peroneus longus and brevis muscles may be transferred to the tendo-Achilles.

TARSAL COALITION

In this condition there is fusion which is either bony, cartilaginous or fibrous between two or more bones of the tarsus. The commonest forms are talocalcaneal and calcaneonavicular fusions although other types such as talonavicular, naviculocuboid and naviculocuneiform have been described. In many instances the condition is perfectly symptom-free, but may be associated with peroneal spastic flat foot in which there is a painful stiff flat foot with marked spasm of the peroneal muscles.

Special radiographic projections may be necessary to demonstrate the bony bar (Harris & Beath 1948). An oblique radiograph of the foot is also very useful (see Chapter 12). Excision of the bar connecting the bones may be helpful if the patient has severe symptoms (Mitchell & Gibson 1967). Braddock (1961) in a long term review showed that the presence or absence of tarsal coalition on a radiograph was no guide to the prognosis or response to treatment of a peroneal spastic flat foot. In some cases there is a family history which appears to be of autosomal dominant type (Wynne Davies 1973). Treatment is symptomatic. Frequently a medial arch support is all that is required. If acute peroneal spasm develops, a below-knee walking plaster for six weeks followed by an outside iron and inside T-strap for 3–6 months may be necessary. Braddock (1961) showed that only 10% of cases developed persistent disability requiring surgical treatment by excision of the bony bar or triple arthrodesis. Cain and Hyman (1978) advocate medial wedge osteotomy of the os calcis as an alternative to triple arthrodesis.

CONGENITAL CURLY (VARUS) TOES AND OVERLAPPING TOES

Minor deformities of the second, third, fourth and fifth toes are very common in children and cause considerable parental anxiety (Fig. 5.21). The child is

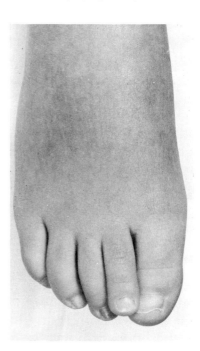

Fig. 5.21 Anterior view of a child's foot showing overlapping of the second toe and curly third, fourth and fifth toes.

frequently brought to the out-patient department in the first year of life before walking or standing are established and before any form of shoe is worn. The condition is nearly always symptom-free but the parents are worried that problems may be encountered when walking and shoe-wear starts. A family history of foot or toe problems is very common in these cases. In the so-called varus or curly toe, the toe is flexed at the interphalangeal joints and rotated medially. The condition is commonest in the fourth and fifth toes and in over 20% of cases a similar condition is present in a close relative.

Conservative treatment by 'over and under' strapping is often advised. Trethowan (1925) advised that such treatment should be pursued with patience and assiduity. However, Sweetnam (1958) in a long-term review of the value of such treatment showed that there was no evidence that treatment by strapping or splintage had any effect on the condition, which did not tend to deteriorate, and improved spontaneously in many cases. It seems, therefore, that parents should be advised that the deformity normally improves with time and no form of conservative treatment is of any value. The condition is nearly always asymptomatic and in the rare case of fixed deformity causing symptoms, surgical correction is necessary. If possible surgical correction should be delayed until maturity.

Overlapping or dorsal displacement of the second or third toe is also common (Fig. 5.21). It is frequently associated with minor degrees of syndactyly and hypoplasia of the two toes. Again, there is very little evidence that conservative treatment by strapping or splintage has any effect. Usually the condition is fully correctable passively and on weight-bearing the toes spread apart and do not cause symptoms. If there is a serious degree of syndactyly then appropriate plastic surgical procedures are necessary. In the rare event of a fixed deformity causing symptoms, surgical correction is advisable.

Overlapping or overriding fifth toe is common (Fig. 5.22) but unlike the other deformities the toe is often fixed in the overriding position and does not correct on weight-bearing. When shoes are worn this can cause considerable problems. Conservative attempts at strapping the toe down in the normal position are rarely

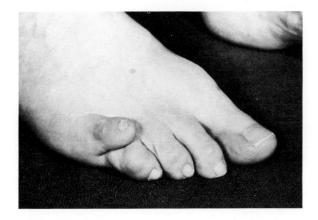

Fig. 5.22 Congenital overriding fifth toe (varus deformity).

successful but operative correction either by Butler's operation described by Cockin (1968) or V–Y correction (Wilson 1953) give good results.

PAIN IN THE FOOT

Pain in the foot is a common presenting symptom in children. There are a number of clear-cut entities which should be considered when examining a child with a painful foot. It is very important to try and localize the site of the pain as accurately as possible as certain conditions occur in specific sites.

PAIN IN THE HINDFOOT

Calcaneal apophysitis or Sever's disease

This was formerly thought to be a form of osteochondritis of the calcaneal apophysis (Fig. 5.23). The radiological appearance of increased density and fragmentation of the apophysis is nearly always bilateral and the condition is now thought to be simply a chronic strain of the attachment of the tendo-Achilles at the apophysis, similar to Osgood–Schlatter's disease of the tibial tubercle. The patient is nearly always between the ages of seven and thirteen years and gives a history of pain at the back of the heel, particularly after exercise. On examination there is local tenderness over the apophysis and often a slight limp. The condition recovers spontaneously with time. Frequently all that is necessary is a short rest from games and other physical activities. Sometimes elevation of the heel with a heel pad is of help and occasionally, in severe cases, a below-knee walking plaster is required for a few weeks. There are no long-term sequelae of the condition.

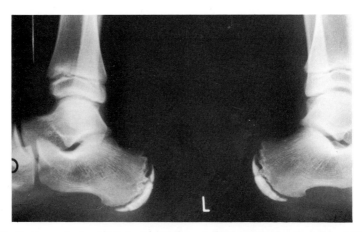

Fig. 5.23 Radiograph of a child's heels with Sever's disease affecting the left heel. Note that there is increased density and fragmentation of the apophysis of both heels. This is a strain of the insertion of the tendo-Achilles rather than a true apophysitis.

PAIN IN THE HEEL PAD

This may occur in children after trauma such as jumping from a height or inadvertent penetration of the heel by a foreign body. True plantar fascitis is rare. The condition usually settles with the use of a felt or rubber pad to cushion the heel, or the discovery and removal of the foreign body.

Acute osteomyelitis can occur in any bone in the foot but should be considered in the differential diagnosis of pain in the heel. In the calcaneum it may be mistaken for apophysitis until the abscess cavity is visible on the radiograph. In the child under four years the rare case of osteomyelitis of the talus is often misdiagnosed as a ligamentous injury or sprain in a patient who refuses to bear weight on the foot until there is evidence of bony infection on the radiograph (Antoniou & Connor 1974) associated with a raised erythrocyte sedimentation rate.

JUVENILE CHRONIC ARTHRITIS

Juvenile chronic arthritis may present as a monarticular arthritis more commonly in the lower limb joints than the upper. The most common sites are the ankle and knee and sometimes the subtalar joint. Therefore, a child who presents with a stiff swollen ankle or subtalar joint in the absence of any history of trauma or infection should be investigated for this disorder. Foot deformities are common in the established case.

Tumours of the foot in childhood are rare but can of course present as a painful swelling in the foot. Usually clinical and radiological examination will suggest the diagnosis which can be confirmed by biopsy. An osteoid osteoma should always be considered when investigating the cause of persistent and puzzling pain. The talus and calcaneum are more common sites than other bones in the foot, although any may be involved (Jaffe 1964).

PAIN IN THE MIDTARSAL REGION

Osteochondritis of the navicular (Kohler's disease)

This condition presents as a painful tender area, often with some local swelling over the tarsal navicular in a child between the age of three and six years with a limp. Radiography shows increased density of the navicular, often with flattening of the bone and sometimes fragmentation (Fig. 5.24). The condition recovers spontaneously (Waugh 1958) and there do not appear to be any long term sequelae (Cox 1958). Specific treatment is often unnecessary, but if symptoms are severe a short period of 3–6 weeks in a below-knee plaster is all that is required.

A strain of the insertion of the tibialis posterior tendon or tenosynovitis of the tibialis posterior may give rise to a painful flat foot. This should respond to rest, the

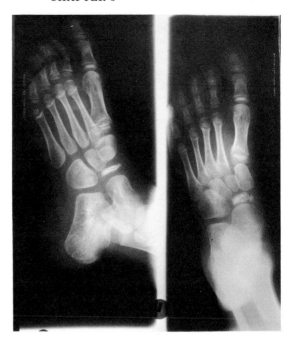

Fig. 5.24 Antero-
posterior and lateral
radiograph of a child
aged 5 years with
osteochondritis of the
tarsal navicular
(Kohler's disease).

use of a valgus insole for a short period or occasionally a walking plaster. The
condition may be associated with an accessory tarsal navicular which, if
persistently painful or causing a troublesome prominence on the medial side of the
foot, can be excised, taking care not to injure the insertion of the tibialis posterior
tendon (Fig. 5.25).

PAIN IN THE FOREFOOT

Metatarsalgia

This is uncommon in children unless there is severe clawing of the toes. If this fails
to respond to a metatarsal insole or bar, surgical correction by flexor to extensor
tendon transfer can be performed. Osteochondritis of the head of the second
metatarsal (Freiberg's disease) can occur and is probably an infraction of the
metatarsal head. It usually occurs over the age of thirteen and is more common in
girls than boys. The symptoms can nearly always be treated by a metatarsal pad or
bar but in adult life they may warrant surgery because of a deformed metatarsal
head.

Hallux rigidus

Painful hallux rigidus does occur in children and can be troublesome to treat. It
frequently follows stubbing of the big toe. The condition may also be associated
with elevation of the first metatarsal (Lambrinudi 1938).

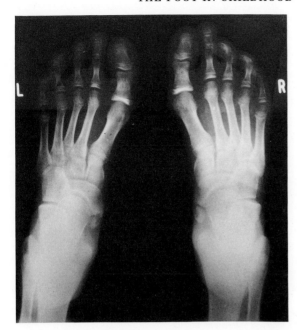

Fig. 5.25 Radiograph showing an accessory navicular on both feet.

Radiographs may show the appearance of osteochondritis of the head of the first metatarsal. If conservative treatment fails extension osteotomy at the base of the proximal phalanx (Bonney & MacNab 1952) gives good results (see Chapter 6).

REFERENCES

ANTONIOU D. & CONNOR A.N. (1974) Osteomyelitis of the calcaneus and talus. *Journal of Bone and Joint Surgery* **56A,** 338–45.

ATTENBOROUGH C.G. (1966) Severe congenital talipes equinovarus. *Journal of Bone and Joint Surgery* **48B,** 31–9.

BANKART A.S.B. (1921) Metatarsus varus. *British medical Journal* **2,** 685.

BASMAJIAN J.V. & STECKO G. (1963) The role of muscles in arch support of the foot. *Journal of Bone and Joint Surgery* **45A,** 1184–90.

BERMAN A. & GARTLAND L.J. (1971) Metatarsal osteotomy for correction of adduction of the fore part of the foot in children. *Journal of Bone and Joint Surgery* **53A,** 498–505.

BLOCKEY N.J. & SMITH M.G.H. (1966) The treatment of congenital club foot. *Journal of Bone and Joint Surgery* **48B,** 660–65.

BONNEY G. & MACNAB I. (1952) Hallux valgus and hallux rigidus. *Journal of Bone and Joint Surgery* **34B,** 366–85.

BRADDOCK G.T.F. (1961) A prolonged follow-up of peroneal spastic flat foot. *Journal of Bone and Joint Surgery* **43B,** 734–7.

BREWERTON D.A., SANDIFER P.H. & SWEETNAM D.R. (1963) The aetiology of pes cavus. *British medical Journal* **2,** 659–61.

BROCKMAN E.P. (1930) *Congenital Club Foot.* John Wright, Bristol.

Browne R.S. & Paton D.F. (1979) Anomalous insertion of the tibialis posterior tendon in congenital metatarsus varus. *Journal of Bone and Joint Surgery* **61B**, 74–6.

Cain T.J. & Hyman S. (1978) Peroneal spastic flat foot—its treatment by osteotomy of the os calcis. *Journal of Bone and Joint Surgery* **60B**, 527–9.

Cholmeley J.A. (1953) Elmslie's operation for the calcaneus foot. *Journal of Bone and Joint Surgery* **35B**, 46–9.

Clark J.M.P. (1968) Early detection and management of the unreduced club foot. *Proceedings of the Royal Society of Medicine* **61**, 779–82.

Cockin J. (1968) Butler's operation for an overriding fifth toe. *Journal of Bone and Joint Surgery* **60B**, 78–81.

Colton C.L. (1973) The surgical management of congenital vertical talus. *Journal of Bone and Joint Surgery* **55B**, 566–74.

Cox M.J. (1958) Kohler's disease. *Postgraduate medical Journal* **34**, 588–91.

Crego C.H. Jr. & Ford L.T. (1952) An end result study of various operative procedures for correcting flat feet in children. *Journal of Bone and Joint Surgery* **34A**, 183–95.

Davis L.A. & Hatt W.S. (1955) Congenital abnormalities of the foot. *Radiology* **64**, 818–25.

Drennan J.C. & Sharrard W.J.W. (1971) The pathological anatomy of convex pes valgus. *Journal of Bone and Joint Surgery* **53B**, 455–61.

Duckworth T. & Smith T.W.D. (1974) The treatment of paralytic convex pes valgus. *Journal of Bone and Joint Surgery* **56B**, 305–13.

Dwyer F.C. (1963) Osteotomy of the calcaneum for pes cavus. *Journal of Bone and Joint Surgery* **45B**, 67–75.

Dwyer F.C. (1976) Causes, significance and treatment of stiffness of the subtalar joint. *Proceedings of the Royal Society of Medicine* **68**, 97–102.

Evans D. (1961) Relapsed club foot. *Journal of Bone and Joint Surgery* **43B**, 722–33.

Evans D. (1975) Calcaneovalgus deformity. *Journal of Bone and Joint Surgery* **57B**, 270–8.

Eyre-Brook A.L. (1967) Congenital vertical talus. *Journal of Bone and Joint Surgery* **49B**, 618–27.

Fitton J.M. & Nevelos A.B. (1979) The treatment of congenital vertical talus. *Journal of Bone and Joint Surgery* **61B**, 481–3.

Freeman E.A. & Sheldon J.H. (1938) Cranio-carpo-tarsal dystrophy. An undescribed congenital malformation. *Archives of Disease in Childhood* **13**, 277.

Fripp A.T. & Shaw N.E. (1967) *Club Foot.* E. & S. Livingstone Ltd, Edinburgh.

Garceau G.J. & Palmer R.M. (1967) Transfer of the anterior tibial tendon for recurrent club foot. *Journal of Bone and Joint Surgery* **49A**, 207–31.

Gianestras N.J. (1973) Foot Disorders. *Medical and Surgical Management*, 2nd edition. Henry Kimpton, London.

Grice D.S. (1952) An extra-articular arthrodesis of the subastragular joint for correction of paralytic flat feet in children. *Journal of Bone and Joint Surgery* **34A**, 927–40.

Harris R.I. & Beath T. (1948) Etiology of peroneal spastic flat foot. *Journal of Bone and Joint Surgery* **30B**, 624–34.

Harrold A.J. (1967) Congenital vertical talus in infancy. *Journal of Bone and Joint Surgery* **49B**, 634–43.

Helfet A.J. (1956) A new way of treating flat feet in children. *Lancet* **i**, 262–4.

Herndon C.H. & Heyman C.H. (1963) Problems in the recognition and treatment of congenital convex pes valgus. *Journal of Bone and Joint Surgery* **45A**, 413–29.

Heyman C.H., Herndon C.H. & Strong J.M. (1958) Mobilization of the tarsometatarsal and intermetatarsal joints for the correction of resistant adduction of the fore-part of the foot in congenital club foot or congenital tarsus varus. *Journal of Bone and Joint Surgery* **40A**, 299–310.

Jaffe H.L. (1964) *Tumours and Tumorous Conditions of Bones and Joints*, p. 94. Henry Kimpton, London.

JAHSS M.H. (1980) Tarso-metatarsal truncated wedge arthrodesis for pes cavus and equino varus deformity of the fore-part of the foot. *Journal of Bone and Joint Surgery* **62A,** 713–22.

JAPAS L.M. (1968) Surgical treatment of pes cavus by tarsal-V osteotomy. *Journal of Bone and Joint Surgery* **40A,** 927–44.

KITE J.H. (1967) Congenital metatarsus varus. *Journal of Bone and Joint Surgery* **49A,** 388–97.

KOUTSOGIANNIS E. (1971) Treatment of the mobile flat foot by displacement osteotomy of the calcaneus. *Journal of Bone and Joint Surgery* **53B,** 96–100.

LAAVEG S.J. & PONSETI I.V. (1980) Long-term results of treatment of congenital club foot. *Journal of Bone and Joint Surgery* **62A,** 23–31.

LAMBRINUDI C. (1938) Metatarsus primus elevatus. *Proceedings of the Royal Society of Medicine* **31,** 1273.

LLOYD-ROBERTS G.C. & SPENCE A.J. (1958) Congenital vertical talus. *Journal of Bone and Joint Surgery* **40B,** 33–41.

LLOYD-ROBERTS G.C. & PILCHER M.F. (1965) Structural idiopathic scoliosis in infancy. *Journal of Bone and Joint Surgery* **47B,** 520–3.

LLOYD-ROBERTS G.C. & CLARK R.C. (1973) Ball and socket ankle joint in metatarsus adductus varus. *Journal of Bone and Joint Surgery* **55B,** 193–6.

MAIN B.J., CRIDER R.J., POLK M., LLOYD-ROBERTS G.C., SWANN M. & KAMDAR B.A. (1977) The results of early operation in talipes equinovarus. *Journal of Bone and Joint Surgery* **59B,** 337–41.

MITCHELL G.P. & GIBSON J.M.C. (1967) Excision of calcaneonavicular bar for painful spasmodic flat foot. *Journal of Bone and Joint Surgery* **49B,** 281–7.

MORLEY A.J.M. (1957) Knock-knee in children. *British medical Journal* **2,** 976–9.

NISSEN K.I. (1957) In Rob C. & Smith, R. (eds.) *Operative Surgery.* Vol. 5, p. 348. Butterworth, London.

OSMOND-CLARKE H. (1956) Congenital vertical talus. *Journal of Bone and Joint Surgery* **38B,** 334–41.

PONSETI I.V. & BECKER J.R. (1966) Congenital metatarsus varus. The results of treatment. *Journal of Bone and Joint Surgery* **48B,** 702–11.

ROSE G.K. (1962) Correction of the pronated foot. *Journal of Bone and Joint Surgery* **44B,** 642–7.

RUSHFORTH G.F. (1978) The natural history of hooked fore-foot. *Journal of Bone and Joint Surgery* **60B,** 530–2.

RYERSON E.W. (1923) Arthrodesing operations on the feet. *Journal of Bone and Joint Surgery* **5,** 453–71.

SEYMOUR N. (1967) The late results of naviculo-cuneiform fusion. *Journal of Bone and Joint Surgery* **49B,** 558–9.

SILK F.F. & WAINWRIGHT D. (1967) The recognition and treatment of congenital flat foot in infancy. *Journal of Bone and Joint Surgery* **49B,** 628–33.

SINGER M. & FRIPP A.T. (1958) Tibialis anterior transfer in congenital club foot. *Journal of Bone and Joint Surgery* **40B,** 252–5.

SWANN M., LLOYD-ROBERTS G.C. & CATTERALL A. (1979) The anatomy of uncorrected club feet. *Journal of Bone and Joint Surgery* **51B,** 263–9.

SWEETNAM D.R. (1958) Congenital curly toes. An investigation into the value of treatment. *Lancet* **ii,** 398–400.

TAYLOR R.G. (1951) The treatment of claw toes by multiple transfers of flexor into extensor tendons. *Journal of Bone and Joint Surgery* **35B,** 539–42.

TRETHOWAN W.H. (1925) The treatment of hammer toe. *Lancet* **i,** 1257–8.

TURCO V.J. (1971) Surgical correction of the resistant club foot. *Journal of Bone and Joint Surgery* **53A,** 477–9.

TURCO V.J. (1979) Resistant congenital club foot—one stage postero-medial relase with internal fixation. *Journal of Bone and Joint Surgery* **61A,** 805–14.

WALKER G. (1972) Minor orthopaedic problems of childhood. *The Practitioner* **208,** 227–38.

WALTON J.N. (1956) Amyotonia congenita. A follow-up study. *Lancet* **i,** 1023–7.

WAUGH W. (1958) The ossification and vascularisation of the tarsal navicular and their relation to Kohler's disease. *Journal of Bone and Joint Surgery* **40B,** 765–77.

WILSON N.N. (1953) V–Y correction for varus deformity of the fifth toe. *British Journal of Surgery* **41,** 133–5.

WYNNE-DAVIES R. (1964) Family studies and the cause of congenital club foot. *Journal of Bone and Joint Surgery* **46B,** 445–63.

WYNNE-DAVIES R. (1973) *Heritable Disorders in Orthopaedic Practice.* Blackwell Scientific Publications, Oxford.

6

Hallux Valgus and Associated Conditions

M.A. EDGAR

Hallux valgus and hallux rigidus may be conveniently grouped together since they have a number of aetiological factors in common and several operative procedures are applicable to both. Nevertheless they are distinct entities with quite different pathology, and it is interesting to note that despite their common features it is unusual for the conditions to coexist.

Some of the relevant terminology in the literature has been confusing. McMurray (1936) considered hallux valgus to be an adduction deformity of the great toe; anatomically this is a correct description. In contrast Rocyn-Jones (1948) observed that in hallux valgus, 'the greater the adduction of the first metatarsal, the greater the abduction of the phalanx'—thus implying a reverse deformity. Simmonds and Menelaus (1960) suggest the term metatarsus adductus for an anatomically abducted first metatarsal bone. Confusion can best be avoided by using only clinical terms to describe these deformities—namely varus and valgus.

The 'exostosis' of the first metatarsal head was originally thought to arise from new bone growth, but this is clearly untrue, except for osteophytes. The term 'medial prominence' of the metatarsal head, although more clumsy, is to be preferred.

Metatarsus primus varus has led to differences of interpretation. Truslow (1925) coined the term specifically to mean a varus of the first metatarsal, and not to imply that such a varus was of primary importance in the pathogenesis of hallux valgus. If this were the case then the term would be 'metatarsus varus primus' as suggested by Lapidus (1934).

Hallux flexus is a severe form of hallux rigidus. Metatarsus elevatus refers to a raised distal end of the first metatarsal bone in association with supination of the forefoot, or it may be secondary to hallux flexus.

HALLUX VALGUS

This may be defined as a 'complex progressive deformity affecting the forefoot in which lateral deviation of the great toe is the most obvious feature' Stamm (1957). 'The complex' may involve the following conditions: rotation of the hallux, metatarsus primus varus, overriding of the hallux and second toe, overriding of the lateral toes, metatarsalgia, hammer and claw deformities of the lateral toes and bunionette of the fifth metatarsal.

Aetiology

Despite a number of papers putting forward a single cause for hallux valgus there is little doubt that the condition has multiple aetiology.

Hereditary factors

Mitchell and his colleagues (1958) noted that 58% of patients reviewed with hallux valgus gave a family history of the condition. Hardy and Clapman (1951) gave a comparable figure of 63% in contrast to their controls with normal feet who had a family history of only 1%. This is an impressive difference, although for the control group it may be an artificially low figure simply because these subjects had no reason to enquire into any of their relevant family history. Johnston (1956) described the pedigree of one family with the condition, and concluded that the hereditary pattern was autosomal dominant with incomplete penetrance. Bonney and MacNab (1952) found that patients with a family history presented earlier. While this points to a hereditary basis it may be that such patients are simply alerted to the condition earlier.

90% of cases coming to surgery are female. Although this suggests a genetic pattern with a sex-linked factor, Hardy and Clapman (1951) found in a large series of adolescents that the sexes were involved equally and Johnston (1956) was unable to find differences in the incidence between the two sexes. This discrepancy is probably answered by the differences between the sexes concerning other factors, in particular shoes.

Metatarsus primus varus

It is well established that hallux valgus is associated with a varus deformity of the first metatarsal. There is also a close relationship between the extent of these two deformities (Hardy & Clapman 1951; Fig. 6.1). Considerable difference of opinion exists as to which deformity is the primary one. This debate is largely academic but it does have some bearing on the indications for operative treatment, particularly metatarsal osteotomy, and therefore the main points will be considered briefly.

Truslow (1925) felt that metatarsus primus varus preceded hallux valgus in many cases. He noted that an oblique first cuneometatarsal joint was often present and thought that it might be associated with a retrogression to the simian type of foot which has a short varus first metatarsal. Morton (1935) and Ross-Smith (1952) supported this. However, it has since been shown that there is no correlation between a short first metatarsal and hallux valgus (Hardy & Clapman 1951). In addition obliquity of the first cuneometatarsal joint, when it occurs, is probably a

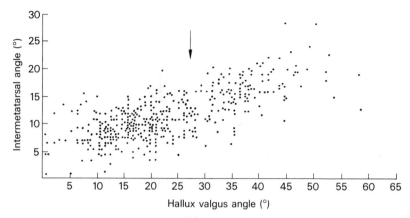

Fig. 6.1 The correlation of hallux valgus with angle of metatarsus primus varus (expressed the intermetatarsal angle). The arrow indicates the region where the morbid group and normal range meet in a series of 101 patients with hallux valgus and 41 controls (after Hardy & Clapham 1951).

secondary development. Although there has been a great deal of support for the metatarsus primus varus aetiology, there would appear to be three main objections to this concept:

1 It is difficult to explain the reason why the first metatarsal should swing into varus of its own accord without influence of the lateral deviating hallux (Piggott 1960). Certainly there is no muscle inserted into the metatarsal head to produce this effect. Splay forefoot due to the laxity of the ligaments binding the metatarsal heads together, which affects principally the first intermetatarsal angle and to a lesser extent the metatarsal angle in the fourth and fifth rays, occurs in later life, very often after the age at which hallux valgus becomes apparent. There is also little evidence to suggest varus growth at the epiphyseal plate at the proximal end of the first metatarsal is ever a factor. Kelikian (1965) discussed the possible contribution of a curved first cuneometatarsal joint in allowing metatarsus primus varus, but this finding is not consistent in hallux valgus.

2 Simple osteotomy of the base of the metatarsal which attempts to correct the so-called primary deformity is associated with a high recurrence rate (Bonney & MacNab 1952). This is in contrast to distal metatarsal osteotomy, where the results are much better and where other factors are corrected.

3 An epidemiological study of 3642 children's feet by Hardy and Clapman (1952) showed that both the first metatarsal angle and hallux valgus angle increased during adolescence. The hallux valgus displacement occurred mainly before 14 years whilst the varus swing of the first metatarsal occurred generally after 14 years of age. This difference was found to be highly significant when analysed statistically.

Over the last decade or so, support for the metatarsus primus varus theory of aetiology has declined. It would appear that metatarsus primus varus occurs *pari passu* with hallux valgus or in fact is secondary to the hallux deformity.

Muscle imbalance

McBride (1935) pointed out that the adductor hallucis has considerable mechanical advantage over its antagonist muscle the abductor hallucis. This imbalance tends to pull the great toe into valgus (Fig. 6.2). Stein (1938) also stressed the important place of adductor hallucis contracture in the aetiology of hallux valgus. The extent to which this contributes to the primary development of the deformity is doubtful but it seems probable that the imbalance is important in the further development of an already established hallux valgus. Miller (1975) described the displacement of the abductor hallucis to the plantar aspect of the great toe transferring its effect from an abductor to that of a flexor tending to maintain the deformity. The tendons of the extensor hallucis longus, flexor hallucis longus and flexor hallucis brevis become bow-strung across the valgus angle and further contribute to an increasing deformity.

Girdlestone and Spooner (1937) noted that the first metatarsal head has no

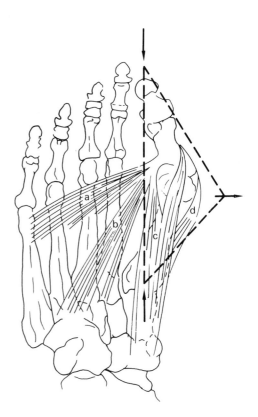

Fig. 6.2 A diagram to illustrate the imbalance of the muscles inserted into the hallux (after McBride 1955). (a) transverse belly of adductor hallucis; (b) oblique belly of adductor lucis; (c) flexor hallucis; (d) abductor hallucis. The arrows indicate the direction of the forces involved.

muscular insertions. Various groups of muscles which surround it and support it in fact insert into the base of the phalanx, which sits like a cap on the metatarsal head. The latter may deform medially in hallux valgus because of pressure from the phalangeal base.

Foot pronation

A high proportion of patients with hallux valgus have flat valgus feet. Rogers and Joplin (1947) quote an incidence of 83%. In such feet the medial side of the forefoot takes more weight than normal and this is transmitted to the great toe. In addition, lateral deviation of the forefoot causes more pressure to be applied to the medial aspect of the hallux during the push-off phase of walking (Fig. 6.9).

Shoes

Sir Robert Jones (1924) commented on the importance of shoes in the aetiology of hallux valgus. 'The demands of fashion are to blame. It is a question of boots; they are the exciting cause, ligaments and muscle joints are merely their victims!' The case which incriminates shoe fashion is based on two arguments: the great number of females affected, and the remarkably low incidence of the condition amongst unshod people compared with shoe-wearers in the same communities.

There is little doubt that in the past tight-toed shoes into which women forced their feet were a potent factor in producing hallux valgus. The present shoe design with a broad toecap and a straight inner border is preferable by far. Of course if the shoe factor is as important as has been suggested, then the incidence of hallux valgus presenting for surgical treatment among the adolescent and young adult population should fall. As already mentioned, both Hardy and Clapman and Johnston could detect no sex difference in the incidence of hallux valgus. Cleveland and Winnant (1950) observed that there are a preponderance of women coming to surgery, and felt that this was due to an increased bunion pain arising from their tighter shoes.

Barnicot and Hardy (1955) found that the hallux valgus angle of Europeans was much higher when compared with the West Africans in Nigeria. Moreover, the European women were more affected than the men, whereas Africans showed no sex difference. They concluded that shoes were a most important factor. A similar comparative study in the Solomon Islands reached the same conclusions (James 1939). Sim Fook and Hodgson (1958) have shown that clinical hallux valgus is seventeen times more common among shoe-wearers in the Chinese of Hong Kong as compared with the unshod members of the community (Table 6.1). More recently, Shine (1965) in a study among the partially shoe-wearing community of the island of St Helena showed similar striking differences between the shod and unshod. In Japan where the Western style shoe is replacing the older open-thonged sandal, the incidence of hallux valgus is increasing.

Table 6.1 A comparison of the incidence of hallux valgus and other conditions among the shod and unshod members of a Chinese community (from Sim Fook & Hodgson 1958).

	Shod	Unshod
Hallux valgus	33%	1.9%
Metatarsus primus varus	6%	24.3%
Hypermobility of 1st metatarsal	9.9%	13.1%
Hallux rigidus	17%	10.3%
Female	39	90
Male	79	17
Total	118	107

Cholmeley (1958) is more cautious about the effect of shoes in view of the fact that a relatively high proportion of cases coming to surgery are unilateral.

Other factors

Rheumatoid arthritis is commonly associated with hallux valgus. Joint erosion and weakening of the capsular structures, particularly on the medial side, lead to deformity. Similar changes can occur in other collagen disorders (Boyle & Buchanan 1971).

Congenital hallux valgus is extremely rare. It has been described by Heller (1928) and Giannestras (1973). Obesity was observed in 30% of Rogers and Joplin's series and considered to be an important factor. However, there were no controls and it may be that this was not a grossly abnormal incidence of obesity.

Cleveland (1927) made the interesting observation that 93% of his cases of hallux valgus had tightness of the Achilles tendon preventing a normal range of foot dorsiflexion. Although the association of these two conditions is mentioned in the literature, no figures to support Cleveland's work can be found in other series.

Os intermetatarsium occurs rarely as an accessory ossicle between the bases of the first two metatarsals. Henderson (1961, 1963) described four cases associated with metatarsus primus varus and hallux valgus. McMurray (1936) concluded that this anomaly was a coincidental finding as he had observed it in normal feet.

The length of the first metatarsal has been regarded as an important factor. Although Morton (1935) felt that a number of foot problems may arise from a short first metatarsal. Harris and Beath (1949) were unable to find a higher incidence of forefoot problems in patients with a short first metatarsal, and Wood-Jones (1949) noted that the first metatarsal is often shorter than the second metatarsal in the normal foot. By contrast, Hardy and Clapman (1952) observed in their series that the first metatarsal is longer than the second in hallux valgus feet by a small but significant amount compared with controls. In some cases the hallux was also long.

Finally, mention must be made of iatrogenic hallux valgus following amputation of the second toe (Fig. 6.3).

Pathology

This subject has been investigated in detail by Haines and McDougall (1954). Changes in the various structures involved are best considered separately.

The first metatarsophalangeal joint

The base of the proximal phalanx first deviates laterally and then later subluxates on the head of the first metatarsal (Piggott 1960). In addition the proximal phalanx rotates into pronation. On the medial aspect of the articular surface of the metatarsal head there is a vertically orientated groove which separates the functional articular area laterally from the medial prominence. This is termed the sagittal groove (Fig. 6.4) which, when marked, can give the medial prominence the appearance of an exostosis. Degenerative changes are usually present just medial to the groove, including osteophytes and cystic changes within the metatarsal head. On the plantar aspect this sagittal groove usually merges into the articular groove for the medial sesamoid. The groove may arise by moulding from the medial edge of the proximal phalangeal base or it may represent an area immediately medial to this articulation where the articular cartilage has atrophied from disuse. The groove can usually be defined on x-rays and this suggests that it is widespread

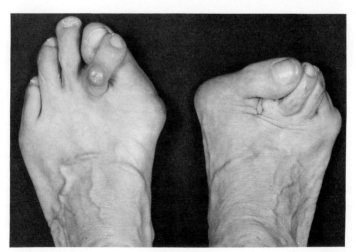

Fig. 6.3 A case of hallux valgus in which there is an overriding second toe on the left. The deformity on the right is associated with previous amputation of the second toe, as a result of which the hallux valgus has increased.

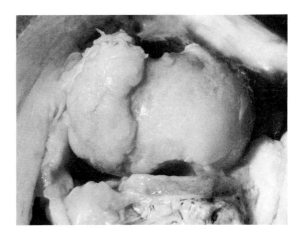

Fig. 6.4 An operative
photograph of the first
metatarsal head in a
case of hallux valgus.
The sagittal groove is
well marked and defines
the articular surface
from the exostosis.

in adult cases, including articular erosions and bony eburnation of the metatarsal
head.

The two sesamoid bones subluxate laterally in relation to the metatarsal head,
and this is proportional to the amount of deformity. During this process they
maintain their relationship to the proximal phalanx of the hallux and to the lateral
metatarsals, while the first metatarsal head 'swings' away medially. The sesamoids
(Fig. 6.5) are situated in the tendons of the short muscles which themselves form
part of the plantar pad of the first metatarsophalangeal joint. The plantar pad and
the tendons are inserted into the phalangeal base, thus anchoring the sesamoids to
the proximal phalanx. The plantar pad and sesamoids are attached to the second
metatarsal heads by means of the strong deep transverse plantar ligament. The
medial sesamoid ligament attaches the plantar pad to the medial aspect of the
metatarsal head. This is the weakest structure amongst those considered and in
hallux valgus it stretches, allowing the metatarsal head to move into varus.

Haines and McDougall describe three stages of sesamoid displacement (Fig.
6.5, B–D). In the first stage of subluxation the medial sesamoid articulates with the
medial aspect of the sesamoid ridge which lies between the two sesamoid articular
areas on the metatarsal head. Erosions may develop at these sites of contact and
the sesamoid ridge may develop osteophytes. In the second stage further
subluxation causes the medial sesamoid to articulate on the sesamoid ridge with
further bony erosion. The transition from stage 2 to stage 3 occurs when the ridge is
destroyed and the medial sesamoid dislocates. There is evidence that this ridge is
important in preventing varus displacement of the first metatarsal (Ing &
Fergusson 1933). There may be less erosion in stage 3 than earlier on. Fig. 6.5 shows
that the lateral sesamoid also progressively displaces during the three stages and
that its final position in stage 3 may be between the first and second metatarsal
heads having rotated through 90°. In this position it blocks any attempted

reduction of the metatarsus varus and shortening of the lateral sesamoid ligament prevents its reduction to a more plantar position.

The metatarsals and the first cuneometatarsal joint

Separation of the metatarsal heads is prevented in the normal foot by the deep transverse plantar ligament. This is a strong band which connects the plantar pads of the five metatarsophalangeal joints. A number of important structures pass in relation to it and it separates the lumbricals and neurovascular bundles from the interosseous muscles and conjoined tendon of the adductor hallucis. The transverse head of the adductor hallucis takes its origin from the ligament. The plantar pad of the metatarsophalangeal joint of the big toe contains the two sesamoid bones already referred to. That part of the plantar pad which connects the medial sesamoid to the metatarsal head is termed the ligament of the medial sesamoid. It is the weak link in the chain of ligamentous structures holding the metatarsal heads together and by stretching it allows the varus deformity of the first metatarsal (Fig. 6.5).

In forefoot splaying (Fig. 6.6) it would appear that a similar process occurs, added to which the fifth metatarsal becomes valgus as a result of stretching of the plantar pad of the lateral ligament to the fifth metatarsophalangeal joint. In

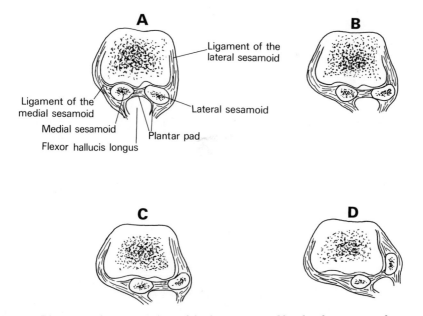

Fig. 6.5 Diagrammatic cross-sections of the first metatarsal head to demonstrate the stages of sesamoid displacement in hallux valgus (after Haines & McDougall 1954). (A) Normal relationship of sesamoids and metatarsal head; (B) to (D) Stages in medial and lateral sesamoid displacement.

forefoot splaying it is principally the first and fourth intermetatarsal angles which are widened. The relationship between the three intermediate metatarsal heads is unchanged because of bracing by the strong deep transverse plantar ligament.

The plane of the first cuneometatarsal joint is usually more obliquely situated in hallux valgus with metatarsus primus varus than in the normal foot, but this is not a consistent finding and it is thought by Haines and McDougall to be a secondary effect. Lapidus (1960) commented that obliquity of the first cuneometatarsal and the tendency for it to become curved was a sign of its retroversion to the ball and socket joints of the primates. However, the curved joint is an unusual finding. Hauser (1950) observed that the first metatarsal rotates about its longitudinal axis into supination or inversion in hallux valgus. This observation is quoted by Kelikian but is not otherwise referred to in the literature.

Bunion

This swelling on the medial aspect of the forefoot is produced by three structures. Superficially there is a callosity or occasionally ulceration of the overlying skin. The subcutaneous tissues contain a bursa which may become inflamed as a result of trauma or infection. Finally the increased medial prominence of the metatarsal head results from the varus deformity of the first metatarsal and subluxation of the metatarsophalangeal joint.

Muscular imbalance

This has already been considered in relation to aetiology. In established hallux valgus the transverse and oblique heads of the adductor hallucis increase their

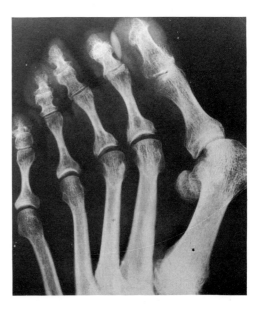

Fig. 6.6 X-ray appearances of hallux valgus with marked splaying of the forefoot (from Sir Reginald Watson-Jones', Collection).

potential leverage on the hallux as a result of its valgus position. In addition, there is little opposition to their action since the abductor hallucis comes to lie on the plantar aspect of the metatarsophalangeal joint.

Stein (1938) stressed the importance of changes in the action of the abductor hallucis contributing to the pathology of hallux valgus. The muscle no longer acts as a medial guide-rope supporting the metatarsophalangeal joint, and the gap which it leaves in the medial side allows the metatarsal head to 'escape' further into varus. Another effect of the altered position of the abductor hallucis is the rotational effect which it exerts on the base of the proximal phalanx.

The two heads of the short flexor of the big toe, together with the flexor hallucis longus, and the extensor hallucis longus on the dorsal aspect, all become bow-strung and shortened across the hallux valgus deformity. Obviously contraction of these muscles tends to increase the deformity.

Hallux rotation

In hallux valgus, to a variable extent, the hallux 'pronates' or rotates into eversion at the metatarsophalangeal joint. The amount to which this occurs is directly related to the extent of the hallux valgus (Hardy & Clapman 1951). Rotation results from the altered direction of forces from muscles inserted into the hallux, as shown in Fig. 6.7. It would appear that the most important factor is a change in the action of the abductor hallucis due to its more plantar position (Miller 1975).

Lateral toes

The hallux which has become valgus may override or more commonly underride

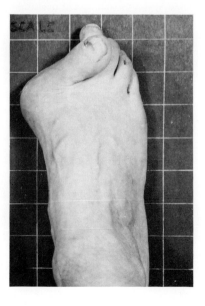

Fig. 6.7 Photograph of hallux valgus with an underriding second toe.

the second toe (Fig. 6.3, 6.7). Alternatively, the second toe itself may be pushed into valgus and come to override or underride the third toe. Generally the lateral toes become crowded together and in addition often show hammer or claw deformities (Fig. 6.8). A varus first metatarsal causes increased weight-bearing through the middle metatarsal heads (Harris & Beath 1949), and this may progress to troublesome metatarsalgia. Clawing of the lateral toes can enhance this condition.

If the hallux valgus is associated with splaying of the forefoot, valgus deformity of the fifth metatarsal may produce a lateral prominence of the head, forming a bunionette (see below).

Clinical features

The condition may present during adolescence from the age of 13 onwards or any time during adult life. The juvenile form and congenital hallux valgus are extremely rare. 90% of patients presenting for surgery are female, although the sex incidence of the condition is probably equal. Generally the condition is bilateral but it is usually worse on one side and about 50% of surgical cases have unilateral procedures. There is a strong family history present in 60% of cases.

Symptoms

These may be related to pain, the deformity, or both.

Pain

This may be felt on different aspects of the metatarsophalangeal joint of the big toe. Bunion pain is felt medially and is related to an inflamed bursa or pressure from a

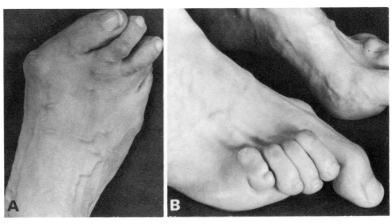

Fig. 6.8 Conditions of the lateral toes associated with hallux valgus. (A) Bunching of the lateral toes with hammer deformity; (B) Clawing of the lateral toes which fail to reach the ground on standing.

callosity in the overlying skin. Alternatively a discomfort may be felt mainly on the plantar aspect where it is related to metatarsalgia of the first metatarsal head or to osteoarthritis of the sesamoid articulation (Ing & Fergusson 1933). Less commonly, pain may be felt mainly on the dorsal aspect arising from the pressure of dorsal osteophytes, but this is more usually the case in hallux rigidus. In addition Stamm (1957) drew attention to a less well-defined pain arising within the first metatarsophalangeal joint caused by degenerative changes.

Not uncommonly symptoms arising from the lateral toes may be the main complaint and should always be enquired about. Such symptoms may be related to metatarsalgia, or to dorsal callosities or claw toes.

Shoe problems

One of the most common complaints is the difficulty of purchasing a shoe which is wide enough to contain the forefoot comfortably. When the lateral toe deformities are present the toe of the shoe needs to be deep as well as wide. Such shoes are often difficult to obtain and tend to be cosmetically unacceptable for the female sufferer.

Cosmetic complaints

These are close allied to shoe problems. In the adolescent group, however, the appearance of mild hallux valgus or shoe problems may cause the patient to seek advice. In particular, it has been shown that in cases where the patient's mother has suffered from hallux valgus, she often seeks advice early, concerned that the child's feet may deteriorate cosmetically.

Stiffness

This is occasionally complained of, particularly if degenerative changes are present. However, a true hallux valgorigidus is uncommon.

Physical signs

On inspection the extent of the deformity should be observed. This is best done with the patient standing. The hallux valgus angle can be judged clinically, though this usually underestimates the x-ray angle. The amount of metatarsus primus varus can be roughly gauged from the width of the forefoot. In addition the amount of hallux rotation and the deformities affecting lateral toes should be recorded.

On palpation sites of tenderness are noted. Tenderness around the first metatarsophalangeal joint may be related to the metatarsal prominence medially, or to degenerative changes of the joint dorsally, or the sesamoid articulation on the plantar aspect. It is important to test for metatarsalgia, and tenderness under a particular metatarsal head is often associated with a plantar callosity. Subluxation or dislocation of the metatarsophalangeal joints can usually be detected by careful palpation.

The range of movement of the interphalangeal and metatarsophalangeal joints of the big toe, or any pain during this procedure should be noted. Similarly, mobility of the lateral toe joints should be assessed. Passive dorsiflexion of the metatarsophalangeal joint of the big toe is an important movement, and it is interesting that even in gross hallux valgus a range varying from 30–90° is often present. The amount of interphalangeal movement of the big toe is important, particularly if metatarsophalangeal arthrodesis is being considered. Finally the range of movement at the midtarsal, subtalar and ankle joints should be tested. With regard to this, hallux valgus is commonly associated with a pronated foot. Apart from a mobile pes planus, a spastic type of flat foot has been observed (Fig. 6.9). In addition, a tight tendo-Achilles may be present.

During walking the foot is watched to see if the hallux is used in its normal push-off function and whether the lateral toes reach the ground. Lastly, the quality of skin, the state of peripheral circulation and any distal infection, whether fungal or related to an ingrowing toenail, should be noted, especially if surgery is planned.

X-rays

Anteroposterior and lateral films are taken in the standing position. The angle of the tube can be standardized and this provides greater accuracy in comparison studies (Hardy & Clapman 1951; Piggott 1960).

Hallux valgus may be measured on the films as the angle between the axes of

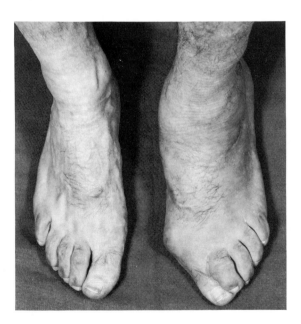

Fig. 6.9 Unilateral hallux valgus association with a left spastic flat foot due to tarsal coalition. The right foot is normal.

the first metatarsal and proximal phalanx, similarly metatarsus primus varus (m.p.v.) may be measured as the angle between the axes of the first two metatarsals. Hardy and Clapman (1951) found that the mean m.p.v. angle in normal adolescents was 7.4° and in adults 8.5°. The upper limit of normal for metatarsus primus varus is generally accepted at 9° (Mitchell *et al* 1958; Carr & Boyd 1968). There is less certainty about the normal limit of hallux valgus. Hardy and Clapman (1951) found a mean angle in adolescents of 12.0° and in adults of 15.7°. Angles of over 20° can be considered as pathological and likely to cause symptoms. The relative protrusion of metatarsal heads may be measured on x-rays (Harris & Beath 1949; Hardy & Clapman 1951). However, it is difficult to be certain about these measurements and their interpretation is doubtful.

Other features of importance include displacement of the first metatarso-phalangeal joint and associated degenerative changes, the extent of sesamoid displacement, dislocation of the lateral toe metatarsophalangeal joints and abnormalities of the tarsometartarsal joints. Occasionally x-rays show evidence of erosions as in rheumatoid arthritis, periosteal thickening or a stress fracture affecting the second or third metatarsals, calcification of the distal arteries and (rarely) an os intermetatarseum.

Piggott (1960) usefully classified hallux valgus in adolescents and young adults into three radiological groups according to the congruity of the first metatarsophalangeal joint (Fig. 6.10). In the congruous group the mild hallux valgus is due to an angulation of the articular surface perpendicular with the shaft axis. The deformity here is not progressive. In contrast, the deviated and subluxed groups are different stages of the same process. The deviated joints when followed up, tend to become subluxed. Cases with subluxed joints generally had the largest

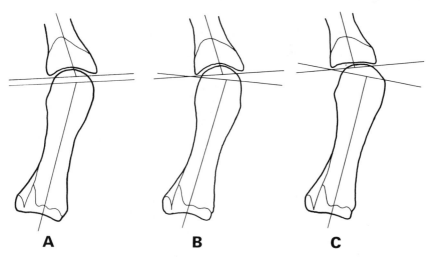

A   **B**   **C**

Fig. 6.10 Piggott's radiological classification of adolescent hallux valgus into three types (Piggott 1960). (A) congruous; (B) deviated; (C) subluxated.

amount of hallux valgus and a much greater tendency to progress. This third group therefore, has a radiological indication for treatment.

Conservative management

Splints, insoles and physiotherapy have been well tried in the past with uniform lack of success (Platt 1957; Cholmeley 1958). Surgical shoes which have a broad deep toe, however, have a definite place in conservative management. They are of value especially where a hallux valgus is associated with marked forefoot splaying and lateral toe deformity, as in rheumatoid arthritis, or where there is a contraindication to surgical intervention. Chiropody deserves a mention as a useful adjunct to treatment, particularly if symptoms arise from painful callosities.

Surgical treatment

A host of surgical procedures for hallux valgus fills the literature. Some are well-established and have a definite place in correcting the deformity. Others are difficult to assess because no long-term results have been reported following the initial description and they tend to be largely of historical interest. The results of different procedures are difficult to correlate in the absence of a standardized method of subjective and objective follow-up assessment. Bonney and MacNab's (1952) method of study is perhaps the most useful of the many suggested.

The operations to be described will be classified according to the structure and site operated on. Operative policy and indications are considered later.

Soft tissue procedures

McBride's conservative operation. The object of this procedure described by McBride in 1928 is to release the contracted structures on the lateral side of the first metatarsophalangeal joint. The released conjoined adductor hallucis tendon is then re-attached to the lateral side of the metatarsal head to prevent further varus deformity of the first metatarsal (see Figs. 6.11, 6.12). Where there is sesamoid displacement or fixed valgus contracture at the first metatarsophalangeal joint, the lateral sesamoid is excised and tight structures on the lateral side of the joint released. Gripping the sesamoid with a simple towel clip makes filleting out of this bone a less irksome procedure. In the younger patients (under the age of 30) where the lateral sesamoid is undisplaced, McBride (1967) suggests a modified procedure in which the common adductor hallucis tendon is divided from its insertion into the lateral sesamoid, leaving the lateral sesamoid and the lateral head of the flexor hallucis *in situ*. This avoided the occasional complication of hallux varus (Miller 1975). Although the indications for this procedure were set out by McBride (1935) its place is now generally restricted to the mild adolescent case (Cholmeley 1958).

Joplin's sling procedure   Joplin developed his operation after reviewing unsatis-

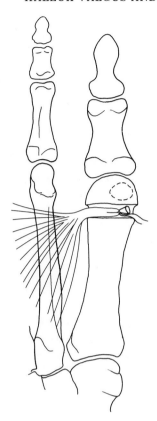

Fig. 6.11 A modified McBride procedure—the lateral sesamoid has been removed and the adductor tendon has been brought through one drilled hole in the metatarsal head to be secured to the medial capsule.

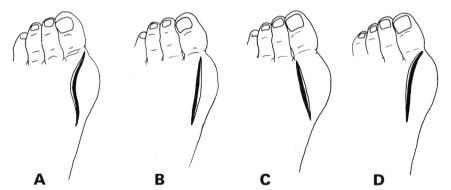

Fig. 6.12 Diagram of the incisions used in some of the operations for hallux valgus. (A) Mitchell's osteotomy; (B) Keller's arthroplasty; (C) McBride's procedure; (D) Wilson's osteotomy.

factory long-term results of Keller's arthroplasty (Rogers & Joplin 1950). The aim of this procedure is to correct splaying of the forefoot, which in associated with metatarsalgia formed a large proportion of the failures in his review of Keller's operation.

The procedure is complex and time-consuming. No recent long-term results have been reported in the literature and its mention is largely of historical interest. The first step of the operation consists of transferring the conjoined adductor hallucis tendon to the metatarsal neck, as in the McBride procedure. The extensor tendon of the fifth toe is then divided at the level of the ankle and brought through a third incision over the dorsum of the fifth metatarsophalangeal joint and the distal end of this tendon is tenodesed to the head of the fifth metatarsal. In addition the abductor digit minimi is brought to the dorsum of the little toe to act as an extensor. The free strip of extensor tendon is then passed as a sling from the fifth metatarsal across the plantar aspects of the other metatarsal necks to be secured through a hole drilled in the first metatarsal head. Suture here is performed after reducing the forefoot spread.

Silver's procedure   Silver (1923) described his operation which consists of three steps. Firstly, the adductor hallucis insertion is divided by percutaneous tenotomy. Secondly through a medial longitudinal incision a V–Y capsulorrhaphy of the medial capsule corrects the valgus deformity. Prominence of the metatarsal head may be trimmed at this stage. Lastly, the abductor hallucis is removed from its plantar position and restored to a more medial position by suture to the base of the V-flap of the medial capsule. Giannestras (1973) recommends that the adductor tenotomy is best done as an open procedure.

Silver's operation by itself is not widely performed. Its main importance is that the V–Y capsulorrhaphy forms an essential part of Mitchell's osteotomy.

Osteotomy procedures

The different types of operation which have been described under this heading are enormous. They may be classified according to the osteotomy site, namely: basal osteotomy, oblique osteotomy of the shaft, and distal osteotomy.

Basal osteotomy   Corrective wedge excision of the base of the first metatarsal was advocated by Lapidus (1934) (Fig. 6.13). His rationale is based on the assumption that metatarsus varus is the primary abnormality and correction should be at the fulcrum of the deformity. In addition to the wedge excision of the metatarsal base he excised the joint surface of the first cuneiform so that correction was stabilized by arthrodesis. Stamm (1957) was concerned about its effect on the mechanics of the midtarsal region, and was also critical of this tarsometatarsal fusion. A more recent account of the procedure was given by Lapidus in 1960 but no figures from a follow-up study were reported.

Rocyn-Jones (1948) performed a cuneiform osteotomy at the base in which a peg was fashioned on the distal fragment to provide stability by its insertion into the base fragment (Fig. 6.13). Baker (1953) and Golden (1961) devised similar basal osteotomies but with different shapes to the osteotomy line.

In their review of basal osteotomies performed at the Royal National Orthopaedic Hospital, Bonney and McNab (1952) found that there was a high recurrence rate of the deformity and this finding was supported by Cholmeley (1958). Bonney and McNab suggested a method in which a bony wedge is inserted at the basal osteotomy site and the first two metatarsal heads fixed together by means of a screw. The results from this modification have not been published. Trethowan (1923), Stamm (1957) and Simmonds and Menelaus (1960) similarly proposed basal opening osteotomies in which a wedge of bone graft is inserted (Figs. 6.13, 6.20).

Lateral stapling of the basal epiphysis of the first metatarsal in adolescent hallux valgus was described by Ellis (1951) and may be conveniently considered here. In the few cases reviewed by Helal *et al* (1974) it would appear the procedure was done too late in growth to make a difference to the deformity. Haines and McDougall (1954) observed that the first cuneiform rapidly adapts to growth

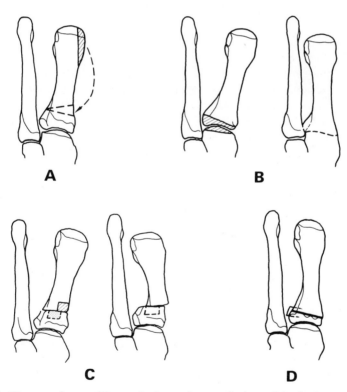

Fig. 6.13 Diagram of some of the surgical procedures to the base of the first metatarsal used to correct metatarsus primus varus. (A) Trethowan 1923; (B) Lapidus 1934; (C) Rocyn-Jones 1948; (D) Ellis 1951.

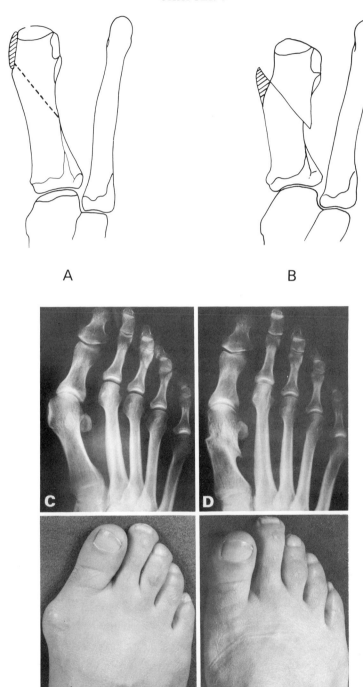

A   B

changes involving the first metatarsal. In view of this, it is doubtful if earlier stapling would be effective either. Joplin (1958) advocated an opening wedge osteotomy of the first cuneiform to correct an oblique first cuneometatarsal joint associated with metatarsus primus varus.

Oblique osteotomy of the metatarsal shaft This procedure was described by Wilson (1963) (Figs. 6.12, 6.14). Displacement at the oblique osteotomy line allows correction of the varus position of the metatarsal, slackens the conjoined adductor tendon and the slight shortening relaxes other tight structures. Union occurs more quickly than in the transverse osteotomies. In Wilson's review (1963) and in a more recent follow-up by Helal *et al* (1974) no cases of non-union have been reported. Other advantages are the simplicity of the procedure and the minimal soft tissue trauma. Stiffness of the first metatarsophalangeal joint is not a problem and at least 30° of dorsiflexion were regained in all patients in Wilson's series. The main complication, as with all distal osteotomies, concerns mal-union of the osteotomy site, in which the distal fragment is dorsiflexed producing a metatarsus elevatus. This causes weight to be shifted on to the lateral metatarsal heads with consequent metatarsalgia. Helal has largely overcome this complication by modifying the Wilson osteotomy so that the saw cut is not vertical but oblique, so that the distal fragment comes to lie beneath as well as lateral to the proximal fragment. This prevents the distal fragment from displacing upwards and further increases the area of bone in contact with the osteotomy site.

The Wilson procedure has a definite place in the correction of adolescent and young adult hallux valgus. In Wilson's series the ages ranged from 14 to 49 years.

Distal osteotomy The development of this operation has been reviewed by Cholmeley (1958). Distal osteotomy was established by Hohmann in 1923 although it was probably first described by Reverdin in 1881. Hohmann's technique consisted of the excision of a medially-based wedge and the lateral displacement of the distal fragment (Fig. 6.15). The aim of the procedure was to correct hallux valgus and not metatarsus primus varus, and to slacken soft tissue structures. The main problem concerned the stability of the displaced fragment. In 1931 Peabody modified the operation by leaving a lip of the medial cortex on the distal fragment to provide some stability on displacement, and the fragments were internally fixed with catgut. The medial capsule was repaired after trimming of the medial prominence.

Hawkins *et al* (1945) carried out a similar procedure to the Peabody operation, in which a transverse osteotomy was performed, with the removal of a transverse section one eighth of an inch thick on the medial side of the metatarsal neck (Figs.

Fig. 6.14 Wilson's oblique osteotomy of the first metatarsal shaft. (A) and (B) diagram of the procedure; (C) and (D) pre-operative and follow-up radiographs corresponding to (E) and (F) respectively. (E) pre-operative photograph of the foot of female aged 30 years; (F) follow-up photograph taken 12 years later showing the good result has been maintained. (By kind permission of Mr J.N. Wilson ChM, FRCS.)

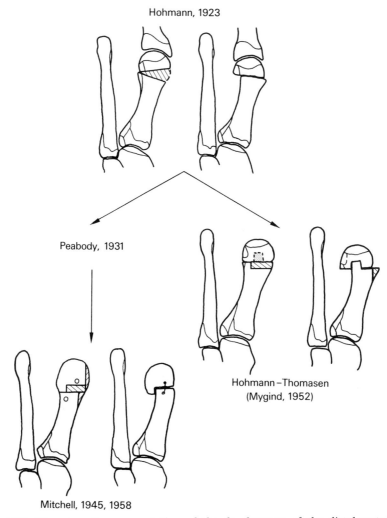

Fig. 6.15 Diagrammatic representation of the development of the distal metatarsal osteotomy.

6.15, 6.16). The distal fragment was displaced until the lateral peg hooked over the proximal shaft and internal fixation with catgut followed. The medial prominence was also trimmed and the medial capsular structures repaired and tightened by means of Silver's capsulorrhaphy (p. 100). Mitchell *et al* (1958) have reported satisfactory results from this procedure.

The rationale of Mitchell's osteotomy is primarily that the metatarsus primus varus is corrected. Although in theory this deformity is best corrected as close to its points of origin, correction in practice is much more effective just proximal to the metatarsophalangeal joint. This view is at variance with that of Lapidus (1934;

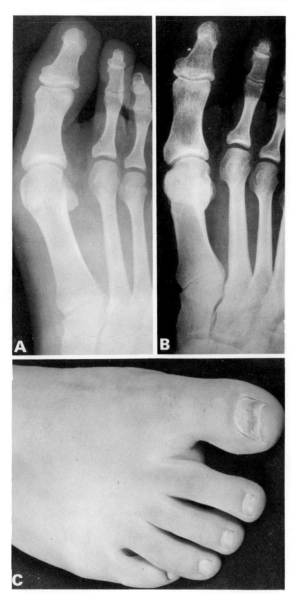

Fig. 6.16 Mitchell osteotomy. (A) and (B) pre-operative and follow-up radiograph; (C) follow-up photograph 8 years after operation.

1960). The slight shortening relaxes the soft tissues that are bow-strung across the hallux valgus deformity and lateral displacement slackens the adductor hallucis. Hallux valgus is further corrected by the medial capsulorrhaphy. Trimming of the exostosis gives added narrowing to the forefoot.

Mitchell's procedure is indicated mainly in the adolescent and the young adult case. Waugh (1963), from the results of a short-term review, suggested it was best used in the female patient under the age of 25 with moderate hallux valgus and a mobile metatarsophalangeal joint, and where there is no lateral toe deformities or metatarsalgia. In their longer follow-up studies Mitchell *et al* (1958) and Hart and Bentley (1976) found that 80% of patients had a satisfactory or excellent result. Carr and Boyd (1968), Miller (1974) and Glynn *et al* (1980) found 90% in this category. Failure in these series was due to recurrence of the deformity, stiffness of the first metatarsophalangeal joint and lateral metatarsalgia. The incidence of non-union was about 0·5%. Metatarsalgia of the lateral toes is related to either dorsal angulation of the distal fragment or to excessive shortening of the metatarsal length at the osteotomy site. Carr and Boyd considered that 4 mm is the maximum amount of shortening that is acceptable. Mitchell *et al* recommended that the osteotomies should be cut so that the distal fragment lies in a position of slight plantarflexion, after correction. The technique of this operation is clearly seen from Mitchell's drawings (Mitchell *et al* 1958). Union is slower than in the Wilson's oblique osteotomy and it may be that a wire loop provides better internal fixation than the chromic catgut suggested by Mitchell.

The Mitchell and Peabody procedures described above may be considered as modifications of the Hohmann operation. A different modification to the original operation was devised by Thomasen (Fig. 6.15), in which stability is achieved by retaining a lateral peg on the proximal fragment at the osteotomy site. A hole consistent with the size of the peg is then drilled, such that on insertion of the peg the distal fragment is fixed in a position of lateral and plantar displacement. Mygind (1952) from Denmark, and Crawford Adams (1974) from this country, reported good results with this technique. A long-term follow-up by Gibson and Piggott (1962) produced results similar to those found in Mitchell's osteotomy, 90% being classified as good. The few failures were due to lateral toe metatarsalgia, dorsal angulation of the distal fragment and non-union of the osteotomy which occurred in one case only (less than 1%). The amount of shortening of the metatarsal caused by the procedure was not related to their poor results. They argue that this can be compensated for by adequate plantar displacement.

The Chevron osteotomy has recently been described (Johnson *et al* 1979; Bargman *et al* 1980). In this procedure a V-osteotomy is performed through the distal metatarsal with the point facing distally. This is a variation on the same theme of the distal metatarsal procedures described above. The shape of the osteotomy prevents dorsal angulation of the distal fragment when this is displaced medially (Fig. 6.17). The site of the osteotomy prevents interference with the capsular attachment of the metatarsophalangeal joint and in theory should lead to less joint stiffness.

Osteotomy of the proximal phalanx   Steelenfreund and Fried (1973) presented adequate results in the correction of hallux valgus by excising a medially based wedge from the proximal phalanx of the big toe, a procedure originally described by Allen (1940). This was combined with a trimming of the medial metatarsal

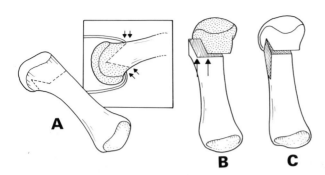

Fig. 6.17 Further development of the distal osteotomy as illustrated by the 'Chevron' or 'V' shaped osteotomy carried out in the head of the metatarsal. (Reproduced by kind permission of the editor of *Foot and Ankle* and Dr J. Bargman and co-authors.)

prominence. However, the series reviewed was small and extended over a few years only. Their failures were due to recurrence of the deformity, metatarsophalangeal joint stiffness and metatarsalgia of the lateral toes. Contraindications to the procedure included a hallux vagus deformity over 40°, a stiff first metatarsophalangeal joint and lateral toe metatarsalgia.

Arthrodesis of the first metatarsophalangeal joint

A number of different techniques have been devised for shaping the joint and for providing fixation until fusion has taken place. The main types are illustrated in Fig. 6.27 and further details are considered in the section of hallux rigidus. The main advantage of arthrodesis is that the correction of hallux valgus is combined with a consistent reduction in metatarsus primus varus (Harrison & Harvey 1963). The result is accompanied therefore by a narrowed forefoot. This is particularly valuable for the patient with a very marked hallux valgus.

Arthrodesis appears to have a definite place in the surgical management of hallux valgus patients who also have metatarsalgia. This was emphasized by Raymakers and Waugh (1971) who found that arthrodesis combined with trimming of the middle metatarsal heads improved or cured metatarsalgia in 25 out of 30 cases.

Arthroplasty of the first metatarsophalangeal joint

Keller's operation   This has been the most widely used surgical procedure in the treatment of hallux valgus (Figs. 6.12, 6.18). Despite this, considerable controversy exists as to its value and the indications for its use.

Resection of the proximal part of the proximal phalanx of the big toe and excision of the medial prominence of the first metatarsal head was described by Keller in 1904 and the results reported by him in 1912. A long time elapsed before it was used widely. Galland and Jordan (1938) advocated the procedure in the treatment of hallux valgus, and Cleveland and Winnant (1950) in their review, found that both patient and surgeon were satisfied with the result in more than

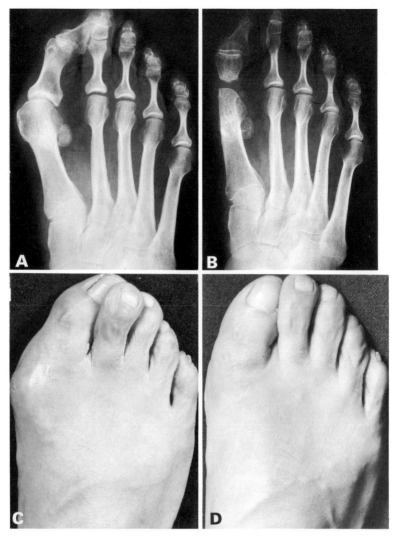

Fig. 6.18 Keller's arthroplasty. (A) and (B) pre-operative and follow-up radiographs corresponding to the photographs; (C) pre-operative photograph in a 52-year-old female; (D) follow-up photograph 3 years after operation.

90% of cases. They pointed out that at least half the proximal phalanx should be removed and that subperiosteal resection of the bone should be avoided to prevent bony reformation. Jordan and Brodski (1951) supported these findings in a large series of patients followed up for twelve years. 98% of cases had a satisfactory result. Their few poor results were due to insufficient proximal phalanx excision and they advocated that at least two-thirds should be removed. Lateral toe deformities and metatarsalgia were treated surgically at the same time, and they found considerable improvement in the incidence of metatarsalgia postoperatively. In contrast to these two reports Rogers and Joplin (1947) seemed to consider the procedure in an unfavourable light following a review of their cases. Although bunion pain was relieved in 91%, other symptoms were unchanged or in fact made worse in over 70% of cases by the operation. They noted that the flexion power of the big toe was made worse in over 50% of patients, that the metatarsus primus varus generally deteriorated postoperatively. They concluded that Keller's operation could throw 'upon the rest of the foot a burden greater than that of the deformity for which the operation was performed'.

Bonney and MacNab (1952) were more impressed with the results of the operation than Rogers and Joplin. Their comments are pertinent in selection of the patient. They found that arthritic joints in the old age group tended to give rise to poor results. They found that if the patient's occupation required him to be on his feet all day, then an unsatisfactory outcome could be expected. In cases with a very broad forefoot, even after a Keller's procedure, the wearing of normal shoes could not be guaranteed. They could find no constant effect on metatarsalgia which preceded the operation.

Gilmore and Bush (1957) and Thomas (1963) recommended the use of a Kirschner wire to keep the arthroplasty site distracted during the healing phase, and they both found that this produced better muscular control and a longer great toe. They recommended that the wire should be removed at the end of the third week. In the author's experience, if it is left in any longer during the mobilizing phase, there is a tendency for it to break at the level of the arthroplasty.

It should be emphasized that Keller's procedure should not be used in the adolescent or young adult.

The rationale of the operation is that by shortening the hallux, the tight longitudinal structures such as the extensor hallucis longus and the flexor hallucis longus, which are bow-strung across the deformity, become relaxed. Excision of the base of the proximal phalanx in addition releases the lateral capsular structures and the adductor hallucis. Trimming of the medial metatarsal prominence narrows the forefoot and helps bunion pain. Theoretically, once the pressure of the proximal phalangeal base on the first metatarsal head has been released, then improvement in the metatarsus primus varus should also occur. However, opinions vary as to the effect of Keller's operation on the metatarsus primus varus. In cases where there is considerable varus deformity an intermetatarsal suture between the first two metatarsal necks may improve the cosmetic and functional result (see below).

Postoperative physiotherapy to restore the function of the flexor hallucis longus is of paramount importance in obtaining a good result to this operation. Otherwise a non-functioning dorsiflexed hallux is produced which takes no part in the push-off phase of walking and may not touch the ground (Fig. 6.19). Another complication can occur when the second toe is long. In such a patient Keller's operation may produce a hammer toe deformity, which in turn gives rise to other

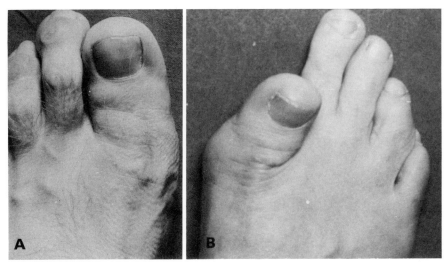

Fig. 6.19 Complications following Keller's arthroplasty. (A) hammer second toe with a painful callosity caused by shortening of the big toe by operation; (B) 'cocked-up' big toe.

symptoms (Fig. 6.19). An effect of the operation is to displace the sesamoids proximally but this does not appear to be the cause of any complication.

Mayo's arthroplasty In 1908 Charles Mayo described an operation for hallux valgus in which the first metatarsal head is excised and a medial capsular flap based distally on the proximal phalanx is turned in to separate this from the cut surface of the metatarsal bone. By shortening the toe, the tight structures tending to maintain the hallux valgus are released and in addition the prominence is excised from the metatarsal head, thereby narrowing the forefoot.

Subsequently the operation was criticized because removal of the weight-bearing part of the first metatarsal was alleged to transfer excess weight bearing to the lateral metatarsal heads, resulting in metatarsalgia. McMurray (1936) reported good results from the Mayo operation, but admitted his concern over excising the metatarsal head. Blundell Bankart at The Middlesex Hospital expressed similar doubt over the effects of this excision, but subsequently admitted to the excellent results of the operation (Kelikian 1965). Lloyd (1936) treated a series of bilateral hallux valgus cases in which he performed a Keller's procedure on one foot and a Mayo on the other. He could make no distinction between the results on the two sides and overall the outcome was satisfactory. Subsequent follow-up studies by Bonney and MacNab (1952) and Rix (1968) have also shown that the results of Keller's and Mayo's operations are similar, and in particular there does not appear to be a higher incidence of postoperative metatarsalgia in the Mayo's procedure, compared with the Keller's operation.

The Mayo's operation is not widely used today but it has a place in association with forefoot arthroplasty, particularly in rheumatoid arthritis. After excision of the lateral metatarsal heads during forefoot arthroplasty hallux valgus is corrected by excising the first metatarsal head (Kates *et al* 1967).

Combined operations

Combined osteotomy and arthroplasty Stamm (1957) and Simmonds and Menelaus (1960) described operations which involve a basal osteotomy with the insertion of a wedge of bone to correct the metatarsus primus varus, added to which there is an arthroplasty of the first metatarsophalangeal joint. In Stamm's procedure (Fig. 6.20) the arthroplasty consists of both a Keller's and a McBride's operation. Added to this the medial capsule is plicated and the abductor tendon brought round to a more medial position. By carrying out this elaborate technique Stamm overcomes the main disadvantages of the simple opening wedge basal osteotomy by relaxing the medial tight soft tissue structures, as well as tightening the lateral capsule. Whether the McBride procedure adds to the value of the operation is debatable.

The arthroplasty in Simmonds and Menelaus' operation is less complex. A similar McBride procedure is carried out and after trimming of the medial prominence a capsulorrhaphy of the medial capsule is added. The Simmonds procedure has the advantage over the Stamm procedure of being a simpler method and yet still achieves some relaxation of the tight lateral soft tissues. However, tension in the extensor and flexor hallucis longus is increased.

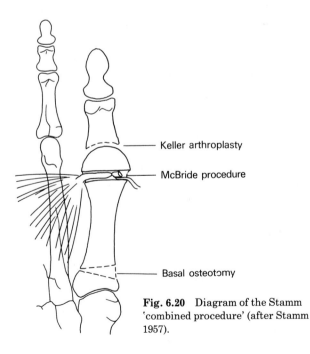

Keller arthroplasty

McBride procedure

Basal osteotomy

Fig. 6.20 Diagram of the Stamm 'combined procedure' (after Stamm 1957).

It is difficult to see a routine place for these two complex methods when the oblique and distal metatarsal osteotomies are much simpler and achieve the same percentage of good results (Simmonds & Menelaus 1960).

Girdlestone's operation (combined arthroplasty and arthrodesis)   This procedure was described by Girdlestone and Spooner in 1937 and is mainly of historic interest. Excision of the distal part of the proximal phalanx relaxes the long flexor and extensor tendons. The rationale of arthrodesing the proximal phalangeal base to the metatarsal head is that the conjoined adductor tendon attached to the phalangeal base prevents further varus displacement of the metatarsal. The phalangeal base is fixed with a Kirschner wire which is removed when fusion has occurred. It is therefore similar in principle to the McBride operation. Following operation is it difficult to restore the function of the hallux and the distal phalanx tends to become dorsiflexed.

Miscellaneous procedures

Excision of exostosis   Trimming of the medial prominence of the first metatarsal or 'exostectomy' as an isolated procedure may have a very limited place as a simple method of treatment in the elderly patient but generally it is to be avoided as a routine operation. The hallux valgus and metatarsus varus consistently deteriorates postoperatively (Fig. 6.21) and the results are often poor (MacNab 1952; Mygind 1952; Stamm 1957). Medial capsulorrhaphy in association with trimming of the prominence may halt deterioration of the hallux valgus but such a procedure is best accompanied by release of the tight lateral structures (i.e. Silver's procedure).

Intermetartarsal suture   A number of different methods have been employed in holding the first two metatarsal heads together to maintain correction of

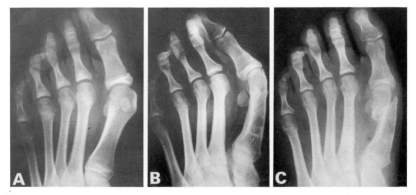

Fig. 6.21   Effect of 'exosteotomy', i.e. simple removal of exostosis. (A) pre-operative radiograph from a 15 year old female; (B) radiograph one year after operation; (C) Wilson osteotomy used as a salvage procedure.

metatarsus primus varus. Leggenhager (1935) used an intermetatarsal wire loop, Petri (1940) transferred a strip of fascia lata similarly, and McBride (1950; 1952) advocated circumferential number 2 chromic catgut as an intermetatarsal suture. Kelikian (1965) doubted the durability of these materials from his own experience of them. Bonney and MacNab (1952) suggested an intermetatarsal screw, but this gives an artificial rigidity to the forefoot. Recently the author has been involved in a review of cases where metatarsus primus varus has been corrected and held with an intermetatarsal suture of doubled strong silk. This has been combined with a Keller's procedure in the treatment of hallux valgus associated with marked metatarsus varus in the older patient. Over a period of up to ten years after operation the suture held in 30 out of 32 feet with only slight notching of the metatarsal necks. Metatarsalgia was improved in 14 out of 23 feet.

Silastic replacement of the metatarsophalangeal joint of the great toe   The Swanson finger prosthesis has been used in the great toe and reviewed by Whalley and Wenger (1975). Good results in patients with hallux valgus and hallux rigidus were found in 80% overall. When these figures were broken down, the hallux rigidus cases were found to do better. Keller's procedure has been modified with the use of a silastic replacement for the phalangeal base (Swanson *et al* 1979). This has the advantage of maintaining the length of the great toe. Initial results again suggest that it is of more value with hallux rigidus (Sethu *et al* 1980). Swanson has also introduced a larger version of the finger prosthesis for use in the great toe, for patients with rheumatoid arthritis and senile hallux valgus.

Lateral toe operations   Deformities of the lateral toes causing symptoms should be treated surgically at the same time as the hallux valgus and considered on their own merits. When this is done, the incidence of complications which affect the lateral toes, particular metatarsalgia, does appear to be lower (Jordan & Brodski 1951; Raymakers & Waugh 1971). Most operations give rise to some shortening of the big toe postoperatively. If the second toe is already the longest, and if there is early second hammer toe deformity, then operation for hallux valgus may tip the balance and give rise to postoperative symptoms in the second toe. At surgery consideration should therefore be given to shortening the second toe, either by proximal interphalangeal arthrodesis, or if there is subluxation at the metatarso-phalangeal joint, by partial or total proximal phalangectomy.

An oblique osteotomy in the distal part of the shaft of one or more lateral metatarsals has been suggested as a useful procedure in patients with metatarsalgia (Helal 1975).

Policy of surgical treatment

Adolescent patients   The majority of early cases of mobile hallux valgus in this group do not require surgical treatment, and indications for operating need to be well considered. Cholmeley (1958), Simmonds and Menelaus (1960), and more recently Helal *et al* (1974), have given detailed thought to the place of treatment in adolescent hallux valgus. Surgery is indicated partly for symptoms, but is largely prophylactic. There are good grounds for surgery when there is a family history and serial x-rays show deterioration in the hallux valgus and metatarsus primus varus. Marked bunion pain and difficulty with shoe-fitting are also indications. Piggott's (1960) radiological classification (Fig. 6.10) is a most useful radiological guide and generally surgery is indicated in the subluxed type or where a deviated joint has recently become subluxated.

The ideal operation should correct metatarsus primus varus and relax the soft tissue structures, allowing the hallux valgus to correct also. The Wilson oblique osteotomy or the Mitchell distal osteotomy are the simplest and most proven methods now recommended in the adolescent needing surgery.

Occasionally in an adolescent with mild hallux valgus and a strong family history the McBride procedure is useful to correct the deformity and also to act as a prophylactic measure. As the operation is entirely a soft tissue one, the postoperative period is short and the patient can be walking free after a month.

Young adults   The Mitchell or Wilson osteotomy is the operation of choice providing there is no element of hallux rigidus and no metatarsalgia.

Uncommonly when there is associated stiffness of the metatarsophalangeal joint, an arthrodesis ensures a more reliable result. Similarly when there is metatarsalgia of the lateral toes, results from arthrodesis of the first metatarsophalangeal joint appear more favourable than from a metatarsal osteotomy. However, as mentioned previously, lateral toe deformities should be treated on their own merits. As a rule there is no place for arthroplasty in this age group unless the condition is association with a disabling polyarthropathy.

Older patients   Occasionally in the older adult who has a mobile first metatarsophalangeal joint without degenerative changes on x-ray, oblique or distal metatarsal osteotomy can still be the operation of choice. Osteotomy has been shown to be successful in patients up to the age of 60 years (Carr & Boyd 1968) but as a rule its value is limited to a decade before this. Where degenerative changes are present or when the patients are elderly, a simple Keller's procedure has yet to be bettered. If there is lateral metatarsalgia present in addition, an oblique osteotomy (Helal) can be useful. Otherwise a partial proximal phalangectomy of the lateral toes with trimming of the plantar aspect of the metatarsal heads is of value (Jordan & Brodski 1951). When the metatarsalgia is associated with splaying of the forefoot and a wide metatarsal angle, an intermetatarsal suture using number 2 silk can give considerable benefit. In the rheumatoid foot where there is dislocation of most metatarsophalangeal joints and generalized metatarsalgia, a forefoot arthroplasty of the Kessel–Kates type, in which the hallux valgus is corrected as well, should be considered.

Salvage procedures

These can be kept to a minimum if patients are carefully selected for surgery. One of the main problems which can require a major salvage procedure is when Keller's operation is performed in a young active adult. Disabling pain at the base of the big toe can be treated by an arthrodesis. The arthrodesis may still be of the screw type if there is some of the proximal metaphyseal lip of the proximal phalanx remaining, but usually arthrodesis needs to be of the cone type or performed using a Charnley compression principle (Hulbert 1955). If only a small amount of the phalangeal base was removed at the original operation, a radical excision of some two-thirds of the phalanx and the use of a Kirschner wire to maintain distraction during the postoperative period is of benefit.

Postoperative metatarsalgia following Keller's procedure can also be disabling and in the young adult there is similarly a place for arthrodesis of the proximal phalanx to the metatarsal head, especially if there is a dorsiflexion deformity of the great toe.

Non-union at the Mitchell osteotomy site is a rare complication, which can best be treated by a sliding bone graft from the metatarsal shaft or by the application of cancellous bone chips. If union is then successful the first metatarsophalangeal joint is invariably stiff and a Keller's type arthroplasty may be required as yet another procedure. Lateral metatarsalgia following distal metatarsal osteotomy may be corrected by an oblique osteotomy of the neck of the affected metatarsal (Helal 1975).

BUNIONETTE

Bunionette, or tailor's bunion, is an uncommon cause of symptoms which arise from prominence of the fifth metatarsal head in association with an overlying bursa and callosity. The prominence is due to valgus of the fifth metatarsal, usually with splaying of the forefoot. The condition is to be distinguished from symptoms relating to an overriding fifth toe.

A number of operations have been described to treat the condition. Wilson (1953) suggested soft tissue correction by means of a V–Y plasty as for the overriding fifth toe, and this has a small place in treating young patients. More recently Leach and Igou (1974) recommended a distal osteotomy of the fifth metatarsal of the Mitchell type, and they claimed excellent results from this technique. However, it would appear to be a relatively difficult procedure. Alternatively, trimming of the lateral prominence of the fifth metatarsal head, as described by DuVries (1973), combined with partial or complete proximal phalangectomy of the fifth toe is probably the simplest and most reliable procedure. Care must be taken that not too much of the fifth metatarsal head is removed or metatarsalgia may result.

A simple and satisfactory technique is an oblique osteotomy of the fifth metatarsal shaft, which is carried out immediately proximal to the neck of the bone. The line of the osteotomy is from lateral to medial (a reverse of the Wilson procedure on the first metatarsal shaft). A useful amount of medial displacement is thus obtained and good cosmetic correction is achieved (Spansel 1976).

HALLUX RIGIDUS

Hallux rigidus is a painful limitation of dorsiflexion of the metatarsophalangeal joint of the big toe. This limitation of movement, which can also affect plantarflexion, may be due to spasm or contracture of the flexor musculature, tightness of the plantar capsule of the joint or to osteoarthritic changes within the joint.

Patients may be separated into the adolescent group where females predominate, and the adult group where apparently the sex incidence is equal or the male tends to predominate (Bingold & Collins 1950). Giannestras (1973) divides hallux rigidus into a primary type due to a localized arthritic process, and a secondary type where it occurs in association with rheumatoid arthritis, gout or a generalized metabolic condition.

Aetiology

Osteochondritis dissecans of the first metatarsal head

Kessel and Bonney (1958) found this condition in two out of ten cases of adolescent hallux rigidus. They were uncertain whether the osteochondritis dissecans had a primary or secondary role. Goodfellow (1966) considered that it was a relatively common finding among the adolescent group and that x-ray films in the early case could be normal. Goodfellow thought that osteochondritis dissecans is the primary factor in aetiology to which the joint initially responds by flexor muscle spasm and joint swelling. Secondary osteoarthritis results from the incongruity of a flattened metatarsal head which develops when the avascular fragment is soft (Fig. 6.22). It may be that the first metatarsal head is particularly susceptible to minor stubbing injuries at a particular stage in its growth. Braddock (1959) has demonstrated experimentally that this is true for the second metatarsal head at an age which matches the incidence of Freiberg's infraction. Hallux rigidus could be regarded as a parallel process. This concept has been further elaborated by McMaster (1978).

Trauma

Repeated minor stubbing injuries to the big toe has been put forward as a cause of hallux rigidus. This may produce traumatic synovitis in the joint, associated with muscle spasm, subsequent capsular contraction, and possible degenerative changes, or such trauma may cause osteochondritis dissecans, as already

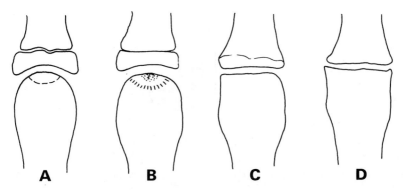

Fig. 6.22 Diagrammatic representation of the development of osteoarthritis from osteo-chondritis dissecans of first metatarsal head (after Goodfellow 1966). (A) early lesion in childhood, probably not detectable on radiographs; (B) healing lesion in adolescence visible on radiographs; (C) flattening of the head following healing in the adult; (D) secondary osteoarthritis.

discussed. Jack (1940) noted that the first metatarsal and the hallux tended to be longer than average in cases of hallux rigidus. He considered that the greater length of the first ray increased susceptibility to trauma.

Foot shape

Long, narrow, pronated feet which have a flat longitudinal arch tend to predominate (McMurray 1936; Bingold & Collins 1950; Jordan & Brodski 1951). It would appear that the increased pressure transmitted through the first metatarsal and big toe leads to hallux rigidus in some, and hallux valgus in others.

Metatarsus elevatus

There is some dispute as to whether an elevated first metatarsal (Fig. 6.23) is due to a developmental abnormality or is secondary to plantarflexion of the first metatarsophalangeal joint resulting from marked flexor spasm in association with hallux rigidus. To some extent this is an argument parallel to that which concerns the precedence of metatarsus primus varus or hallux valgus.

   Lambrinudi (1938) considered that congenital metatarsus elevatus was the primary abnormality in hallux rigidus. Kessel and Bonney (1958) demonstrated two cases with iatrogenic metatarsus elevatus, both following surgery, which subsequently developed a secondary hallux rigidus. Jack (1940) considered that metatarsus elevatus causes an increase of pressure of the dorsal part of the proximal phalangeal articular surface on the metatarsal head. This could lead to an erosion and osteoarthritis. Of course it could be argued that this localized area of pressure produced the site of the osteochondritis dissecans on the metatarsal head.

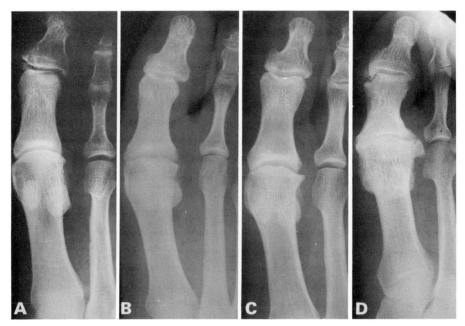

Fig. 6.23 Radiographs of hallux rigidus showing the variation in appearances. (A) normal, apart from a medial osteophyte; (B) flattening of the metatarsal head with a central area suggestive of osteochondritis dissecans; (C) further squaring of the metatarsal head due to osteophytes; (D) marked osteoarthritis. These radiographs correspond to the stages represented in Fig. 6.22.

Bingold and Collins (1950) reflect the general view that in the majority of cases metatarsus elevatus is secondary to flexor spasm of the joint. They noted also that it tends to be associated with hypermobility of the first metatarsal. Whatever may be the relation of these two factors with regard to aetiology, their association generally is a sign of poor prognosis for the joint.

Other factors

A familial pattern to the condition was observed by Bonney and MacNab (1952) although the hereditary factors are not clear. A secondary hallux rigidus may result from polyarthritis, such as rheumatoid or gout. DuVries (1973) referred to a rare congenital type caused by an anomalous flattening of the first metatarsal head.

Osteochondritis of the epiphysis of the proximal phalanx causing sclerosis on the x-ray was originally considered to be associated, but this was excluded as a factor by Bingold and Collins. Miller and Arendt (1940) considered that hallux rigidus arises as a proximal displacement of the sesamoid bones. However there has been no confirmation of this in the literature.

The author has seen two patients with hallux rigidus secondary to tightness of the flexor hallucis longus tendon, in whom plantarflexion of the foot allowed dorsiflexion of the first metatarsophalangeal joint. Both cases followed ankle fractures.

Pathology

Although there has been much speculation about the pathogenesis of hallux rigidus, little has been written on the actual pathological changes at the various stages of the condition. Bingold and Collins (1950) observed the microscopic and histological changes in the synovium and joint surfaces in a number of patients. Synovial hypertrophy, together with fibrillation or erosion of the articular cartilage over the dorsal part of the proximal phalangeal articular surface, is a consistent finding in both the adolescent and adult group. As mentioned above, Goodfellow and McMaster have observed flattening of the first metatarsal head in association with osteochondritis dissecans. Certainly in the established case the square flattened head of the first metatarsal is a characteristic appearance on x-ray (Fig. 6.25). Osteophytes form at the articular margin of the metatarsal and these can become large enough to cause symptoms, especially on the dorsum.

Clinical features

The adolescent patient typically presents with intermittent acute bouts of pain at the base of the big toe aggravated by walking, particularly in high heeled shoes. As already noted, females predominate in this group. In adults, the sex incidence tends to be equal and symptoms of pain and stiffness are more continuous in pattern. In addition, in the advanced case, a dorsal bunion may give rise to pain and tenderness (Fig. 6.24).

On examination the big toe is typically straight at the metatarsophalangeal joint and very often there is a dorsal callosity and bony prominence in contrast to the medial bunion of hallux valgus. In cases with marked osteoarthritis considerable bony swelling may exist. A callosity on the medial aspect of the plantar surface at the base of the distal phalanx is a consistent finding. Dorsiflexion by definition is noticeably reduced. Its range should be assessed with the ankle in a plantargrade position and then fully plantarflexed position. The amount of plantarflexion at the first metatarsophalangeal joint is important and this may vary from a normal to a very restricted range. In the acute phase all attempts at movement produce pain, and commonly the joint is held in a position of plantarflexion due to flexor muscle spasm (hallux flexus). It is important to record movements at the interphalangeal joint.

The lateral toes and hindfoot should be examined and polyarthropathy excluded from general examination. On standing and walking the typical case has a narrow, pronated flat foot in which the first ray is often the longest. The foot is

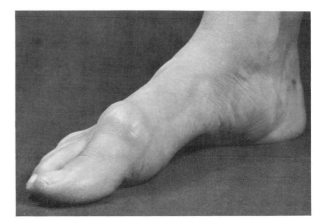

Fig. 6.24 Foot with
hallux ridigus showing
typical dorsal bunion.

inverted on push-off during walking and typically the shoe is worn on the outer
part of the heel and sole (Milgram 1964).

X-ray appearance

This can vary from normal to a gross osteoarthritic joint (Fig. 6.25). In the
adolescent, the x-rays may be normal or slight narrowing of the joint space may be
present. Osteochondritis dissecans should be excluded and a lateral view is useful
for this. Later there is flattening of the metatarsal head and early osteophyte

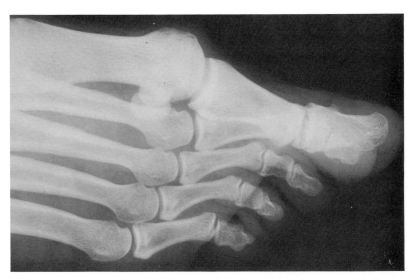

Fig. 6.25 Lateral radiograph in a case of hallux rigidus with flexor spasm showing hallux
flexus and metatarsus elevatus.

formation produces the typical square appearance at the metatarsal head characteristic of the established young adult case.

In the secondary hallux rigidus, due to gout or rheumatoid arthritis, there is usually erosions at the articular margins associated with some local osteoporosis and some joint space narrowing. A more punched-out erosion on the articular surface may be due to a tophus in gout, but this is an uncommon finding.

Treatment

Conservative management

As a first line of treatment, modification of the shoe with a rocker sole allows the patient to be comfortable during acute bouts of the condition, although it is difficult to persuade the female adolescent towards its use. During an acute flare-up an intra-articular injection of hydrocortisone (25 mg) combined with a local anaesthetic occasionally proves of value. A below-knee walking cast to rest the metatarsophalangeal joint can be used as a last resort in settling an acute bout (Kessel & Bonney 1958).

Surgical treatment in adolescent patients

Hallux rigidus in this group is characterized by intermittent episodes of pain. Surgery should be reserved for cases where exacerbations are increasing in severity or where there are persistent symptoms.

Osteotomy of the proximal phalanx   This was advocated by Bonney and MacNab (1952), in which a dorsally based transverse wedge is excised from the base of the proximal phalanx (Fig. 6.26). Satisfactory results from this technique have been reviewed by Kessel and Bonney (1958) and Heaney (1970). It is important that there is 30° of plantarflexion present, and x-rays show minimal changes. A dorsal longitudinal incision is made and care taken not to open the joint. In their paper Kessel and Bonney provide an illustrative graph from which the size of the wedge base can be calculated from a knowledge of the diameter of the bone and the angle of osteotomy required. Postoperatively the foot is immobilized in plaster for six weeks, with the big toe held dorsiflexed in order to keep the osteotomy closed.

It is generally held that arthroplasty of the Keller's type is not to be recommended in the adolescent patient (Bonney & MacNab 1952), even though Severin (1948) claimed good results in patients as young as 16 years of age. There is probably little place either for arthrodesis in this group. Metatarsal osteotomy has been recommended in the past for metatarsus elevatus (McMurray 1936; Lambrinudi 1938; Bonney & MacNab 1952). However, its long-term value is doubtful.

Surgical treatment in young adults

Osteotomy of the proximal phalanx is again to be recommended, especially in the female, provided there is an adequate range of plantarflexion at the first metatarsophalangeal joint and radiological changes are slight.

Arthrodesis This is the operation of choice, in cases where there is increasing pain and stiffness and where there is radiological deterioration, particularly in the male patient. Many different techniques have been described and recent follow-up studies on a number of these have shown good results (Harrison & Harvey 1963; Moynihan 1967; Wilson 1967; Wilson & Fitzgerald 1969). Generally no attempt was made in these reviews to separate its value in hallux rigidus from that in hallux valgus.

Position of arthrodesis is important; 20–30° of valgus is optimum (Fitzgerald 1969). Opinions as to the correct angle of dorsiflexion vary considerably and some estimates would appear to be too large. The best position in the male is 10–15° of dorsiflexion and in the female 15–20°. The latter will allow a maximum heel height of $1\frac{1}{2}$ inches.

Long-term postoperative complications concern mal-position at the site of fusion and osteoarthritis of the interphalangeal joint. The latter occurred in 25% of Fitzgerald's series and was usually accompanied by a valgus deformity at the interphalangeal joint. Mal-union of the arthrodesis occurred in 16% and included unacceptable position of valgus, dorsiflexion and rotation.

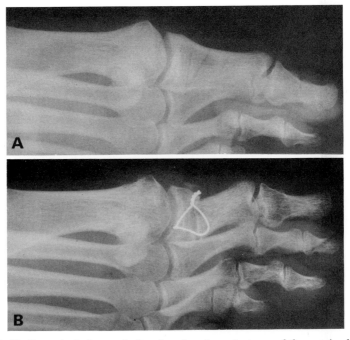

Fig. 6.26 Radiographs before and after dorsal wedge osteotomy of the proximal phalanx (Kessel & Bonney 1958).

Methods of arthrodesis fall broadly into three groups (Fig. 6.27):

1   Shaped arthrodesis include the cone procedures of Marin (1960) and Wilson (1967). Special reamers ensure a good fit between the adjacent bone surfaces. The main difficulty concerns the direction of reaming as this determines the final position of fusion. The Brockman fusion (Harrison and Harvey 1963) in which a chisel-shaped metatarsal head is fitted into a wedge in the phalangeal base and the mortise and tenon method of Favreau and LaBelle (1957), where the shaped base of the phalanx fits into a slot in the metatarsal head, may also be considered in this group. Stability of the fitted surfaces in these operations is enhanced by internal fixation such as the wire-loop in the Wilson technique (Fig. 6.27).

2   Compression arthrodesis was favoured by Harrison and Harvey (1963) because of its high rate of union. Hulbert (1955) devised small compression clamps which he removed at four weeks when fusion had occurred. In this method the articular cartilage is removed from the joint surfaces, the bones are then drilled transversely before inserting the pins to prevent bone splitting, and then compression is applied after the joint has been adjusted to its optimum position. The compression system is cumbersome and this does interfere partially with the postoperative mobilization.

3   Screw fusion (Figure 6.27) has been shown to produce excellent results (McKeever 1952; Moynihan 1967), and is probably the method of choice. It may be carried out through a longitudinal dorsomedial incision. The articular cartilage is excised from both surfaces which can then be put into the optimum position before

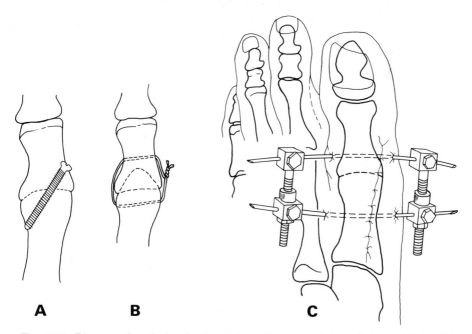

A   B   C

Fig. 6.27 Diagram of methods of arthrodesis of the first metatarsophalangeal joint. (A) screw fusion; (B) Wilson's cone arthrodesis; (C) compression technique.

drilling and the insertion of the screw. A 1 or $1\frac{1}{4}$ inch screw is directed proximally through the medial side of the base of the proximal phalanx into the metatarsal. Its direction of insertion is such that it just engages the lateral cortex of the metatarsal (Fig. 6.27). After insertion the head of the screw comes to rest against the flare of the phalangeal base. Postoperatively a below-knee walking cast or plaster bootee is applied for six weeks.

Arthroplasty of the Keller's type relieves pain but can cause disability from weakness and lateral metatarsalgia in this age group. It occasionally has a place in the female providing the patient is rehabilitated with well-supervised physiotherapy to restore the flexor function of the big toe.

Surgical treatment in the older patient

In this group Keller's arthroplasty is the operation of choice. It should be noted that its use in hallux rigidus was originally described by Davies-Colley in 1887 and therefore should strictly be called the Davies-Colley operation. Keller's name should be restricted to the treatment of hallux valgus. There is no medial prominence to excise, but trimming of the osteophytes of the metatarsal head is important. Nilsonne (1930) and Severin (1948) both advocated its use. Mobilization is quicker than with other procedures and the overall results are good.

REFERENCES

ALLEN F.G. (1940) Hallux valgus and hallux rigidus. *British medical Journal* i, 579.

BAKER L.D. (1953) Diseases of the foot. *American Academy of Orthopaedic Surgery Instruction Course Lectures* **10**, 327–43.

BARGMAN J., CORLESS J., GROSS A.E. & LANGER F. (1980) A review of surgical procedures for hallux valgus. *Foot and Ankle* **1**, 39–43.

BARNICOTT N.A. & HARDY N.H. (1955) Position of the hallux in West Africans. *Journal of Anatomy* **89**, 355–61.

BINGOLD E.C. & COLLINS D.H. (1950) Hallux rigidus. *Journal of Bone and Joint Surgery* **32B**, 214–22.

BONNEY G. & MACNAB I. (1952) Hallux valgus and hallux rigidus—critical survey of operative results. *Journal of Bone and Joint Surgery* **34B**, 366–85.

BOYLE J.A. & BUCHANAN W.W. (1971) *Clinical Rheumatology*, p. 971. Blackwell Scientific Publications, Oxford.

BRADDOCK G.T.F. (1959) Experimental epiphyseal injury and Freibergs disease. *Journal of Bone and Joint Surgery* **41B**, 154–9.

CARR C.R. & BOYD B.M. (1968) Correctional osteotomy for metatarsus primus varus and hallux valgus. *Journal of Bone and Joint Surgery* **50A**, 1353–67.

CHOLMELEY J.A. (1958) Hallux valgus in adolescents *Proceedings of the Royal Society of Medicine* **51**, 903–6.

CLEVELAND M. (1927) Hallux valgus. *Archives of Surgery* **27**, 1125–35.

CLEVELAND M. & WINNANT E.M. (1950) An end result study of the Keller operation. *Journal of Bone and Joint Surgery* **32A**, 163–75.

CRAWFORD-ADAMS J. (1974) Personal communication.

DAVIES-COLLEY J.N.C. (1887) Contraction of the metatarso-phalangeal joint of the great toe. *British medical Journal* **1**, 728.

DuVRIES H.L. (1973) In Inman, V.T. (ed.) *Du Vries Surgery of the Foot.* C.V. Mosby, St Louis.

ELLIS V.H. (1951) Method of correcting metatarsus primus varus. *Journal of Bone and Joint Surgery* **33B**, 415–17.

FAVREAU J.C. & LABELLE P. (1957) Hallux valgus and hallux rigidus *Journal of Bone and Joint Surgery* **39B**, 792–3.

FITZGERALD J.A.W. (1969) A review of Long-Term Results of Arthrodesis of the First Metatarsophalangeal Joint. *Journal of Bone and Joint Surgery* **51B**, 488–93.

GALLAND W.I. & JORDAN H. (1938) Hallux valgus. *Surgery, Gynaecology and Obstetrics* **66**, 95–9.

GIANNESTRAS N.J. (1973) *Foot Disorders—Medical and Surgical Management,* 2nd edition. Lea & Febiger, Philadelphia.

GIBSON J. & PIGGOTT H. (1962) Osteotomy of the neck of the first metatarsus in the treatment of hallux valgus. *Journal of Bone and Joint Surgery* **44B**, 349–55.

GILMORE G.H. & BUSH L.F. (1957) Hallux valgus. *Surgery, Gynaecology and Obstetrics* **104**, 524–8.

GIRDLESTONE G.R. & SPOONER H.J. (1973) A new operation for hallux valgus and hallux rigidus. *Journal of Bone and Joint Surgery* **19**, 30–5.

GLYNN M.K., DUNLOP J.B. & FITZPATRICK D. (1980) The Mitchell distal metatarsal osteotomy for hallux valgus. *Journal of Bone and Joint Surgery* **62B**, 188–91.

GOLDEN G.N. (1961) Hallux valgus, the osteotomy operation. *British medical Journal* **1**, 1361–5.

GOODFELLOW J. (1966) Aetiology of hallux rigidus. *Proceedings of the Royal Society of Medicine* **59**, 821–4.

HAINES R.W. & McDOUGALL A. (1954) The anatomy of hallux valgus. *Journal of Bone and Joint Surgery* **36B**, 272–93.

HARDY R.H. & CLAPMAN J.C.R. (1951) Observations on hallux valgus. *Journal of Bone and Joint Surgery* **33B**, 376–91.

HARDY R.H. & CLAPHAM J.C.R. (1952) Hallux valgus—predisposing anatomical causes. *Lancet* **i**, 1180–3.

HARRIS R.I. & BEATH T. (1949) The first short metatarsal. *Journal of Bone and Joint Surgery* **31A**, 553–65.

HARRISON M.H.M. & HARVEY F.J. (1963) Arthrodesis of the first metatarsophalangeal joint for hallux valgus and hallux rigidus. *Journal of Bone and Joint Surgery* **45A**, 471–86.

HART J.A.L. & BENTLEY G. (1976) Metatarsal osteotomy in the treatment of hallux valgus. *Journal of Bone and Joint Surgery* **58B**, 260.

HAWKINS F.B., MITCHELL C.L. & HENDRICK D.W. (1945) Correction of hallux valgus by metatarsal osteotomy. *Journal of Bone and Joint Surgery* **27**, 387–94.

HEANEY S.H. (1970) Phalangeal osteotomy for hallux rigidus. *Journal of Bone and Joint Surgery* **52B**, 799.

HELAL B. (1975) Metatarsal osteotomy for metatarsalgia. *Journal of Bone and Joint Surgery* **57B**, 187–92.

HELAL B., GUPTA S.K. & GOJASENI P. (1974) Surgery for adolescent hallux valgus. *Acta Orthopaedica Scandinavica* **45**, 271–95.

HELLER E.P. (1928) Congenital bilateral hallux valgus. *Archives of Surgery* **88**, 798–800.

HENDERSON R.S. (1961) Os intermetatarseum and a possible relationship to hallux valgus. *Journal of Bone and Joint Surgery* **43B**, 610.

HENDERSON R.S. (1963) Os intermetatarseum and a possible relationship to hallux valgus. *Journal of Bone and Joint Surgery* **45B**, 117–24.

HULBERT K.F. (1955) Compression clamp for arthrodesis of the 1st metatarsophalangeal joint. *Lancet,* **1**, 597.

INGE G.A.L. & FERGUSON A.B. (1933) Surgery of the sesamoid bones of the great toe. *Archives of Surgery* **27**, 466–89.

JACK E.A. (1940) The aetiology of hallux rigidus. *British Journal of Surgery* **27**, 492–7.

JAMES C.S. (1939) Footprints and feet of natives of the Solomon Islands. *Lancet* **ii**, 1390–93.

JOHNSON K.A., COFIELD R.H. & MORREY B.F. (1979) Chevron osteotomy for hallux valgus. *Clinical Orthopaedics and Related Research* **142**, 44–7.

JOHNSTON O. (1956) Further studies of the inheritance of hand and foot anomalies. *Clinical Orthopaedics* **8**, 146–59.

JONES SIR ROBERT (1924) Discussion on the treatment of hallux valgus and rigidus. *British medical Journal* **2**, 651–4.

JOPLIN R.J. (1950) Sling procedure for correction of splay foot, metatarsus primus varus and hallux valgus. *Journal of Bone and Joint Surgery* **32A**, 779–85.

JOPLIN R.J. (1958) Some common foot disorders amenable to surgery. *American Academy of Orthopaedic Surgery* **15**, 144–58.

JORDAN H.H. & BRODSKI A.E. (1951) Keller operation for hallux valgus and hallux rigidus. *Archives of Surgery* **62**, 586–90.

KATES A., KESSEL L. & KAY A. (1967) Arthroplasty of the forefoot. *Journal of Bone and Joint Surgery* **49B**, 552–7.

KELIKIAN H. (1965) *Hallux valgus allied deformities of the forefoot and metatarsalgia.* W.B. Saunders, Philadelphia.

KELLER W.L. (1904) Surgical treatment of bunions and hallux valgus. *New York Medical Journal and Philadelphia Medical Journal* **80**, 741–2.

KELLER W.L. (1912) Further observations on the surgical treatment of hallux valgus and bunions. *New York Medical Journal* **95**, 696–8.

KESSEL L. & BONNEY G. (1958) Hallux rigidus in the adolescent. *Journal of Bone and Joint Surgery* **40B**, 668–73.

LAMBRINUDI C. (1938) Metatarsus primus elevatus. *Proceedings of the Royal Society of Medicine* **31**, 1273.

LAPIDUS P.W. (1934) Operative correction of metatarsus varus primus. *Surgery, Gynaecology and Obstetrics* **58**, 183–91.

LAPIDUS P.W. (1960) Author's bunion operation 1931–1959. *Clinical Orthopaedics* **16**, 119–35.

LEACH R.E. & IGOU R. (1974) Metatarsal osteotomy for bunionette deformity. *Clinical Orthopaedics* **100**, 171–5.

LEGGENHAGER K. (1935) In Kelikian, H. (1965) *Hallux Valgus Allied Deformities of the Forefoot and Metatarsalgia.* W.B. Saunders, Philadelphia.

LLOYD E.I. (1936) Hallux valgus—a comparison of the results of two operations. *British Journal of Surgery* **24**, 341–5.

McBRIDE E.D. (1928) A conservative operation for bunions. *Journal of Bone and Joint Surgery* **10**, 735–9.

McBRIDE E.D. (1935) Conservative operation for bunions. *Journal of the American Medical Association* **105**, 1164–8.

McBRIDE E.D. (1950) Discussion of sling procedure for correction of splay foot. *Journal of Bone and Joint Surgery* **32A**, 785.

McBRIDE E.D. (1967) McBride bunion and Hallux valgus operation. *Journal of Bone and Joint Surgery* **49A**, 1675–83.

McKEEVER D.C. (1952) Arthrodesis of the first metatarsophalangeal joint for hallux valgus and metatarsus primus varus. *Journal of Bone and Joint Surgery* **34A**, 129–34.

McMASTER M.J. (1978) The pathogenesis of hallux rigidus. *Journal of Bone and Joint Surgery* **60B**, 82–7.

McMURRAY T.P. (1936) Treatment of hallux valgus and rigidus. *British medical Journal* **2**, 218–21.

MARIN G.A. (1960) Arthrodesis of the first metatarso-phalangeal joint for hallux valgus and hallux ridigus. *Guy's Hospital Report* **109**, 194.

Mayo C.H. (1908) Surgical treatment of bunion. *Annals of Surgery* **48**, 300–2.

Milgram J.E. (1964) Relief of the painful foot. *Journal of Bone and Joint Surgery* **46A**, 1100.

Miller J.W. (1974) Distal first metatarsal displacement osteotomy. *Journal of Bone and Joint Surgery* **56A**, 923–31.

Miller J.W. (1975) Acquired hallux varus: a preventable and correctible disorder. *Journal of Bone and Joint Surgery* **57A**, 183–8.

Miller L.F. & Arendt J. (1940) Deformity of the first metatarsal head due to faulty foot mechanics. *Journal of Bone and Joint Surgery* **22**, 349–53.

Mitchell C.L., Fleming J.L., Allen R., Glenney C. & Sandford G.A. (1958) Osteotomy-bunionectomy for hallux valgus. *Journal of Bone and Joint Surgery* **40A**, 41–59.

Morton D.J. (1937) Foot disorders in general practice. *Journal of the American Medical Association* **109**, 1112–9.

Moynihan F.J. (1967) Arthrodesis of the metatarsophalangeal joint of the great toe. *Journal of Bone and Joint Surgery* **49B**, 544–51.

Mygind H. (1952) Operations for hallux valgus: Report of Danish Orthopaedic Association. *Journal of Bone and Joint Surgery* **34B**, 529.

Nilsonne H. (1930) Hallux rigidus and its treatment. *Acta Orthopaedica Scandinavica* **1**, 295.

Peabody C.W. (1931) The surgical cure of hallux valgus. *Journal of Bone and Joint Surgery* **13**, 273–82.

Piggott H. (1960) Natural history of hallux valgus in adolescence and early adult life. *Journal of Bone and Joint Surgery* **42**, 749–60.

Platt H. (1957) Hallux valgus. *Journal of Bone and Joint Surgery* **39B**, 787.

Raymakers R. & Waugh W. (1971) The treatment of metatarsalgia with hallux valgus. *Journal of Bone and Joint Surgery* **53B**, 684–7.

Reverdin J. (1881) Anatomie et operation de hallux valgus. *International Medical Congress* **2**, 408–12.

Rix R.R. (1968) Modified Mayo operation for hallux valgus and bunion—a comparison with the Keller procedure. *Journal of Bone and Joint Surgery* **50A**, 1368–77.

Rocyn-Jones A. (1948) Hallux valgus in the adolescent. *Proceedings of the Royal Society of Medicine* **41**, 392–3.

Rogers W.A. & Joplin R.J. (1947) Hallux valgus weak foot and Keller operation—an end result study. *Surgical Clinics of North America* **27**, 1295–1302.

Ross-Smith N. (1952) Hallux valgus and rigidus treated by arthrodesis of the metatarsophalangeal joint. *British medical Journal* **ii**, 1385–7.

Seelenfreund M. & Fried A. (1973) Correction of hallux valgus deformity by basal phalanx osteotomy of the big toe. *Journal of Bone and Joint Surgery* **55A**, 1411–15.

Sethu A., D'Netto D.C. & Ramakrishna B. (1980) Swanson's silastic implant in great toes. *Journal of Bone and Joint Surgery* **62B**, 83–5.

Severin E. (1948) Removal of the base of the proximal phalanx in hallux rigidus. *Acta Orthopaedica Scandinavica* **18**, 77–87.

Shine I.B. (1965) Incidence of hallux valgus in a partially shoe-wearing community. *British medical Journal* **i**, 1648.

Silver D. (1923) The operative treatment of hallux valgus. *Journal of Bone and Joint Surgery* **5**, 225.

Sim-Fook L. & Hodgson A.R. (1958) A comparison of foot-forms among the non-shoe and shoe-wearing Chinese population. *Journal of Bone and Joint Surgery* **40A**, 1058–62.

Simmonds F.A. & Menelaus M.B. (1960) Hallux valgus in adolescents. *Journal of Bone and Joint Surgery* **42B**, 761–8.

Sponsel K.H. (1976) Bunionette correction by metatarsal osteotomy: preliminary report. *The Orthopaedic Clinics of North America* 809–19.

Stamm T.T. (1957) Surgical treatment of hallux valgus. *Guy's Hospital Reports* **106**, 273; also *Guy's Hospital Reports* **112**, 21–6.

Stein H.C. (1938) Hallux valgus. *Surgery, Gynaecology and Obstetrics* **66**, 889–98.

SWANSON A.B., LUMSDEN R.M. & SWANSON G.G. (1979) Silicone implant arthroplast of the great toe. *Clinical Orthopaedics and Related Research* **142,** 30–43.

THOMAS F.B. (1963) Keller's arthroplasty modified. *Journal of Bone and Joint Surgery* **44B,** 356–65.

TRETHOWAN J. (1923) *A system of surgery*, p. 1046. P.B. Hoeber, New York.

TRUSLOW W. (1925) Metatarsus primus varus or hallux valgus? *Journal of Bone and Joint Surgery* **7,** 98–108.

WAUGH W. (1963) Mitchell's operation for hallux valgus. *Proceedings of the Royal Society of Medicine* **56,** 159–62.

WHALLEY R.C. & WENGER R.J.J. (1975) Total replacement of the first metatarsophalangeal joint. *Journal of Bone and Joint Surgery* **57B,** 398.

WILSON J.N. (1953) V–Y Correction for varus deformity of the fifth toe. *British Journal of Surgery* **41,** 133–5.

WILSON J.N. (1963) Oblique displacement osteotomy for hallux valgus. *Journal of Bone and Joint Surgery* **45B,** 552–6.

WILSON J.N. (1967) Cone arthrodesis of the first metatarsophalangeal joint. *Journal of Bone and Joint Surgery* **49B,** 98–101.

7

Common Causes of Pain in the Region of the Foot

L. KLENERMAN, K.I. NISSEN & H. BAKER

In this chapter disorders affecting the heel, sole and toes are discussed. The last section is an outline of the common problems affecting the skin and nails of the foot and has been written by a dermatologist.

Painful bursae around the heel

At the level of the insertion of the tendo-Achilles there are two bursae. One lies deep to the tendon between it and the posterior smooth surface of the os calcis and the tendo-Achilles (retrocalcanean bursa) and the other is an adventitious bursa superficial to the insertion of the tendon.

The deep retrocalcanean bursa is not a common cause of symptoms. It is likely that the cause is underlying inflammation (Keck & Kelly 1965). It is suggested that it may be an early symptom of rheumatoid arthritis. The treatment is essentially conservative. Carefully placed local anaesthetic and elevation of the heel usually suffice. If operation is indicated, excision of the posterosuperior angle of the bone is the procedure of choice.

Symptoms from the subcutaneous bursae tend to become worse in winter, hence the alternative name of 'winter heel'. This bursa is usually situated just lateral to the midline and the site coincides with the upper edge of the back of the heel of the shoe, hence a further alternative term 'pump bumps' (Fig. 7.1). Many patients are adolescent girls. Examination reveals a bony prominence with a variable covering of soft tissue. If the symptoms are severe, relief can be obtained by surgery. At operation the posterosuperior angle of the calcaneum is excised freely (Nissen 1957).

Sometimes in persons involved in long distance running or in a considerable amount of walking, a thickening of the tissues around the subcutaneous part of the tendo-Achilles occurs (peritendinitis). It may disappear with the use of shock-absorbing insole, local physiotherapy such as ultrasonics, but when chronic and persistent is best treated by local excision (Kvist & Kvist 1980). Hydrocortisone injections are not recommended as if the tendon itself is injected necrosis may occur (Balasubramaniam & Prathrap 1972).

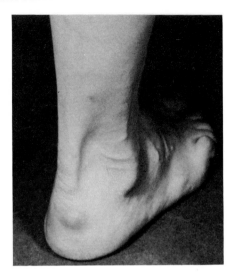

Fig. 7.1 Winter heel ('heel bump').

Ossification of the tendo-Achilles

This is a relatively rare condition. A hard mass is palpable in the line of the tendon. It may occur either in the main body of the tendon or at its insertion into the calcaneum. The ossified mass is usually asymptomatic and does not require treatment unless it becomes painful due to a fracture of the ossified segment (Lotke 1970). Local excision may then be indicated and has to be very carefully performed to avoid rupture of the tendon and to prevent recurrence.

Xanthoma of the tendo-Achilles

The occurrence of xanthomatosis of the tendo-Achilles is a local manifestation of a generalized disorder of lipid metabolism. It is hereditary and the primary effect is an increase in the body pool of cholesterol. The appearance of localized deposits first takes place in middle life. These xanthomas tend to occur bilaterally and are usually painless.

Tarsal tunnel syndrome

This condition, which is analogous to the carpal tunnel syndrome in the upper limb, was first described in 1962 (Keck 1962; Lam 1962). It is uncommon and is probably misdiagnosed as 'foot strain' or 'plantar fasciitis'. The symptoms are mainly burning on the sole of the foot in line with the distribution of the medial plantar nerve, especially at night. On examination there may be a positive Tinel sign over the posterior tibial nerve immediately behind the medial malleolus. Nerve conduction tests show evidence of delay at the level of the flexor retinaculum. Treatment consists of operative decompression of the posterior tibial nerve at the ankle by dividing the flexor retinaculum.

Chronic non-specific tendovaginitis of tibialis posterior

This is a relatively infrequent cause of pain on the inner side of the ankle. The onset is gradual. Pain may become worse after strenuous activities such as sport. Diagnosis may be delayed unless it is noted that the swelling does not involve the whole ankle region, but is specifically localized to the medial side (Fig. 7.2). On examination there is a swelling in the line of the distal part of tibialis posterior.

Active inversion and passive eversion cause pain. Radiographs of the ankle do not show any abnormality. The sedimentation rate and latex tests are normal. Conservative measures such as hydrocortisone injections, a valgus insole or immobilization in a below-knee plaster may bring relief but it is usually necessary to decompress the tendon sheath. At operation the tendon sheath is found to be thickened and there is evidence of inflammation of the synovial sheath. After operation, persistent local swelling may be troublesome. Histological sections show non-specific inflammatory changes (Williams 1963).

Disease of the calcaneum

Paget's disease may occur in the heel. When present in the foot it is usually found in other bones as well. It does not always cause symptoms (Murray 1952; Fig. 7.3). Infections such as pyogenic osteomyelitis or tuberculosis may involve the cal-

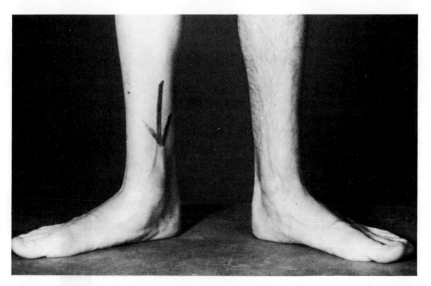

Fig. 7.2 On the right side there is obvious swelling related to the tendon sheath of tibialis posterior. At operation, the diagnosis of chronic non-specific tendovaginitis was confirmed.

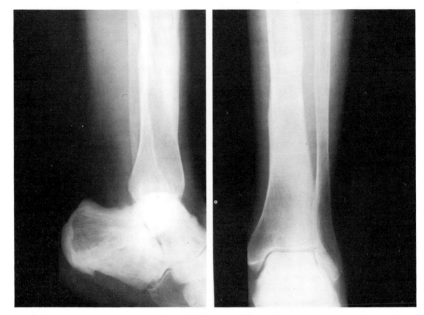

Fig. 7.3 Paget's disease of the calcaneum.

caneum and are difficult to eradicate because of its cancellous structure. Similarly this bone may be the site of a benign tumour such as a solitary cyst or a metastatic deposit. Stress fractures are an occasional source of pain.

The subtalar joint

A consideration of pain in the hindfoot is incomplete without mention of the subtalar joint. One of the commonest disorders affecting the joint is a tarsal anomaly such as a calcaneonavicular or talocalcanean bar. (See section tarsal coalition in Chapter 11.)

Juvenile chronic arthritis and rheumatoid arthritis frequently involve this joint. Osteoarthritis is common after fractures of the calcaneum. The treatment depends on the cause of the symptoms and the range includes insoles, calcaneal osteotomies, subtalar fusion and triple arthrodesis.

Rupture of the tendo-Achilles

Complete rupture

This is the commonest tendon to rupture spontaneously in the region of the foot and ankle. It occurs most frequently during some unaccustomed strenuous physical activity, such as the fathers' race in the school sports. It also occurs when the muscle is exhausted (Barfred 1973) and this may account for the injury in trained athletes. It has been described in several patients on oral corticosteroid therapy where rupture occurred spontaneously (Melmed 1965). There is usually sudden severe pain and occasionally an audible noise. Examination will often reveal a gap in the continuity of the tendon. The site of rupture is commonly localized to a site three to four centimetres from the calcaneum. Confusion in diagnosis often occurs because of mistaken interpretation of the power of plantarflexion due to the effect of the deep flexor group. Confirmation is provided by Thompson's squeeze test (Fig. 7.4; Thompson & Doherty 1962). The patient kneels on a chair with the feet and ankles over the edge. On squeezing the normal calf, plantarflexion is produced which is in marked contrast to total absence of movement on the injured side. It is not uncommon for diagnosis to be delayed and in a series of 28 patients reported by Hooker (1963), 14 came to surgery after at least one month had elapsed, including four where the diagnosis was made after one year. In the late cases the extent of the rupture is not realized until the swelling and bruising subside. The gap between the tendon ends is then very obvious.

The treatment is either operative or conservative. The theoretical objections to surgery are complications such as wound sepsis, delayed healing due to skin sloughing and damage to the sural nerve. Non-operative treatment carries the risk of re-rupture (about 10%), immobilization in plaster is necessary for 8 rather than 6 weeks and it is also necessary to wear a raised heel for 4 weeks after immobilization has been completed (Lea & Smith 1972). Surgical repair is an absolute indication in the late case. Often there is a persistent gap which has to be bridged by using the plantaris tendon and strips of aponeurosis of gastrocnemius and soleus turned distally and passed through the distal stump of tendons (Fig. 7.5).

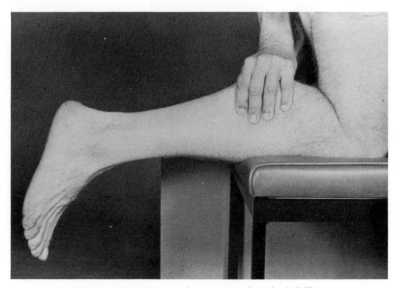

Fig. 7.4. Squeeze test for rupture of tendo-Achilles.

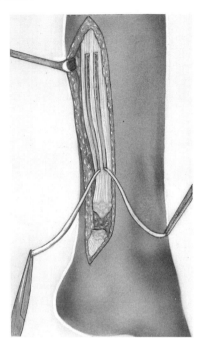

Fig. 7.5 Bridging the gap of an old
ruptured tendo-Achilles with the aid
of two strips of aponeurosis, while the
gap in the tendon is narrowed by
holding the foot in full equinus.

When sutures are used for repair of the tendo-Achilles, it is wise always to use absorbable material which does not require removal at a later date nor produce additional foci of localized infection should sepsis occur.

Partial rupture

For a long time the very existence of this injury has been denied. The majority of these injuries are produced playing sport. There is pain and tenderness in the tendo-Achilles. On examination, there is a small gap or dent in the tendon like a fusiform thickening. There may be atrophy of the gastrocnemius and increased dorsiflexion at the ankle due to tendon lengthening.

Treatment is only effectively performed surgically. The damaged area is excised and the local damage repaired by suture. This is followed by a period of 3 weeks in plaster with the foot in equinus (Ljungquist 1968).

DISORDERS OF THE SOLE OF THE FOOT

The skin of the sole, apart from its thickness over the weight-bearing area, is notable in several respects. Sebaceous glands are absent, sebaceous cysts therefore do not occur, though an epidermoid inclusion cyst is often thought to be one. Hair follicles are also absent, but a small lesion rather like an ingrowing hair of the beard may be caused by a short piece of fibre driven into the skin from walking on rough carpet or a rug. Sweat glands, however, are abundant. Hyperidrosis is due to their oversecretion; it demands a rigorous toilet and, whenever possible, an open type of footwear to allow ventilation of the sole. When a plaster cast is retained for two or three months under humid conditions, a normal level of sweating may be enough to cause maceration of the epidermis and almost total desquamation, leaving the sole pink in colour and very tender.

The overall thickness of the epidermis varies greatly with the amount of weight-bearing. Thinning may result from prolonged bed rest and contribute to acute discomfort when weight-bearing is resumed. This can be avoided by including a short spell of firm friction on the sole in routine care of such patients.

General thickening of the epidermis is found in people who habitually walk barefoot. By itself this affords little protection from thermal burns. An Indian fire-walker, however, can go barefoot across a bed of glowing embers after prolonged immersion of the feet, which allows the thick layer of keratin to absorb a minimal amount of water.

Callosities

Callosities are local areas of keratosis overlying subcutaneous tissue thinned by continual undue pressure, and usually occur under one or more of the downward bony prominences of the forefoot. If neglected they are liable to break down centrally, when they resemble verrucae. The pain of a callosity may be almost negligible or quite crippling.

The formation of all callosities is favoured by long hours of work standing on hard surfaces, and footwear with thin soles; such factors can often be reduced. The risk of ulceration is greatly increased when the nutrition of the tissues is impaired as in diabetes or peripheral vascular disease, or when the sole is insensitive as in lesions of the sciatic nerve or peripheral neuropathy; any callosity in the presence of such a disorder demands meticulous care.

The cause of the undue pressure is often a fault in the bony architecture of the foot. This may be quite obvious, as when pes cavus leads to a row of callosities across the tread, or incomplete correction of a club foot to a long callus under the fifth metatarsal. Usually, however, the fault is a local one and some common examples will be given.

Downward prominence of an enlarged medial sesamoid of the great toe is not infrequent and can be treated most successfully by dissecting it out of the tendon of the flexor brevis through a short incision. Depression of the head of the first metatarsal causes a more extensive callosity; the basis of surgical treatment is an osteotomy of the base of the metatarsal with removal of a dorsal wedge to permit elevation of the head, or if there is a cavus element, a Robert Jones operation to transfer the extensor hallucis longus tendon to the neck of the first metatarsal and arthrodesis of the proximal interphalangeal joint.

A callosity exactly under the condyles of one of the three middle metatarsal heads is often associated with conditions such as dorsal subluxation or dislocation of the metatarsophalangeal joint and hammer toe. Sometimes the callosity is more diffuse and may extend across the area beneath the second, third and fourth metatarsal heads. Conservative measures, supports, improved footwear and better working conditions may succeed in controlling the discomfort. Plastazote insoles, which are moulded to the contour of the patients feet so that the prolapsed metatarsal heads tend to produce depressions and the surrounding normal areas have a greater role in weight-bearing, have been found to be useful (Lindahl & Nilsson 1974). Patients troubled with pain in the anterior part of the foot are often heard to complain that new shoes cause them discomfort for weeks and months until they have been worn in. Inspection of the old shoes invariably discloses small depressions in the sole, corresponding to the metatarsal heads; this bears out the logic of the treatment with a Plastazote insole.

If surgical treatment is clearly indicated because of failure of non-operative measures, correction of toe deformities may be sufficient to relieve symptoms. However, Helal (1975) advocates a telescoping or sliding osteotomy at the level of the metatarsal neck to elevate the heads out of the forefoot; at the same time it produces shortening of the metatarsals and spontaneous repositioning of the weight-bearing fibro-fatty tissue behind the metatarsal heads. It is advisable to operate on all three middle metatarsal heads at the same time, but Helal states that it is not necessary to specifically deal with fixed deformities of the toes which may be present, other than by attempting to manually correct the interphalangeal joints. Thomas (1974) has advised a basal wedge osteotomy for those patients who have callosities but undeformed toes.

In hallux rigidus a callosity under the head of the fifth metatarsal may develop from transference of weight to the outer border of the foot; an associated callosity may be seen under the hyperextended interphalangeal joint of the hallux. The ball of the great toe is atrophied and the outer border of the sole of the shoe is worn down.

The subcutaneous tissues of the sole

Numerous fibrous bands bind the skin to the strong plantar fascia and form compartments filled by firm lobulated fat. This tough arrangement, so well marked under the heel, resists many of the disorders to be seen on the dorsum—contusion, haematoma formation, pitting oedema, laceration from moderate direct violence, avulsion, spreading infection. Thus a fall on to the heel may shatter the calcaneum but leave no mark at the point of impact, and an abscess provoked by a foreign body such as a thorn stays well localized with little soft tissue reaction around it.

The subcutaneous tissue can vary greatly in thickness. In some congenital dystrophies it is so thin, and the muscles of the sole so degenerate, that crippling tenderness makes walking a short distance impossible even in the best of surgical footwear; bilateral Symes' amputation may be the only way out. On the other hand, in acromegaly it may be much thicker than normal, rather like a built-in layer of crepe rubber.

A number of special lesions that mainly involve the forefoot will be mentioned later in this chapter.

THE PLANTAR FASCIA

The deep fascia of the sole, often called the plantar aponeurosis, is arranged in three divisions, each covering one of the superficial muscles of the sole and giving partial origin to it. The middle division is much thicker than the other and ends distally in five digital processes; passive hyperextension of the toes therefore renders it taut.

Local strain of the normal fascia may result from direct violence, but frank rupture is rare.

Plantar fasciitis

This is a common cause of pain under the heel of adults of both sexes. The discomfort develops for no obvious reason, is aggravated by weight-bearing, and may become so incapacitating that the patient can only hobble around with the heel held off the ground.

On inspection the general architecture of the foot is normal, contracture of the plantar fascia is conspicuously absent, and locally there is no visible change. On palpation, however, there is generally tenderness of the undersurface of the heel, and firm digital pressure usually discovers a point of acute discomfort just forward of the medial plantar tubercle of the calcaneum, over the attachment of the very dense central portion of plantar fascia and fibrous insertion of flexor digitorum brevis. The nature of the lesion is obscure but appears clinically to be akin to the common variety of tennis elbow.

The findings are so characteristic that the diagnosis is seldom in doubt. In a young adult incipient ankylosing spondylitis may have to be excluded with the aid of an estimation of the sedimentation rate (which is normal in plantar fasciitis) and a radiograph of the sacroiliac joint. The symptoms are usually bilateral.

It is standard practice to take a lateral radiograph of the calcaneum. Some cases show a forward prolongation of the plantar tubercles, enough to be labelled a spur, but the same incidence of spurs is found in random radiographs of painless heels in the same age group, which goes to disprove a causal relationship. In the absence of symptoms a plantar spur should be left alone. The spur may be present with or without any painful symptoms.

Treatment
This is variable. Sometimes a stout stick, a sponge rubber or sorbothane heel pad and restricted weight-bearing are enough. Hydrocortisone injections are often

used for relief although in a controlled trial in a relatively small number of patients there was no statistical proof of its efficacy (Blockey 1956). Rose (1955) advocated an insole extending well back to the heel in the form of a 'convex wedge' to tilt the heel into varus and to relax the plantar fasciae. Freiberg (1957) suggested a transverse pad of felt should be strapped to the heel immediately in front of the tender area and combined with a valgus insole. Others use local physical measures. Radiotherapy has been found to be effective in the resistant case (Martell 1978). Operation is to be avoided.

Plantar fibromatosis (Dupuytren's contracture)

Plantar fibromatosis has many features in common with the palmar type. It is a less serious problem because contractures do not, as a rule, occur (Mackenzie 1970). There may be single or multiple nodules which are not usually painful. The mass in the sole commonly lies under the non weight-bearing area beneath the instep. Of 104 patients reported by Pickren *et al* (1951), 59 had palmar involvement as well. In contrast to the hand, nodules are not seen in relation to the interphalangeal joints of the toes. Surgery should be avoided if possible because of the high likelihood of recurrence (J.I.P. James, pers. comm.).

Fibromatosis of the plantar fascia similar to Dupuytren's contracture in adult life may also occur in childhood. The histological picture of spindle-shaped cells with collagen formation resembles a well-differentiated fibrosarcoma, but the lesion is benign and radical local removal is the treatment of choice.

Contracture

Contracture of the aponeurosis and attached muscles is found in every degree of pes cavus, where it acts as a tie between the two pillars of the elevated long arches. Deep in the sole the strong plantar ligaments of the foot are also contracted. It is possible to correct incipient pes cavus in children before secondary changes in bone have occurred; both contractures must be released before the long arches can be flattened by manipulation and held flat in a plaster cast. At operation the fascia and muscles are detached from the tubercles of the calcaneus and allowed to slide forward; the plantar ligaments are divided where they cross the calcaneocuboid joint. Such release forms the basis of Steindler's operation. In one disorder, arachnodactyly or Marfan's syndrome, it is positively dangerous—complete collapse of the high arches may ensue from the combination of lax ligaments and weak musculature. Steindler's procedure may be combined with the removal of a wedge of bone from the lateral aspect of the calcaneum to correct any varus inclination (Dwyer 1959).

Deep structures of the sole

Various combinations of atrophy, paralysis, fibrosis and contracture of the intrinsic muscles are found in congenital disorders such as arthrogryposis and spina bifida, and in acquired disorders such as poliomyelitis and lesions of the posterior tibial nerve. Two examples of very different aetiology may be cited.

Volkmann's ischaemic contracture in the leg usually follows a closed fracture of the upper tibia with gross swelling from effusion of blood and tissue fluid into the well-defined muscle compartments at that level. If the pressure is not released by one or more timely incisions through the deep fascia, irreversible ischaemic change occurs in the distal musculature; the fibrosis and contracture that develop in the muscles of the sole are most pernicious and difficult to alleviate.

A peripheral neuropathy may cause atrophy of the plantar muscles without contracture, but so gradually that the appearance can easily be mistaken for high medial arches unless the region is carefully palpated. On the dorsum the muscle bellies of the short extensors of the toes, which normally are easy to palpate, may also be atrophied, causing the lateral malleoli to be unduly prominent.

New growths can arise from the various deep tissues but are fortunately uncommon. Two perhaps deserve special mention. A benign synovial tumour may arise from the sheath of a long tendon such as the peroneus longus. It presents as a well-defined soft mass in the line of the tendon; the treatment is excision. The nomenclature used for this type of lesion has changed in recent years. Formerly known as benign synovioma or giant-cell tumour of the tendon sheath, it is now recorded as pigmented villonodular synovitis.

In the series reported by Byers *et al* (1968) two below-knee amputations were performed for foot lesions where the original biopsy specimens had been mistakenly reported as showing malignant synovioma. In a third case a histological diagnosis of malignant synovioma was made following excision biopsy. The patient, a girl of 19 years old, refused amputation and at follow-up showed no evidence of recurrence. It is important therefore to stress the benign nature of pigmented villonodular synovitis.

A synovial sarcoma in the sole, as in the palm, is a sinister lesion. It presents as an invasive mass of firm consistency, fixed to the deep structures. An immediate biopsy is essential; early amputation is the only treatment likely to prolong life.

Middle of the tread

This is the part of the sole beneath the middle three metatarsophalangeal joints. Several disorders of this region can be understood only by a knowledge of some features of the local anatomy.

Structure

The fibrous capsules of the joints incorporate strong lateral and plantar ligaments, but are weak dorsally where there is little resistance to subluxation of the phalanx. Their plantar surfaces are united by the transverse metatarsal ligament, which can be seen as a flat band across the 2–3 and 3–4 interspaces. These two bands strongly resist spreading of the middle metatarsals. Dorsal to each band and lying in a vertical plane is a well-defined bursa separating the stout capsules of each pair of joints. These two intermetatarsophalangeal bursae are small, thin-walled sacs lubricated by a film of synovial fluid. They facilitate a small range of vertical passive movement or 'independent springing' of each metatarsal head, a function which is essential for walking barefoot over uneven surfaces. Despite their modest size, they are of considerable clinical importance.

The intermetatarsophalangeal bursae have been investigated by dissection, radiography and injection (Bossley & Cairney 1980). In the web spaces between the second and third and the third and fourth digits the bursa lies superior to the transverse metatarsal ligament but projects distally to it closely applied to the neurovascular bundle.

Anterior foot strain

The main symptom is vague discomfort in the forefoot from walking a short distance. The physical signs are equally vague, but full passive movement is resented. The previous history often gives some reason to suspect that a minor degree of stiffness has developed, for example from a wrench of the foot, or prolonged bed rest without special care of the feet, or a plaster cast applied round the forefoot without enough padding to allow it to spread. Filmy adhesions across the intermetatarsophalangeal bursae may form under these conditions and limit the 'independent springing' of the metatarsal heads.

The physical treatment consists of passive movement of all the joints of the foot in all directions in order to restore a full range of standard and accessory movements, followed by vigorous active and assisted exercises. The bursae must not be forgotten—each metatarsal head must be firmly pressed up and down separately on every occasion. A resistant case may require manipulation under anaesthesia and the use of a Plastazote insole.

Stress fractures

Stress fractures affecting the second, third and fourth metatarsal shafts are a common cause of pain in the forefoot (Fig. 7.6). There is usually a gradual onset of pain and swelling of the foot, which is aggravated by activity and relieved by rest. One can often palpate a definite swelling in the line of a metatarsal shaft. The initial radiograph, if taken shortly after the onset of symptoms, may appear normal. However, if films are repeated after two or three weeks callus will be clearly visible.

Treatment consists of reduction of the general level of physical activities and supporting strapping or bandages. This is usually sufficient to allow healing of the fracture to occur.

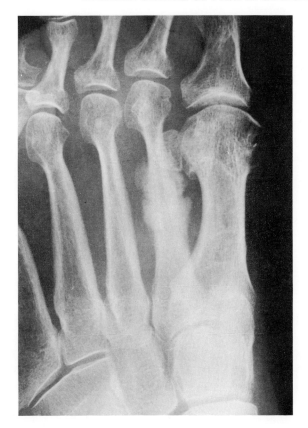

Fig. 7.6 Stress fracture of second metatarsal shaft.

Chronic hypertrophic bursitis

A remarkable degree of thickening of the walls of an intermetatarsophalangeal bursa may develop for no apparent reason; sometimes only a part of one wall is affected. There may be enough new tissue to form a soft swelling visible on the dorsum between the extensor tendons, and even to cause the related metatarsal heads and toes to spread apart on standing.

The symptoms are rather similar to Morton's metatarsalgia because the plantar digital nerve of the interspace is often secondarily involved. The treatment is excision, preferably through the sole to permit inspection of the nerve and neurectomy where necessary.

Rheumatoid bursitis

Rheumatoid changes in the soft tissues of the forefoot, though common, are often overlooked when there are lesions of the joints. An intermetatarsophalangeal bursa may be affected and distended by effusion. A lumpy appearance of the tread may be caused by synovial protrusion from a joint or flexor tendon sheath or even by an isolated cyst in the subcutaneous tissue. All such lesions are painful and hinder conservative treatment, and may become infected.

Morton's metatarsalgia

It is appropriate to discuss this disorder here because the intermetatarsophalangeal bursae and related blood vessels play such an important role in its causation. The following account is based on a series of some 200 cases treated surgically in which an incision across the tread permitted close observation of all the relevant structures in one or both interspaces.

The source of the pain is a lesion of a plantar digital nerve where it divides to supply the adjacent sides of a cleft. The nerve most commonly affected supplies the 3–4 cleft, but the nerve to the 2–3 cleft may also be involved, and sometimes both. The patient is usually a young or middle-aged woman; the age range roughly 17–70 years.

Symptoms

Acute neuralgic pain is felt under the middle of the forefoot, usually with radiation into one or more of the three central toes. In 'Morton's toe' the pain is referred to the end of the fourth toe. The foot is comfortable on rising in the morning, but pain develops after walking or standing for relatively short periods in closed well-fitting footwear. This is an important point. The patient may have no pain at all when wearing loose footwear such as sandals, slippers or wellington boots, or going barefoot. Some patients complain of pain at night causing broken sleep. During the day temporary relief is gained by a few minutes of rest; the patient often takes off the shoe and manipulates the forefoot.

Signs

There is a marked dearth of physical signs. Most commonly the general architecture of the foot is normal.

The cardinal sign is pain on pressure upwards and backwards in the web over the point of division of the nerve. The best way to elicit this pain is alternately to compress and release the forefoot with one hand while maintaining such pressure in the web with one finger of the other. Nearly always this manoeuvre produces a painful click from the lesion being pressed in and squeezed out of the intermetatarsophalangeal bursa. It is known as Mulder's click, and must not be confused with the common painless click produced by similar displacement of a fatty lobule (Mulder 1951).

The radiograph and all tests such as the sedimentation rate are normal.

Pathology

In cases with a short history, the artery and nerve, both slightly swollen, are found to be adherent to the transverse ligament. The typical finding, however, is a fusiform swelling involving the plantar digital nerve and vessels in the region of their bifurcation (Fig. 7.7). In the special case of a Morton's toe, the lesion in the 3–4 space is asymmetrical. The swelling is generally called a neuroma, but this is incorrect; histological sections show that the neural changes are degenerative in nature, not proliferative. The blood vessels show most unusual appearances, the walls being thickened to the point of obliteration, and there is a profusion of small new vessels. The pathogenesis of the neuroma remains an enigma. Nissen (1948) has suggested a vascular cause.

The normal arrangement is as follows: the plantar digital artery and nerve of an interspace meet at the proximal border of the transverse ligament, a flat band about 1 cm wide, and cross it. The artery is in loose contact with the ligament, not adherent to it. At the distal margin of the ligament, where the artery divides to reach the toes, it receives a communicating branch from the dorsum. This small vessel is closely related to the mobile distal wall of the intermetatarsophalangeal bursa. When circumferential pressure is applied to the forefoot, just as in testing for Mulder's click, the bursa bulges distally and renders the communicating artery

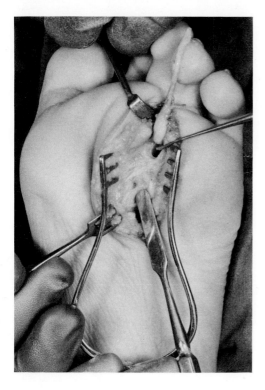

Fig. 7.7 The applied anatomy of Morton's metatarsalgia. The interdigital nerve to the 3–4 space has been divided 2 cm above the 'neuroma' and reflected downwards. The plantar digital vessels are seen entering the neuroma. The end of the flat dissector is on the upper margin of the transverse ligament. The end of the probe points to the intermetatarsophalangeal bursa.

tense. This causes gentle traction on the plantar digital artery near the point of bifurcation, but with little effect because normally it is mobile. No doubt such traction is applied and released with every step taken when spreading of the forefoot is restricted by the upper of a well-fitting shoe. Any tethering of the digital artery must of course enhance the effect of these repeated traction strains. As already noted, an early finding, preceding a fusiform swelling, is adherence of the artery to the ligament. One can only conclude that the subsequent gross changes are the end result of repeated minor traction strains on a tethered artery. In late cases part of the fusiform swelling tends to prolapse into the bursa, where it must suffer further damage. The asymmetrical lesion found in a Morton's toe probably results from asymmetry of the arterial pattern.

Treatment

Minor symptoms may be controlled by open types of footwear and limitation of weight-bearing activities. Injection of the intermetatarsal bursa with hydrocortisone may occasionally help. Otherwise the only treatment is excision. Unless this includes about 2 cm of nerve proximal to the ligament, the inevitable terminal neuroma may adhere to the transverse ligament and cause renewed symptoms.

British surgeons generally follow the example set by Betts of Adelaide and use a plantar incision right across the tread. This gives direct access to all the structures concerned; a slightly longer incision when retracted allows inspection of the next interspace as well. The incision heals well and is barely visible after a few months.

Most American surgeons prefer a dorsal incision in the web, giving limited access to one interspace only. It is difficult to resect a sufficient length of nerve above the transverse ligament without undue traction on the nerve and without division of the ligament. It is also difficult to detect and deal with an unexpected lesion such as a ganglion arising from a flexor tendon tunnel.

Cystic swellings of the sole

Most of these occur under the forefoot, where they enter into the differential diagnosis of metatarsalgia.

A ganglion may arise from the fibrous sheath of the flexor tendons to the second or third toe. It is irregular in outline and has thick walls; the lining contains only a little fluid and no loose bodies. When well developed, the ganglion causes a slight fullness of the sole near the base of the toe which can easily be missed unless the normal foot is used for precise comparison. Palpation in the line of the tendon elicits tenderness and a sense of rough crepitus. The ganglion may involve a plantar digital nerve, most commonly that of the 2–3 cleft; indeed it may be discovered only at exploration of the sole for Morton's metatarsalgia. A small ganglion may be quite difficult to distinguish from the lobulated fat around it.

Treatment

The treatment is complete excision, together with a part of the fibrous sheath from which the cyst stems; otherwise there is a high risk of recurrence. If a digital nerve is involved neurectomy from the usual point 2 cm above the transverse ligament may also have to be performed.

Adventitious bursa

This, under the sesamoids of the great toe, causes a rounded prominence which may attain a large size. It usually contains an effusion and a number of loose bodies, both of which can be detected by careful palpation.

The only treatment is excision. With due care the bursa can be excised intact, leaving the sesamoids and both flexor tendons temporarily exposed. Strangely enough, there is no tendency to recur.

Epidermoid cyst

This may occur anywhere in the sole, and is thought to arise from epidermal cells that have been forced into the subcutaneous tissue. It contains macerated keratin of a caseous nature that may become infected with the formation of a small sinus. The treatment is complete excision, which presents no difficulty.

Rheumatoid cysts

These may develop in the subcutaneous tissue of the forefoot or on one side of the heel, but more obvious lesions are usually present. The treatment is excision as part of the general programme of surgical care of the foot in rheumatoid arthritis.

This short account of disorders of the sole of the foot may well conclude with a few remarks on the plantar incisions that are so often essential for their best treatment. Such incisions are still shunned by surgeons who feel that weight-bearing areas should be avoided at all costs. In 1931, however, the American surgeon Gaenslen (1931) reported his experience of osteomyelitis of the calcaneus by cleaving the bone in twain through a midline incision across the whole pad of the heel, the resultant scars were slightly depressed but gave no trouble. Then in 1940 the Australian surgeon Betts reported a series of cases of Morton's metatarsalgia in which he used a longitudinal incision across the tread. These incisions, which were not infected like Gaenslen's, healed almost without trace. The writers, from a limited experience of Gaenslen's incision but a wide one of Betts' can confirm their favourable observations.

TOES

Deformities of the toes are a common source of discomfort.

Hammer toes

The term 'hammer toe' should be confined to that type of flexion deformity which cannot be overcome by simple stretching. It cannot be straightened by traction because this is prevented by actual contraction of the skin and soft tissue beneath the flexed joint (Higgs 1931). The condition is rarely found in infants and is usually an acquired deformity. The chief factor in its development is an overlong toe which is pressed back into line with the others by tight socks or shoes. The middle three toes are commonly affected.

The typical hammer toe shows a flexion deformity of the proximal interphalangeal joint whilst the metatarsophalangeal and distal interphalangeal joints are hyperextended. The only fixed deformity in this type is of the proximal interphalangeal joint. Occasionally the distal joint is flexed instead of extended and sometimes the distal joint alone is involved ('mallet toe') (Fig. 7.8).

Higgs pointed out that pain occurs in three situations. Firstly in the common type over the prominent proximal interphalangeal joint. A corn and underlying bursa develops and attacks of acute inflammation are not uncommon. Secondly there may be pain in the sole of the foot. The hyperextended proximal phalanx presses down on the head of the corresponding metatarsal producing a callosity in the sole. Lastly, if the terminal joint is flexed a painful corn may develop around the nail at the tip where pressure occurs.

Treatment

Conservative measures have little place in the treatment of the established deformity. Where there is no dislocation of the metatarsophalangeal joint the proximal interphalangeal joint can be arthrodesed after preliminary tenotomy of the contracted extensor tendon, although sometimes a formal capsulotomy of the metatarsophalangeal joint is necessary for full correction. The skin and underlying bursa over the flexed joint are excised. Bony apposition is obtained either by fashioning a square peg out of the distal end of the proximal phalanx and impacting it into a round hole made in the base of the middle phalanx (Fig. 7.9) or by excision of the articular surfaces and the introduction of a Kirschner wire to hold the surfaces together. The use of an intramedullary wire is essential if both interphalangeal joints are to be arthrodesed. Where there is subluxation at the metatarsophalangeal joint excision of the proximal half of the base of the proximal phalanx will allow the toe to drop into normal alignment. Removal of the whole proximal phalanx is unnecessary and results in a very floppy toe. Painful terminal corns are best treated by amputation of the terminal phalanx and the nail. The soft

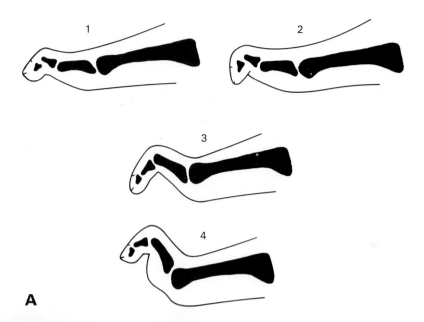

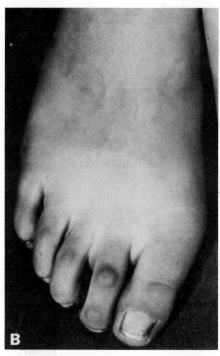

Fig. 7.8   (A) Various types of deformity of the toes. 1, Mallet toes with dorsal pressure on the flexed distal interphalangeal joint. 2, Severe mallet toe with pressure also on the tip of the toe and margin of the nail. 3, Typical hammer toe, as shown in (B). 4, A subluxed hammer toe with depression of the metatarsal head. (B) A typical second hammer toe with dorsal corns over the joints and a mallet deformity distally. The middle toe is similarly affected, but to a lesser extent.

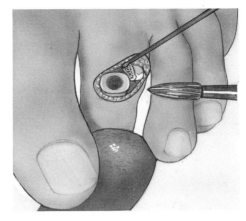

Fig. 7.9 Spike arthrodesis of the second toe. An ellipse of skin including the dorsal corn has been excised and the extensor tendon divided. The condyles of the proximal phalanx have been trimmed, leaving a square peg with a cap of cartilage. A conical hole has been made in the base of the middle phalanx ready for deep impaction of the peg.

plantar pad that is left can then be sewn to the dorsal skin, thus relieving the discomfort.

Claw toes

This pattern of deformity is most commonly but not exclusively found in association with pes cavus. Fixed flexion deformities of the interphalangeal joints may be present in an otherwise normal-looking foot. In the typical case the toes are flexed at both interphalangeal joints and markedly hyperextended at the metatarso-phalangeal joints. At first the toes may be passively correctable. Later the joints become ankylosed and painful callosities develop on the sole of the foot (Fig. 7.10) and also on the tips of the toes and the dorsal aspect of the proximal interphalangeal joint.

Treatment

If the toes are passively correctable the transfer of both flexor tendons to the extensor surface of the lesser toes is usually a reliable method of reproducing the action of the intrinsic muscles as originally proposed by Girdlestone (Taylor 1951; Pyper 1958). For correction of the great toe if there is a cavus element, it is best to carry out Robert Jones' operation. This consists of the transfer of the extensor hallucis longus to the neck of the first metatarsal and the arthrodesis of the proximal interphalangeal joint.

Lambrinudi's operation for claw-toes (Nissen 1957) consisted of excision of all interphalangeal joints and while consolidation of these arthrodeses is taking place the toes are held straight by subcutaneous loops of suture material, such as nylon thread, placed directly over each proximal phalanx and tied down to a special sole-plate. The basis of the operation is the fact that, by arthrodesing the interphalangeal joints, the long flexor muscles are persuaded to exert their main

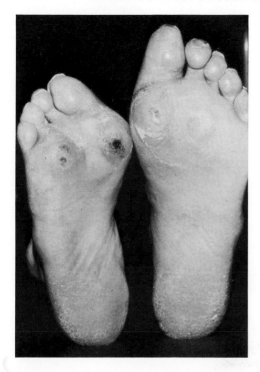

Fig. 7.10 Callosities in association with claw-toes and pes cavus.

action on the metatarsophalangeal joints. Thus it produces a redistribution of the muscle forces which improves both function and appearance.

This operation is rarely performed nowadays. Instead the interphalangeal arthrodeses are stabilized by intramedullary wires and the metatarsophalangeal joints are corrected by extensive soft tissue release (Sandeman 1967). Another variation on this theme (Chuinard & Baskin 1973) consists of the attachment of the long extensor tendons to the neck of each metatarsal in addition to soft tissue release of the metatarsophalangeal joints and the interphalangeal joint arthrodeses described above. The rationale of the operation is to allow the long extensors of the toes to dorsiflex rather than dorsiflexing the toes and depressing the metatarsal heads. Fixed claw-toes due to inflammatory diseases such as rheumatoid arthritis are best treated by filleting operations (Fowler 1959; Kates *et al* 1967). The former procedure is performed from the dorsal surface of the foot, but it is recommended that an ellipse of skin beneath the metatarsal heads be excised from the sole in order to restore the pad of weight-bearing fibro-fatty tissue to its normal pattern. The operation consists of excision of the bases of the proximal phalanges and trimming and re-shaping of the metatarsal heads.

The latter procedure is carried out entirely through the plantar approach. According to Barton (1973), who surveyed a series of patients who had surgery for correction of deformities of the forefoot following rheumatoid arthritis, there was no difference in the results of using the two techniques. It is, however, important to stabilize the medial ray by means of an arthrodesis of the metatarsophalangeal joint in order to prevent a recurrence of the deformity (see Chapter 13).

Subungual exostosis

This condition is most commonly found on the great toe (Fig. 7.11). It presents as a firm swelling below the nail near the tip and gradually displaces the nail. It is often mistaken for a wart but radiographs will establish the diagnosis (Samman 1972). The treatment consists of removal of sufficient nail to allow the protruberance to be completely nibbled away.

Glomus tumour

This is a relatively rare condition. It may arise in the nail bed or the pulp of the toe. The pain may be excruciating. The tumour develops out of normal glomus bodies which are present in large numbers on the palmar surfaces of the soles and feet. Histologically it consists of an arteriovenous anastomosis wrapped in unmyelinated neural filaments (Jaffe 1964).

Sesamoids

The medial and lateral sesamoid bones form part of the insertions of the flexor hallucis brevis into the proximal part of the proximal phalanx of the great toe.

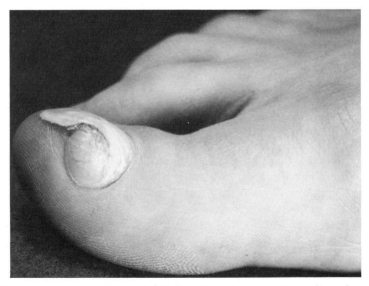

Fig. 7.11   A large subungual exostosis with the nail partly removed in readiness for excision.

They articulate with and rest under the first metatarsal head. Although joined together by strong bands of the joint capsule, they are separated from each other by the tendon of flexor hallucis longus on its path to insert into the base of the distal phalanx, and their articular facets are separated by a bony bridge. Between the sesamoids and the skin there is normally only the thick fibrous pad which forms the ball of the foot, and through which the two small bones may sometimes be palpated. Not infrequently a bursa is interposed between the sesamoids and the skin surface (Inge & Ferguson 1933). Ossification occurs between the eight and eleventh years, often from multiple centres, which may or may not unite subsequently. Failure of the union of these centres gives rise to segmentation of the bones and often the suspicion of a fracture. A bipartite or multipartite sesamoid is not uncommon and occurs in 10% of people. The medial sesamoid is most commonly affected (unilateral in 75%, bilateral in 25%), of those bilateral in 85% the deficiency was symmetrical.

Fracture of a sesamoid is rare and may be difficult to diagnose precisely unless there is evidence of healing. Stress fractures have been reported in athletes. Pain may be due to chrondromalacia or degenerative changes associated with hallux rigidus, which may result in the eventual adherence of the sesamoids to the head of the first metatarsal. Osteomyelitis of a sesamoid has been reported in three juveniles (Colwill 1969). If conservative measures to relieve pain by using supports for the forepart of the foot are unsuccessful, it may be necessary to excise a sesamoid. It should be carefully shelled out of the surrounding tendon to prevent impairment of function. Only the painful sesamoid need be removed, as leaving behind one normal sesamoid does not predispose to recurrence of pain. Pain arising from the sesamoids may be becoming more common with the increased numbers of the jogging population (Scranton & Rutkowski 1981).

DISEASES OF THE SKIN OF THE FOOT

It is not uncommon for symptoms to misdirect certain dermatological problems to the orthopaedic clinic and *vice versa*. The latter is particularly seen where a skin manifestation has an orthopaedic cause, for instance the plantar callosity or the warty subungual hyperkeratosis provoked by a phalangeal exostosis. This short section will therefore be confined to those conditions where the interests of the dermatologist and orthopaedic surgeon overlap.

Plantar warts

Plantar warts are rare before school age but increasingly common thereafter, with a peak incidence in 9–13 year-olds. They are uncommon, but by no means rare, in adults. The cause is a distinct virus of the papova group which infects epidermal cells by direct innoculation. This infection is usually picked up directly from floors, e.g., the bathroom, changing room or swimming pool. A serologically distinct sub-type of human papilloma virus is now known to be responsible for plantar warts.

The wart first appears as a pin-head sago-grain papule. It enlarges into a well defined round or oval lesion up to 1 cm in diameter with a surrounding and overlying zone of hyperkeratotic stratum corneum, which may blur its margins until pared down. The active wart is painful and tender, especially when squeezed laterally. The symptoms vary enormously from the trivial to the disabling. A wart resolving spontaneously is less tender and shows characteristic black punctate spots of purpura.

Most warts are on pressure points either under the metatarsal heads, particularly medially, or on the heels. The toes may be affected. They are often multiple, spread beginning as a satellite process around the first wart. Occasionally a large mass of wart tissue forms a mosaic, usually on the heel. At least half of plantar warts disappear spontaneously within six months but in adults they may persist for years. Mosaic warts in adults are particularly persistent.

Differential diagnosis is from callosity and corn. The latter are both always on pressure points but the wart may not be. Both callosities and corns may be tender on vertical pressure but are less tender than warts when squeezed laterally. The epithelial ridges of the plantar skin are interrupted by a wart but not by a callosity. Paring usually resolves any doubt by defining the wart and, if continued, leading to punctate bleeding in a wart, as the elongated dermal papillae are opened.

Treatment

The single disabling plantar wart is best curretted except in very young children. 2 ml of local anaesthetic are injected directly beneath the wart. The overlying skin is pared and the precise margins defined. A 2 mm incision is then made around the wart deep enough to receive the edge of a sharp curette approximately the size of the lesion, which is then scooped out in a single movement (Fig. 7.12). The cautery can be used lightly on the sides of the cavity but is best avoided in the base lest scarring follows. A firm pressure dressing suffices, for which a 'band-aid' can be substituted on the fourth day.

Multiple plantar warts, if scattered, can be soaked in 1:8 formalin (5% formaldehyde) solution for 15 minutes daily. Grouped warts may be subjected to salicylic acid plasters (30–40%), left on for 48 hours with similar alternate periods of rest.

Single dose cryotherapy with liquid nitrogen is not suitable, being too painful, but frequent paring after light application of liquid nitrogen may sometimes be effective. Radiotherapy and excisional surgery are only rarely justified. Extremely resistant lesions may respond to intra-lesional injections of bleomycin.

Callosities

These are areas of hyperkeratosis induced by friction, pressure or other trauma.

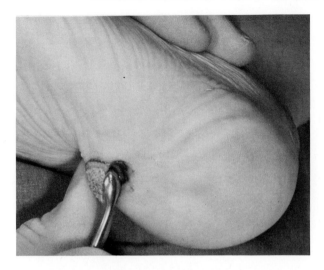

Fig. 7.12 Curettage of a plantar wart.

They are very frequent on the soles in adults, usually beneath the metatarsal heads (see p. 135).

Corns

These are peculiar and very sharply circumscribed callosities usually occurring over the dorsal aspect of a deformed toe joint as a result of pressure. The hyperkeratosis contains a visible central core which presses deeply into the dermis causing pain and sometimes inflammation. They may occur in the interdigital spaces (particularly the most lateral) when maceration and secondary commensal infection produce the typical appearance of 'soft corn'.

Treatment is not always satisfactory. Prevention of pressure, paring, salicylic acid plasters and removal of the core all have a place (see Chapter 15). The last procedure is easiest when the core has been softened by occlusive, keratolytic dressings, but may be complicated by cellulitis if infection is carelessly introduced. Sometimes it is necessary to excise the corn and the underlying bony prominence.

Nail dystrophies

Only a few of the commoner conditions will be described.

Onychogryphosis and nail hypertrophy

These are usually due to trauma, perpetuated by pressure from footwear as the nail lengthens and thickens. The nail may eventually curve like a ram's horn (Fig. 7.13). The great toe nails are usually involved.

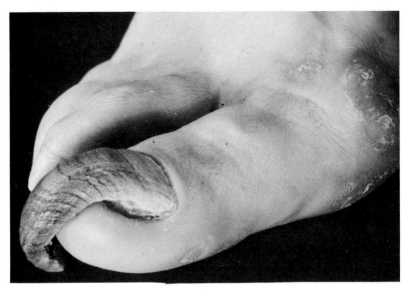

Fig. 7.13   A neglected case of onychogryphosis.

Ingrowing toe nail

This also involves the halluces and is usually due to lateral compression by footwear and inappropriate nail cutting. The lateral nail fold is penetrated by the edge of the nail plate causing first pain then sepsis and subsequently granulation tissue (Fig. 7.14). Conservative treatment is discussed in Chapter 15, but if this is not successful, radical excision of the nail bed using the Zadik technique is indicated (Townsend & Scott 1966).

Treatment, which can be carried out by a well-trained chiropodist, is further elaborated in Chapter 15. The technique of wedge resection is useful if only one border of the nail is affected. The results of wedge resection and radical excision of the nail bed (Zadik 1950) have been improved by the use of 88% phenol applied to the nail matrix for three minutes. The excess is then removed with surgical spirit. Phenol cauterization has a further advantage in that it need not be delayed in infected toe nails (Andrew & Wallace 1979). Indeed, these authors suggest that the need for formal surgical excision of the nail matrix is then unnecessary.

Shedding of big toe nails

This may be repetitive and is usually due to trauma, e.g. by sporting footwear, in persons with a predisposition, sometimes genetic. Nail loss may be preceded by a subcuticular haematoma. A new nail usually grows uneventfully.

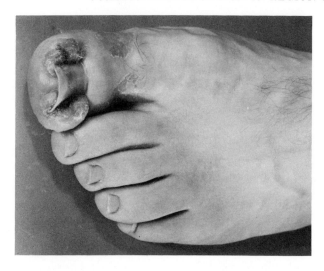

Fig. 7.14 A severe case
of an ingrowing toe nail.

Overcurvature of toe nails

This is sometimes constitutional, but may be due to footwear trauma or psoriasis. It may be complicated by lateral ingrowing. Removal of the nail is the only treatment.

Senile nail

In many old people the toe nails are thickened, opaque and may be split or ridged. Impaired digital circulation may be a factor. Subungual exostoses are responsible for deforming the nail plate (see p. 150).

Tinea unguium

This is produced when dermatophytes (fungi) invade the nail plate. *Trichophyton rubrum, Trichophyton interdigitale* and *Epidermophyton floccosum* are the usual dermatophytes in nail infections in this country. It is rare in children.

The infection usually presents as a well-demarcated, discoloured patch at the side of the nail, initially yellowish-white but later yellow-brown or even black. As the infection spreads, the plate becomes first thickened, then cracked and eventually soft and 'crumbled'.

Frequently, fingers as well as toe nails are involved and there may be associated tinea of the skin of the feet. This may take the form of a simple toe cleft intertrigo with interdigital scaling (especially in the lateral clefts), or there may be a vesicular or pustular and scaly eruption of the feet, often with a well-defined slowly advancing margin. Trichophyton rubrum infections may show a characteristic dry, red branny hyperkeratosis of the plantar skin with whitish accentuation of the skin creases.

The diagnosis is confirmed by microscopy and culture of nail scrapings or clippings. Psoriasis is the important differential diagnosis (see below). Treatment is unsatisfactory. Tinea can be eliminated from the skin often by topical measures alone. These include 1:8000 potassium permanganate compresses if there is acute or sub-acute inflammation, and application of magenta paint, benzoic acid compound (Whitfield's) ointment, clotrimazole cream (Canesten, Bayer) or miconazole cream (Daktarin, Janssen).

Finger nail infections respond to a prolonged course of the antibiotic, griseofulvin, but toe nail infections, especially with *Trichophyton rubrum* can rarely be permanently cured with this drug and attempted eradication from the toe nails is rarely worthwhile. A new oral drug, detoconazole (Nizoral) may be used if griseofulvin cannot be tolerated for any reason.

Psoriasis

In the finger nails, psoriasis produces 'thimble' pitting, ridges and grooves, if the psoriatic inflammation is in the nail matrix and onycholisis (separation of the nail from its bed) or subungual hyperkeratosis if the nail bed or hyponychium is involved. In the toe nails pitting and onycholysis are very unusual and thickening of the plate and subungual keratosis, which may be gross, are generally seen. Psoriasis is rarely confined to the toe nails and if the diagnosis is considered, brief questioning and inspection of the finger nails, knees, elbows and scalp will usually confirm it.

Common inflammatory skin diseases of the feet

The usual differential diagnosis of a rash on the feet is as follows:
1   Tinea
2   Psoriasis (including pustular psoriasis).
3   Endogeneous eczema.
4   Contact eczema (contact dermatitis).

The clinical manifestations of tinea pedis have been briefly described above.

Psoriasis of the feet may take several forms, but it is rarely confined to these extremities. It may be unilateral. Ordinary plaques may occur on the dorsa, toes or soles, showing the characteristic sharply defined margins, the dull red-brown colour and surface scaling, silvery if scratched. Plaques involving a toe cleft may stimulate tinea (Fig. 7.15).

Another pattern produces a diffuse hyperkeratosis of the soles with little scaling. Sometimes hyperkeratosis is gross, especially on the pressure areas under the heels and metatarsal heads, and may lead to painful fissuring (Fig. 7.16). *Trichophyton rubrum* infection may be simulated.

In chronic palmoplantar pustular psoriasis, usually involving the heel or instep, a circumscribed red, scaly area occurs in which erupt indolent 2–3 mm

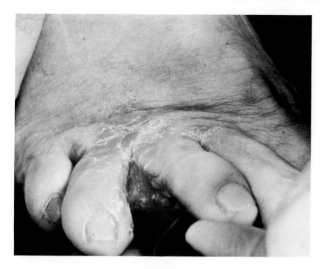

Fig. 7.15 Interdigital psoriasis.

pustules, which slowly dessicate to leave brown stains in the desquamating stratum corneum. The pustules are sterile.

Lastly, Reiter's syndrome may be complicated by keratoderma blenorrhagicum which clinically and histologically is indistinguishable from psoriasis. The lesions usually involve the soles as cone-shaped orange-brown papules whose peaks become scaly. Spread and confluence usually lead eventually to a typical psoriatic appearance. Psoriasis of the nails is described above.

Endogeneous eczema

Endogeneous eczema of the feet may take several forms. Unlike psoriasis, eczema itches and frequently 'weeps', i.e. is exudative. It may be vesicular, as may be tinea, but never psoriasis.

Hypostatic eczema

Hypostatic eczema is due to local venous hypertension and usually starts above the malleoli but may spread on the feet.

Recurrent summer pompholyx

This is an ill-understood pattern of eczema in which intensely pruritic papules and vesicles erupt in an area of erythema and oedema. The subcorneal vesicles may run together to form large blisters and in its fulminating form, pompholyx is completely disabling. Secondary coccal infection may lead to cellulitis or lymphangitis. Pompholyx tends to recur irregularly in summer and may last for weeks or months.

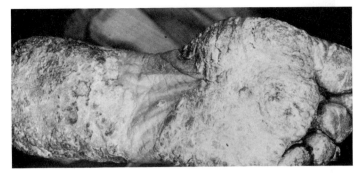

Fig. 7.16 Hyperkeratotic psoriasis of the sole (Skin Department, The London Hospital).

Atopic eczema

This is mainly seen in childhood and frequently involves the feet. In older boys it may take the form of an intractable eczema of the toes.

Peridigital dermatitis of children

This is a common eruption, often in children with an atopic background aged 3–15 years. A dry, scaly fissured dermatitis is confined to the skin on and around the toes. It is chronic and resistant to treatment.

Juvenile plantar dermatosis: forefoot eczema

A dry, glazed less scaly or fissured dermatitis of the distal half of the sole and plantar aspects of the toes has become increasingly common in recent years. Occlusive, synthetic close-fitting slip-on shoes and nylon socks have been blamed (Fig. 7.17).

Contact eczema

This is almost invariably due to footwear. The common causes are chromate or vegetable tans in the leather of the uppers of shoes or sandals, and additives in rubber, used in soles and heels of shoes or slippers or in industrial rubber boots. Rarely dyes and anti-rot chemicals in which the shoes are steeped are allergenic. The pattern of eczema depends upon the cause, the dorsum of the foot being affected by leather uppers and the pressure area of the heels, soles and toes by rubber soles. The diagnosis is confirmed by patch testing.

Pitted Keratolysis (Keratolysis plantare sulcatum)

This common condition is usually seen in hyperhidrotic feet. It is caused by mixed

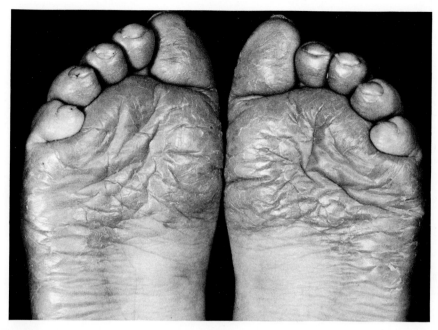

Fig. 7.17   A typical example of juvenile plantar dermatosis (Skin Department, The London Hospital).

filamentous or coccoid micro-organisms including streptomyces and corynebacterium species. The eruption is bilateral and seen on the soles. Irregular erosions on the stratum corneum coalesce to form a patterned network, sometimes with a green or pale brown colour. The feet usually smell foul. The condition is symptomless. Using a Gram stain, filamentous organisms are seen in abundance in superficial scrapings. Improved hygiene and the use of neomycin-containing lotion or cream produce a rapid response.

Tumours of the feet

The three primary invasive tumours of the epidermis are squamous and basal cell carcinomata and malignant melanoma. The first two are rare in the feet. Of dermal malignant tumours, only Kaposi's haemorrhagic sarcoma will be considered, because it usually begins on the skin of the foot.

Malignant melanoma

This arises from melanocytes in the basal layer of the epidermis or from nests of aberrant melanocytes (naevus cells) in the upper dermis close to the dermoepidermal junction. It may or may not be preceded by a benign mole. The tumour may arise anywhere on the foot, but it is more common on the sole than on the dorsum. It may occur in the nail fold or on the nail bed. It is rare in childhood (when benign junctional moles are very common) and the risk increases with age.

Amelanotic melanoma is rare, so the great majority of tumours are pigmented. In previously normal skin, the tumour present as a small area of deep pigmentation (Fig. 7.18).

This either becomes raised and nodular to produce a mass which eventually erodes the epidermis and ulcerates (Fig. 7.19) or spreads laterally to produce a barely palpable plaque. In a pre-existing mole the development of irregularity of contour, profile or pigmentation are the earliest signs. The altered pigmentation is of particular importance. Areas of dark brown or almost black colour are

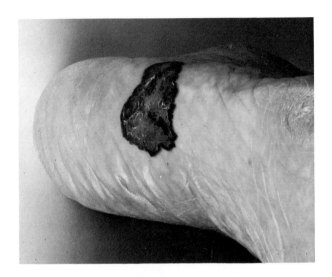

Fig. 7.18 Malignant melanoma. Note irregularity of contour and pigmentation. (Skin Department, The London Hospital).

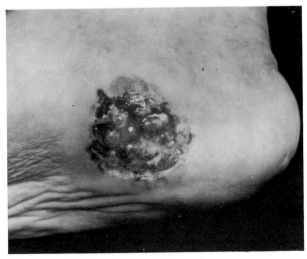

Fig. 7.19 Advanced ulcerated malignant melanoma. Note irregular pigmentation beyond margin of ulceration. (Skin Department, The London Hospital).

intermixed with blue-grey or slate-coloured zones. The edges of the pigmentation may be fuzzy and irregular. It should be emphasized that erosion, ulceration, bleeding and the appearance of satellite papules are late signs, indicating a deeply invasive tumour.

Subungual malignant melanoma may be confused with subungual haematoma. It presents as an area of pigmentation on the nail bed, or an unexplained nail dystrophy or a haemorrhagic and indolent localized paronychia. As the tumour spreads the nail plate is grossly deranged. If the diagnosis is suspected, the nail should be removed and the nail bed biopsied for frozen section before amputation is undertaken (Davis & Little 1974).

Kaposi haemorrhagic sarcoma (Fig. 7.20)

This is a multifocal tumour of avascular and perivascular tissue. It is rare in this country, occurring mainly in elderly male Jews. It is not uncommon in many parts of black Africa. Its pathogenesis is not understood, but it is probably a reticulosis.

The disease usually begins on the feet as multiple reddish-blue plaques which reach a size of 1–3 cm and may coalesce. The tumours may be partially bleached by pressure to leave a brownish plaque. Lesions appear higher on the leg, which may become chronically oedematous. Symptoms are few but eventually lymph nodes and internal organs may become involved.

Histologically the tumour shows bands of spindle cells embedded in a matrix of reticular and vascular spaces. Purpura, haemosiderin-containing macrophages and a lymphocytic inflammatory reaction are superimposed.

Differential diagnosis of a solitary lesion is from dermatofibroma, lichenoid purpura, hypertrophic lichen planus and pyogenic granuloma. Plaques of Kaposi sarcoma may be simulated in chronic venous stasis in the leg.

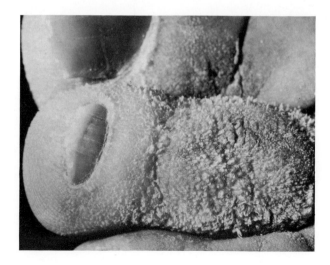

Fig. 7.20 Kaposi sarcoma. Infiltration of toe with overlying 'kettle fur' hyperkeratotis. (Skin Department, The London Hospital.)

Treatment is unsatisfactory but fortunately the disease often progresses only very slowly. Radiotherapy and intra-arterial chemotherapy have been used.

REFERENCES

ANDREW T & WALLACE W.A. (1979) Nail ablation—excise or cauterise? A controlled study. *British medical Journal* 1, 1539.

BALASUBRAMANIAM P. & PRATHRAP K. (1972) The effect of injection of hydrocortisone into rabbit calcaneal tendon. *Journal of Bone and Joint Surgery* **54B**, 729–34.

BARFRED T. (1973) Achilles tendon rupture. *Acta Orthopaedica Scandinavica* (suppl) **152.**

BARTON N.J. (1973) Arthroplasty of the forefoot in rheumatoid arthritis. *Journal of Bone and Joint Surgery* **55B**, 126–33.

BETTS L.O. (1940) Morton's metatarsalgic neuritis of fourth digital nerve. *Medical Journal of Australia* 1, 514–15.

BLOCKEY N.J. (1956) The painful heel. *British medical Journal* 1, 1277–8.

BOSSLEY C.J. & CAIRNEY P.C. (1980) The intermetatarsal bursa—its significance in Morton's metatarsalgia. *Journal of Bone and Joint Surgery* **62B**, 184–7.

BYERS P.D., COTTON R.E., DEACON O.W., LOWY M., NEWMAN P.H., SISSONS H.A. & THOMSON A.D. (1968) The diagnosis and treatment of pigmented villonodular synovitis. *Journal of Bone and Joint Surgery* **50B**, 290–305.

CHUINARD E.G. & BASKIN M. (1973) Claw foot deformity. *Journal of Bone and Joint Surgery* **55A**, 351–62.

COLWILL M. (1969) Osteomyelitis of the metatarsal sesamoids. *Journal of Bone and Joint Surgery* **51B**, 464–8.

DAVIS N.C. & LITTLE J.H. (1974) The role of frozen section in the diagnosis and management of malignant melanoma. *British Journal of Surgery* **61**, 505–8.

DWYER F.C. (1959) Osteotomy of the the calcaneum for pes cavus. *Journal of Bone and Joint Surgery* **41B**, 80–6.

FOWLER A.W. (1959) A method of forefoot reconstruction. *Journal of Bone and Joint Surgery* **41B**, 507–13.

FREIBERG J. (1957) The diagnosis and treatment of common painful conditions of the foot. *American Academy of Orthopaedic Surgeons* **14**, 238.

GAENSLEN F.J. (1931) Split-heel approach in osteomyelitis of os calcis. *Journal of Bone and Joint Surgery* **13**, 759–72.

HELAL B. (1975) Metatarsal osteotomy for metatarsalgia. *Journal of Bone and Joint Surgery* **57B**, 187–92.

HIGGS S.L. (1931) Hammer toe. *Postgraduate medical Journal* **6**, 131–3.

HOOKER C.H. (1963) Rupture of the tendo-calcaneus. *Journal of Bone and Joint Surgery* **45B**, 360–3.

INGE G.A. & FERGUSON, A.B. (1933) Surgery of the sesamoid bone of the great toe. *Archives of Surgery* **27**, 466–89.

JAFFE H.L. (1964) *Tumours and Tumorous Conditions of the Bones and Joints*, p. 254. Henry Kimpton, London.

KATES A., KESSEL L. & KAY A. (1967) Arthroplasty of the forefoot. *Journal of Bone and Joint Surgery* **49B**, 552–7.

KECK C. (1962) The tarsal tunnel syndrome. *Journal of Bone and Joint Surgery* **44A**, 180–2.

KECK S.W. & KELLY P.J. (1965) Bursitis of the posterior part of the heel: evaluation of surgical treatment of eighteen patients. *Journal of Bone and Joint Surgery* **47**, 267–73.

KVIST H. & KVIST M. (1980) The operative treatment of chronic calcaneal paratenonitis. *Journal of Bone and Joint Surgery* **62B**, 353–7.

LAM S.J.S. (1962) The tarsal tunnel syndrome. *Lancet* **2**, 1354–5.

LEA R.B. & SMITH L. (1972) Non-surgical treatment of tendo-Achilles rupture. *Journal of Bone and Joint Surgery* **54A**, 1398–1403.

LINDAHL O. & NILSSON H. (1974) Plantar protrusion of the metatarsal heads. Conservative treatment by a new principle. *Acta Orthopaedica Scandinavica* **45**, 473–80.

LJUNGQUIST R. (1968) Spontaneous partial rupture of tendo-Achilles. *Acta Orthopaedica Scandinavica* (suppl) **113**.

LOTKE P.A. (1970) Ossification of Achilles tendon. *Journal of Bone and Joint Surgery* **52A**, 157–60.

MACKENZIE D.H. (1970) *The Differential Diagnosis of Fibroblastic Disorders*, p. 82. Blackwell Scientific Publications, Oxford.

MARTELL B.S. (1978) Radiotherapy for painful heel syndrome. *British medical Journal* **11**, 90–1.

MELMED E.P. (1965) Spontaneous bilateral rupture of the calcaneal tendon during steroid therapy. *Journal of Bone and Joint Surgery* **47B**, 104–5.

MULDER J.D. (1951) The causative mechanism in Morton's metatarsalgia. *Journal of Bone and Joint Surgery* **33B**, 94–5.

MURRAY J.G. (1952) Tender heel due to Paget's disease. *Journal of Bone and Joint Surgery* **34B**, 440–1.

NISSEN K.I. (1948) Plantar digital neuritis: Morton's metatarsalgia. *Journal of Bone and Joint Surgery* **30B**, 84–94.

PICKREN J.W., SMITH A.G., STEVENSON T.W. JR & STOUT A.P. (1951) Fibromatosis of the plantar fascia. *Cancer* (New York) **4**, 846–56.

PYPER J.B. (1958) The flexor-extensor tendon transplant operation for claw toes. *Journal of Bone and Joint Surgery* **40B**, 528.

SANDEMAN J.C. (1967) The role of soft tissue correction of claw toes. *British Journal of Clinical Practice* **21**, 489–93.

SCRANTON P.E. & RUTKOWSKI R. (1980) Anatomic variations in the first ray: Part II. Disorders of the Sesamoids. *Clinical Orthopaedics and Related Research* **151**, 256–64.

THOMPSON T.C. & DOHERTY J.H. (1962) Spontaneous rupture of tendon Achilles: A new clinical diagnosis test. *Journal of Trauma* **2**, 126–9.

TAYLOR R.G. (1951) The treatment of claw toes by multiple transfers of flexor into extensor tendons. *Journal of Bone and Joint Surgery* **33B**, 539–42.

THOMAS F.B. (1974) Levelling the tread. *Journal of Bone and Joint Surgery* **56B**, 314–19.

TOWNSEND A.C. & SCOTT P.J. (1966) Ingrowing toenail and onychogryphosis. *Journal of Bone and Joint Surgery* **48B**, 354–8.

WILLIAMS R. (1963) Chronic non-specific tendovaginitis of tibialis posterior. *Journal of Bone and Joint Surgery* **45B**, 542–5.

ZADIK F.R. (1950) Obliteration of the nail bed of the great toe without shortening the terminal phalanx. *Journal of Bone and Joint Surgery* **32B**, 66–7.

Further reading

BAKER H. & WILKINSON D.S. (1979) Psoriasis. In Rook A., Wilkinson D.S. & Ebling F.J.G. (eds.), *Textbook of Dermatology*, 3rd edition, p. 1315. Blackwell Scientific Publications, Oxford.

COPEMAN P.W.M., LEWIS M.G. & BLE EHEN S.S. (1973) Malignant Melanoma. In Rook A. (ed.) *Recent Advances in Dermatology* Vol. 3 p. 245. Churchill Livingston, Edinburgh.

SAMITZ M.H. & DANA A.F. (1971) *Cutaneous Lesions of the Lower Extremities*. Lippincott, Philadelphia.

SAMMAN P.D. (1972) *The Nails in Disease*, 2nd edition. Heinemann, London.

8

The Painful Foot in Systemic Disorders

A. ST J. DIXON

All systemic diseases may affect the feet and the feet may provide the first diagnostic clues.

Effects of age

Age can reasonably be accounted as the commonest systemic disorder causing abnormalities of the foot. It is rare indeed for an elderly person to have normal feet. Taking adults, Clark (1969) found that as many as 50% and possibly 80% had something wrong with their feet. Although many of these disorders are relatively trivial, the number who have some minor disorder, such as callosities, hallux valgus, ingrowing toe nails or falling arches increases with age.

History and examination

The history may give important clues. Pain due to arthritis is characteristically worst on first taking weight on the foot after resting—the equivalent of rest stiffness elsewhere. Pain due to arterial insufficiency or peripheral nerve disease is worse at night, troubling the patient when in bed. The patient with bizarre ulcerations and deformities of the feet due to a neuropathic arthropathy characteristically complains little of pain. The history should include the question, 'do you have a problem getting comfortable shoes?'. The answer may well reveal a condition which has led to changes in foot shape or skin sensitivity.

Examination of the foot must be preceded by a general physical examination with the patient stripped and weighed. The urine, haemoglobin and white count must be tested to avoid missing important clues. Foot pain may be a disorder of pain sensibility rather than a disorder of the foot. The foot may be swollen because of heart or kidney disease or because of cancerous blockage of regional lymph nodes. The longitudinal arch of the foot may have collapsed because the patient has gained weight rapidly from some other disorder. The attitude and posture of the rest of the leg and body are also important. The patient with flexed hips or knees must dorsiflex her ankles to stand upright. If the ankles are stiff, very precise adjustment of the height of the heels of her shoes may determine whether or not she can walk without pain. Patients with valgus deformity of the knees also put special strains on their feet and then the valgus deformity of the subtalar joint is often exaggerated.

Arthritis group

Of the named systemic disorders arthritis and allied conditions affect about 2% of the adult population (Clark 1969). The most common of these is rheumatoid arthritis, but all forms of joint disease can involve the feet; this is not surprising since there are over twenty joints in each foot and many synovial bursae and tendon sheaths.

Rheumatoid arthritis

Involvement of the feet is a major cause of crippling in rheumatoid arthritis. In a recent survey two-thirds of the patients with rheumatoid arthritis admitted to hospitals in Bath and Bristol either had to wear, or would have benefited from, surgical shoes. There is no such thing as *the* rheumatoid foot. Many kinds of foot involvement are possible. It is a clinical observation that if the forefoot is severely involved then involvement of the hindfoot is usually absent or mild, and *vice versa*.

Early rheumatoid arthritis   In early rheumatoid arthritis the most indicative physical sign is the transverse tarsal pressure test. Application of gentle pressure across the metatarsophalangeal joints is painless in normal feet, but is painful in early rheumatoid arthritis. Palpation of the individual lateral metatarsophalangeal joints may confirm this, one or two being selectively tender. At this stage one can sometimes demonstrate the 'daylight sign', i.e. swelling around the metatarsophalangeal joints or of the intermetatarsal bursae (Bossley & Cairney 1980) which forces the metatarsal heads apart so that the foot becomes wider and it is possible to 'see daylight' between the individual toes, normally not possible in shoe-wearing peoples in affluent societies. At this stage the patient first finds that her shoes do not fit and that she requires shoes two sizes wider and one size longer than usual in order to obtain sufficient room.

There are few radiological signs at this stage. Osteoporosis of mild degree is not uncommon but erosions of juxta-articular bone are not slow to appear and may do so often before they are visible in the hand x-rays (Thould & Simon 1966). The mid- and hindfoot are not so often affected in early rheumatoid arthritis.

Later rheumatoid disease   In later rheumatoid disease no joint in the foot inevitably escapes but some patterns of joint involvement are more frequent than others. Hallux valgus is very common (Fig. 8.1) and with it subluxation of the lateral metatarsophalangeal joints and usually a bunionette deformity. The dorsal subluxation of the lateral toes implies that they can take no weight in standing and often none in walking (Fig. 8.2). The pressures of posture and gait are concentrated

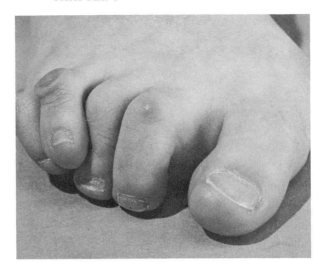

Fig. 8.1 Hallux valgus
and dorsal subluxation
of the lateral toes in
rheumatoid arthritis
with pressure lesions on
the bony prominences.

on the metatarsal heads; painfully, since the normal fibrofatty cushion which
protects these bones will have moved forward with the toes. Callosities form under
the metatarsal heads as a thickening of the cornified layer. The 'centre forward'
callosity is that which occurs under the second or third metatarsal head and is very
characteristic (Fig. 8.3). The patient has pain on walking barefoot and says she
feels as though she is walking on pebbles or marbles.

In favourable circumstances adventitious bursae develop as cushion-like
structures between the skin and the bone and relieve pain, but more often no such
bursa forms and there is nothing between skin and bone. Enormous pressures can
build up locally (see Fig. 8.2) and we have measured them. They may be twenty or
more times as high as in the equivalent place in a normal foot. Not only is the
metatarsal head near the surface, but rheumatoid erosions may leave a downward
pointing spike (Figs. 8.4, 8.5). The latter may generate a sinus (Fig. 8.6) (Bywaters
1953). Where a fluid-filled bursa is formed the pressures of weight-bearing may lead
to tracking widely within the foot. A sinogram or bursagram can be very revealing.

The midtarsal joints are not so frequently affected unless the rheumatoid
arthritis is late and severe. Pain in this area in early disease is usually related to
the insertions of two tendons which together help preserve the longitudinal arch of
the foot—peroneous longus and tibialis posterior—and the associated bursae.
Knowledge of this will lead to more accurate localization of local steroid injections
for midtarsal pain.

The second commonest site of foot crippling due to rheumatoid is at the
subtalar joint. When this is involved the foot has a tendency to twist into valgus—a
self-perpetuating deformity since the weight of the body increases it. The
longitudinal arch flattens and in the worst example of this deformity the head of
the talus may actually bear weight with the formation of a totally abnormal

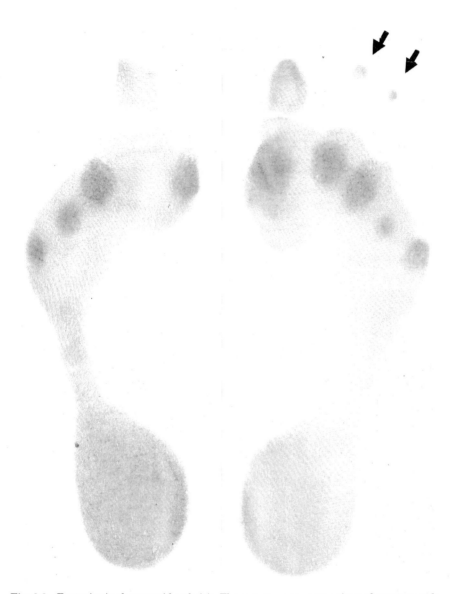

Fig. 8.2 Footprint in rheumatoid arthritis. The enormous concentrations of pressure under the metatarsal heads are well shown. The arrows indicate the only two lateral toes (on the right foot) which take any weight during walking. (Female aged 57 with rheumatoid arthritis of 7 years' duration.)

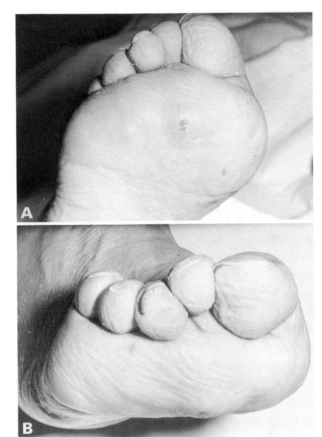

Fig. 8.3 The 'centre-forward' callosity. This is usually due to plantar subluxation of the second metatarsal head and reversal of the anterior arch.

pressure pattern under the sole; the 'rocker-bottom foot' (Fig. 8.7). Much can be done to prevent permanent valgus deformity by giving antivalgus exercises for subtalar joints in early disease. These are of equal importance to the more commonly prescribed quadriceps exercises which are taught to prevent flexion deformities of the knees.

Of the larger foot joints the ankle itself is the least often affected radiologically and clinically. Yet Kirkup and his colleagues (1974) at Bath have been able to recognize characteristic damage. Thinning of joint space and juxta-articular erosions just inside the maleoli are changes similar to those seen in other rheumatoid joints. In patients with severe valgus deformity of the subtalar joint, mechanical strains on the ankle mortice may lead to splaying of the mortice, stretching of the inferior tibio-fibular synostosis or even to stress fractures of the fibula or tibia with remodelling and healing in the new stressed position.

When rheumatoid nodules occur in the foot they are commonest under the

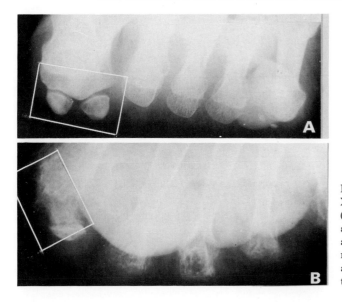

Fig. 8.4 Tangential X-ray of the forefoot; (A) normal, (B) advanced rheumatoid arthritis. *Note* the reversal of the anterior arch and dislocation of the sesamoids.

heel, although it takes a special examination technique to palpate them because of the density of the fibrofatty tissue in which they grow. But they are not rare if sought. Other nodules occur as enlargements of the Achilles tendon, especially where the counter of the shoe provides intermittent pressures. The skin of the foot, like the skin elsewhere, may show thinning, bruising and transparency after prolonged corticosteroid therapy.

Advanced rheumatoid arthritis In advanced, so-called malignant, rheumatoid arthritis there is both arteritis and neuropathy and changes occur which are important to recognize if surgery is being considered. The neuropathy reveals itself to the patient as a nocturnal burning accompanied by a disorder of touch sensation which contributes to the difficulty of finding the patient comfortable shoes. A patient with rheumatoid neuropathy may reject any shoe, however good, because the disorder of sensation interferes with the feeling of a good shoe fit. Local ischaemic changes may manifest themselves as 'geographic' pallor or blueness affecting certain toes only. When arteritis is severe one or both of the major foot pulses may be difficult to palpate, but caution is needed in that persistence of these main pulses, even when strongly pulsating, is no guarantee that the digital circulation is intact. In contrast to atheroma, rheumatoid arteritis tends to affect the small vessels most and may block them without disorder of the larger vessels. The peroneal pulse felt in front of the external malleolus, may be a major source of blood supply in patients with otherwise impalpable pulses. Severe rheumatoid neuropathy affecting the foot is hardly likely to be missed as it is accompanied by foot drop, muscle weakness, loss of ankle jerk and sensory changes.

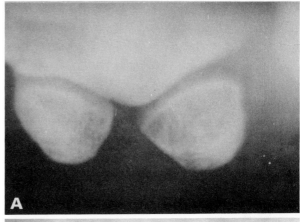

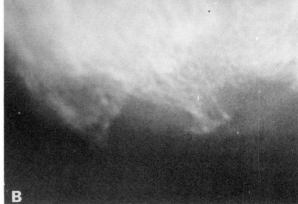

Fig. 8.5 Enlargements of the first metatarsal head from Fig. 8.4. *Note* the loss of the sesamoids and replacement by a sharp downward pointing spicule of bone.

Seronegative arthritis

The seronegative group of arthritides includes chronic Reiter's syndrome, ankylosing spondylitis, psoriatic arthropathy and some varieties of Still's disease. They may all affect the feet. Dorsal subluxation of the lateral toes may be severe. In the hindfoot there is a greater tendency than in seropositive rheumatoid arthritis for massive periosteal reactions to occur around the heel, related especially to the insertion of the long plantar ligament, with the formation of plantar spurs, and also to the sub-Achilles bursa at the back of the calcaneum. Tenosynovitis around the ankle may be associated with periostitis of the lower end of the tibia. Periosteal reactions may be so extreme around the metatarsal bones near affected metatarsophalangeal joints that in the past they have been mistaken for osteosarcomatous changes.

Of interest, but still unexplained, are the curious absorptive changes which are seen in the metatarsophalangeal and interphalangeal joints in the seronega-

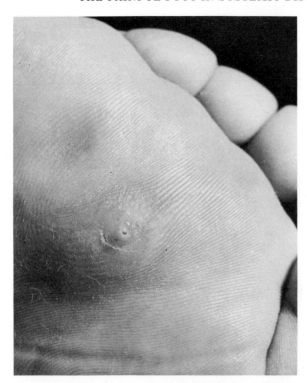

Fig. 8.6 Sinus under the second metatarsophalangeal joint.

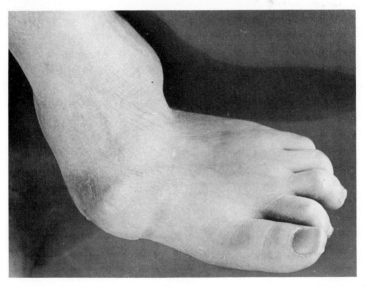

Fig. 8.7 Involvement of the midtarsal and subtalar joints with reversal of the longitudinal arch.

tive arthropathies. They resemble the changes seen in neuropathic joints and may come on quite early in the disease. The toe becomes 'filleted' by a mutilans change, often painless. Sometimes, even more bizarre, they are accompanied by ankylosis in the interphalangeal joints of other toes, again very rare in seropositive rheumatoid arthritis. Clinical involvement of an interphalangeal joint, with swelling and warmth, is not uncommon in the seronegative arthropathies. In *Reiter's syndrome* there is often characteristic coppery discolouration of the skin of the affected toe.

Other systemic disorders of connective tissue

Systemic sclerosis and the rare *Werner's syndrome* are the only ones which commonly give rise to serious foot problems. The hard, rigid feet and poor blood supply need particular care in shoe fitting and are unsuitable for any form of surgery. Plastazote-lined bootees give a combination of moulded internal cushioning and insulation which protects the rigid foot and may lead to healing of previously intractable ulcers.

The relatively good long-term prognosis of Still's disease (juvenile rheumatoid arthritis), combined with considerable protection afforded to the joints by the much greater thickness of articular cartilage in the child's joint, usually means that Still's disease is not a serious foot problem in younger children. Nevertheless, it may be accompanied by a diagnostic deformity when premature closure of a metatarsal epiphysis gives rise to a characteristic shortening of the fourth metatarsal bone.

Gout and pseudo gout

75% of gout sufferers are first attacked in one of the big toes, many of them being initially diagnosed as having cellulitis and treated with an antibiotic. The disease once diagnosed correctly is easily treated with allopurinol by the family doctor. In hospital nowadays acute gout is more often seen in general medical and general surgical wards, particularly where loop diuretics or thiazide diuretics are being given to the elderly for heart conditions, or after prostatectomy where a combination of the metabolic response stress of the operation combined with mild renal disease may lead to urate crystal deposition.

Pseudo gout

This may exactly resemble podagra but is due to the deposition of hydroxyapatite crystals in the capsule or tendons around the big toe. The deposits are opaque to x-rays but rapidly disappear after the acute crystal arthropathy has become established. Pseudo gout of this kind is sometimes a systemic disorder, the patient suffering similar attacks in other periarticular structures, particularly around the knees and shoulders. The serum uric acid level is not raised in pseudo gout.

Osteoarthrosis (osteoarthritis)

Primary osteoarthrosis is not a problem in the feet. There is no foot equivalent, for example, of Heberden's nodes in the terminal interphalangeal joints of the toes, nor of the painful carpometacarpal osteoarthrosis of the thumb base joint. Secondary osteoarthrosis, such as hallux rigidus and valgus from shoe pressures, or at the ankle from previous Pott's fractures are not uncommon. Exuberant bone formation due to shoe pressures may exaggerate a natural bony prominence, particularly at the midtarsal region on the dorsum of the foot.

Haemophilia

Haemophilia and Christmas disease, when severe, cause foot problems, mainly because of haemorrhages in calf muscles with subsequent contracture, or by damage to nerves compressed by bleeding episodes in the knee, calf, thigh or buttock. The seamless shoe technique (see Chapter 14) is adaptable to the problem of the haemophiliac. Hessing braces can be fitted to these shoes. It is of considerable importance to fit the braces so that the centre of rotation of the hinge corresponds as exactly as possible (and this must be checked with x-rays) to the centre of rotation of the ankle. The ordinary below-knee iron with a pin in the heel of the shoe does not do this and may set up shearing stresses in the ankle which can produce further bleeding.

Hyperlaxity syndromes

A short experience in a foot clinic teaches that patients vary enormously in the natural stiffness or mobility of their feet. Often this reflects the degree of generalized hyperlaxity elsewhere.

Miss B, 62 years old, a teacher who retired early on account of precocious cataracts, was diagnosed as having Marfan's syndrome on the basis of loose redundant skin over joints, long patella tendons, generalized hyperlaxity of many joints, a series of fractures after minimal trauma and a metacarpal index (Sinclair 1958) of 9.5. Her feet showed extreme laxity of structure with total collapse of both arches and severe hallux valgus. The deformity superficially resembled that of rheumatoid arthritis.

In other patients the hyperlaxity is familial or racial, in yet others due to prolonged steroid treatment. Conversely, generalized stiffening of foot structure is more common in the elderly, with or without arthritis, and more common in the seronegative and psoriatic arthropathies. An assessment of foot laxity is of importance in shoe fitting. Two feet might have an identical shape if compared in the form of plaster models. Yet if one foot were stiff and the other were comformable they would require quite different shoes to give the same sensation of a comfortable fit. An illustrative experiment is to take the cuff from a packet of 20 cigarettes and open it out as a cylinder when it will be found to hold nearly 50 cigarettes. A conformable forefoot can be squeezed to a more cylindrical cross-section and therefore will fit into a smaller shoe. Indeed, most women's shoes, especially those worn by young women, are narrower than the foot which will go into them, as measured in the weight-bearing position.

Neuropathies and the feet

Central or upper motor neuron neuropathies can affect the feet and cause shoe problems. The commonest is hemiplegia leading to unilateral spastic drop foot, often with a tendency to varus deformity at the subtalar joint and requiring shoes to be fitted with a drop foot stop or a toe-raising spring. A below-knee iron and outside T-strap to counteract the varus tendency may also be needed. In multiple sclerosis weakness and foot drop may be bilateral. The further problem created by intention tremor in the limb may be ameliorated by lead inserts into the heel structure or more simply, by small bags of lead shot tied in under the lacing of the shoe. A simple adaptation such as this may enable an otherwise helpless patient to walk independently. Children with congenital spastic disease such as spina bifida or Little's disease may also present major problems in the feet. The functional and sensory loss may vary from minimal to total with, in the latter case, the legs acting as living prostheses, easily damaged. To the deformities due to growth defects and to the oedema from vascular disturbances are added the problems of dropped foot, loss of proprioception and pain appreciation, incontinence and very often obesity. Bootees made from expanded polyethylene (Plastazote), a mouldable and washable cushioning material, are helpful (Chapter 14).

It is in the lower motor and especially in the sensory neuropathies that some of the worst foot deformities occur. The commonest cause of neuropathic disease in affluent countries is diabetes (see Chapter 9). Tabes, leprosy and the various forms of peripheral familial sensory neuropathy have all been seen in our foot clinic. Since the neuropathies of the foot are seldom completely painless, a man with diabetic sensory neuropathy may walk in complaining of a *painful* foot and the x-ray may reveal a fracture or ischaemic necrosis of one of the tarsal bones. But for the sensory impairment he could not have walked at all!

Penetrating ulcers may lead to deep infections which can involve digital arteries. In turn, gangrene of the toe may threaten. All that is required is local excision of the ischaemic toe but the unwary surgeon may be tempted to a much more extensive amputation, suspecting major arterial involvement. An arteriogram will, of course, decide. In a patient with penetrating ulcers it is wise to feel inside the shoe. A nail or thorn may have pierced the sole unnoticed. In familial sensory neuropathy a very great amount of caution should be exercised before embarking on any surgery. An extensive ulcerated area may be better left to heal naturally. Attempts to debride an ulcer may cause it to enlarge.

Marked pes cavus should always alert the examiner to the possibility of a neurological disorder such as Friedreich's ataxia or old poliomyelitis.

Endocrine problems

Cushing's disease may present as a patient with painful swollen feet due to connective tissue atrophy and osteoporotic stress fractures of the metatarsals. Puffy, firm oedema of the feet, combined with very slow ankle tendon reflex recovery time has given the diagnosis of myxoedema in a patient with otherwise obscure myalgic symptoms. One of the classical presentations of acromegaly is in the shoe shop with the patient demanding an ever-increasing size of shoes.

Treatment

The treatment of pain in the foot which is part of a systemic disorder is only occasionally simple and dependable. In gout the acute stage can be suppressed by an anti-inflammatory drug such as indomethacin and the chronic stage prevented by long term treatment with allopurinol. But in the generalized causes of joint disease the treatment of the inflammatory element is only part of the problem, as there is inevitably some swelling or deformity which means that the patient's foot no longer fits a 'shop' shoe made to a standard commercial last.

Of the two possible solutions to this, that of operating on the foot to obtain a better shape (and hence make it possible for the patient to wear shop-shoes) is increasing in favour. In the common forefoot deformity of rheumatoid arthritis, individually painful callosities can be treated by balancing osteotomies of the metatarsals or, alternatively, operations of the Kates–Kessel type (Kates *et al* 1967) can be very beneficial. Operations may also be needed to amputate stiff, protruding toes which make shoe fitting impossible. In the hind foot operations may be needed to defeat subtalar deformity and pain, for example by the operation of triple fusion.

But for patients medically unsuitable for operation or unwilling to consider it, (and they are still the majority) some form of specially-made shoe or some kind of individualized padding of the foot is essential.

In rheumatoid arthritis and related disorders getting suitable shoes has to be considered as a problem of packaging in light-weight materials, for a delicate object of variable geometry. Shoes made to plaster casts, using modern expanded foams and microcellular rubbers, bonded rather than stitched, in the so-called seamless shoe technique, have provided an answer for many as they cost less than half as much as conventional stitched and welted handcrafted surgical shoes. They are also usually available from initial prescription to acceptable fit in a much shorter time. The last is stored so that repeat prescriptions are easy. They are often much lighter than conventional surgical shoes, a point of considerable importance in disorders such as rheumatoid arthritis where the other joints are damaged and limbs are weak. The technique can be adapted for attachment to leg braces and toe raising springs and to patients whose fingers are too crippled to manage laces. Accessory insocks and chiropody pads are unnecessary.

For other problems, the contribution of a chiropodist (Chapter 15) can be invaluable and there is a lot to be said for doing away with the professional demarcations between the work of the chiropodist and the shoe-fitter and so arrive at the best solution for each patient. Deep lasted shoes providing extra room for the chiropodist's pads and insocks are available commercially and through the Health Service, although not all contractors can provide them.

For the most severe deformities, particularly in diabetics who have required foot surgery, there is no substitute for the highly skilled individual shoemaker who does his own fitting and makes shoes in the traditional way. Once a comfortable pair of shoes has been fitted it is important to make the most of them. Those with outdoor occupations should be advised to buy zip-fronted rubber overshoes to put on top of their surgical shoes in situations such as farming, where they would normally wear rubber boots.

REFERENCES

BOSSLEY C.J. & CAIRNEY P.C. (1980) The intermetatarsophalangeal bursa—its significance in Morton's metatarsalgia. *Journal of Bone and Joint Surgery* **63B,** 184–7.

BYWATERS E.G.L. (1953) Fistulous rheumatism: a manifestation of rheumatoid arthritis. *Annals of Rheumatic Disease* **12,** 114–21.

CLARK M. (1969) *Trouble with Feet.* Bell, London.

KATES A., KESSEL L. & KAY A. (1967) Arthroplasty of the forefoot. *Journal of Bone and Joint Surgery* **49B,** 552–7.

KIRKUP J.R. (1974) Ankle and tarsal joints in rheumatoid arthritis. *Scandinavian Journal of Rheumatology* **3,** 50–2.

SINCLAIR R.J.G. (1958) The Marfan Syndrome. *Bulletin of Rheumatic Diseases* **8,** 153–4.

THOULD A.K. & SIMON G. (1966) Assessment of radiological changes in the hands and feet. Their correlation with prognosis. *Annals of Rheumatic Diseases* **25,** 220–7.

9

The Foot in Diabetes

E.M. THOMAS

As the diagnosis and treatment of diabetes has improved it has become apparent that less than 30% of all diabetics require insulin to prevent the onset of diabetic ketosis. All patients, however, may suffer the long-term complications of the disease, namely retinopathy, nephropathy, neuropathy and vascular disease.

The expectation of life for a diabetic is now approximately 70% of that for non-diabetics. It has improved since the introduction of insulin but little change has occurred in the last 15 years.

Of the complications that can befall a diabetic, those which affect locomotion are amongst the most devastating.

The cause of neuropathy is as yet unknown and with present day therapy the vascular and neurological complications cannot be prevented. The prevalence of diabetes in Britain is of the order of thirteen per thousand and the present high incidence of diabetic foot problems is therefore likely to continue (College of General Practitioners Report 1962).

AETIOLOGY

Oakley (1954) has classified the lesions of diabetics; (a) septic; (b) neuropathic; (c) ischaemic and (d) due to a combination of these causes.

Sepsis

Purely septic lesions are no more common in diabetics than in non-diabetics. Before commencing treatment it is important to exclude the coexistence of neuropathic or ischaemic changes. In the absence of complications the standard surgical principles obtain. Casual treatment, for example by inadequate drainage or the incorrect doses of antibiotic, may lead to the unnecessary loss of a limb. Infection alone does not lead to ketosis unless accompanied by vomiting. It is important to keep strict diabetic control, especially during episodes of infection.

Neuropathy

A number of neurological complications occur in diabetes. The literature is reviewed by Colby (1965). Neuropathy is generally chronic in character and gradual in onset. Acute neuropathy usually follows a period of poor control, due to the patient's lack of care or to generalized infection.

Recent studies (Thomas & Lascelles 1966) suggest that the lesion in most types of neuropathy is in the peripheral nerve. There is an abnormality of Schwann cells, the number of axon cylinders is reduced and there is a loss of anterior horn cells. Nerve conduction abnormalities, with or without clinically apparent neuropathy, exist in nearly all diabetics. A study by Chopra and Hurwitz (1969) has shown that the average amplitude of sensory, mixed sensory and antidromic mixed action potentials in diabetics, both with and without neuropathy, is lower than in controls. It further indicates that the lower amplitudes are more evident in diabetics with neuropathy. Reduction in nerve conduction velocity, however, is a later sign of diabetic neuropathy.

It would appear that neuropathy is due to a metabolic disorder which is part of the diabetic diathesis.

Neuropathy may be conveniently classified (Rackow 1968);

1 Chronic (sensory) neuropathy
2 Subacute neuropathy;
    (a) predominantly sensory,
    (b) predominantly motor.
3 Autonomic neuropathy.
4 Single nerve lesions.

Chronic (sensory) neuropathy

This is the most common form and may be the presenting symptom. Initially the only clinical manifestation is the absence of ankle reflexes. The findings are generally confined to the distal part of the lower limb and are usually symmetrical. Diminution or loss of vibration sense occurs frequently. This should be tested at the toes or foot rather than at the ankle, since the abnormality is essentially distal. Loss of vibration sense at the knee is rare except in advanced cases.

Muscle joint sense, appreciation of pain, heat, cold and light touch are later affected. The pain sense is usually diminished before touch is affected. Hyperaesthesiae, muscle pains and general limb pain described as 'burning', 'aching' or 'gnawing' may occur before the loss of deep pain sensation.

In long-standing cases trophic changes develop which are confined to the feet. The lack of sweating, which occurs in the lower part of the body in diabetics, has been held to be due to changes in the autonomic system. The hyperkeratotic and brittle skin becomes difficult to keep clean. Fissures occur on minor injury in which infection can develop. The toe nails become thickened and deformed (Fig. 9.1).

Clawed toes are no more common in the diabetic than in the non-diabetic, although diabetes is more common in older people, as are claw toes (Fig. 9.2). It was thought that toe clawing followed intrinsic muscle palsy as a part of a peripheral motor neuropathy, however there is no evidence to support this hypothesis. Claw

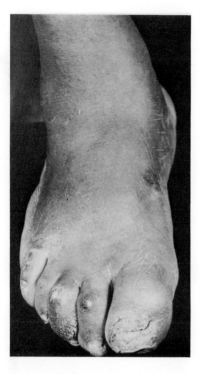

Fig. 9.1 Hyperkeratotic brittle skin.

toes are more easily damaged than normal toes; pressure sores develop on the tips and over the dorsum of the proximal interphalangeal joint and they may also develop over the metatarsal heads. Without care, sores become ulcers. Initially painless, they can rapidly deepen to involve bone or joint with the development of a perforating ulcer or osteomyelitis (Fig. 9.3).

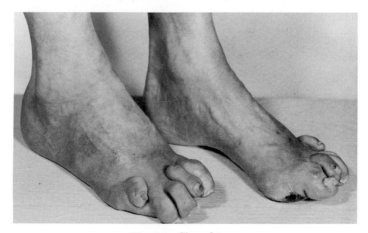

Fig. 9.2 Clawed toes.

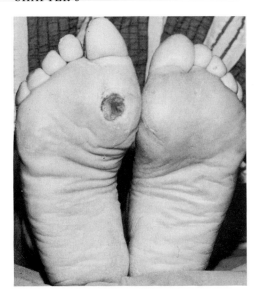

Fig. 9.3 Ulcer under head of
metatarsal.

Neuropathy of long duration results in the development of Charcot joints. The
foot is commonly involved, the ankle seldom but the knee never (Fig. 9.4). Charcot
changes occur only in limbs with sensory and autonomic neuropathy.

Subacute neuropathy

Sensory   Pain and paraesthesiae are prominent symptoms. Lightening pains and
muscle tenderness are common. The signs and symptoms frequently appear in one
limb before the other. The later changes, e.g. trophic skin changes, and Charcot
joints are absent. Peripheral reflexes are frequently lost. Careful examination

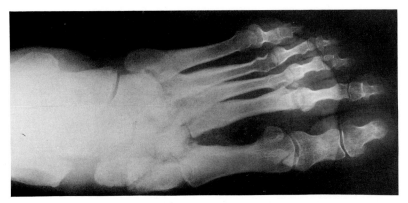

Fig. 9.4   Neuropathic changes in the mid-foot region.

reveals that all forms of sensation are impaired. Curiously, muscle tenderness is often marked, though deep pain may be absent.

Motor (often called diabetic amytrophy)   The characteristic sign is weakness of one muscle group, preceded by pain. The quadriceps group is often affected. Recovery in one site is followed by signs and symptoms in another. The pain may resemble that of a nerve root lesion. The upper limb is occasionally affected. Detailed neurological examination may reveal some sensory changes.

Patients in the predominantly sensory group develop symptoms after a period of poor diabetic control or in association with diabetes of sudden and severe onset. They tend to be younger than those in the predominantly motor group, who are usually 50 years of age or more.

Autonomic neuropathy

This type affects the trunk and lower limbs. Its manifestations include oedema and disturbance of sweating associated with changes in skin texture. Impotence is a common complaint. Diarrhoea, usually worse at night, is sometimes a distressing problem. Postural hypotension may be so incapacitating as to require the administration of mineralocorticoids.

The chronic oedema of the distal part of the lower limbs in many diabetics is due to loss of sympathetic control of arteries and arterioles. Dorsalis pedis arterial pressure can be as high as that in the brachial artery. This has the effect of increasing the amount of tissue fluid present in the foot, and helps to explain why wounds of the feet do not heal unless elevated. The oedema can be reduced by the exhibition of sympathomimetic drugs such as ephidrine, but it is not yet known whether this will be of therapeutic value.

Bladder atony and paralysis can add to the difficulties of nursing, particularly after a major amputation, and should not be misdiagnosed as prostatic obstruction (Ellenberg 1966).

Single nerve lesions

These resemble single nerve lesions in non-diabetics. In the lower limbs the peroneal and posterior tibial nerves are affected. The motor and sensory changes follow the distribution of the nerve. Pain usually precedes paraesthesiae and wasting. Single nerve lesions are considered to be due to local injury of a nerve in which conduction is already impaired (Mulder *et al* 1961).

Arterial disease

It seems to be common knowledge that diabetics are more prone to develop generalized atherosclerosis than the general population. However, the true incidence is difficult to establish since clinical manifestations may depend on the coexistence of neuropathy and sepsis. The matter is further complicated by the facts that diabetes and arterial disease are both more often seen in the elderly.

The incidence of intermittent claudication among men in the fifth decade is similar for diabetic and non-diabetic patients. However, in the sixth decade it is slightly higher in diabetics.

Further, the age at which amputation of the leg for ischaemia was undertaken was found, in a large clinical series to be 71 for diabetics and 73 for non-diabetics (Martin *et al* 1956). The pathological changes are qualitatively the same in the diabetic as in the non-diabetic, though it has been shown that arterial occlusion below the knee is more common in the diabetic (Strandness *et al* 1964). It seems from this study that there is no specific diabetic arterial disease but that atherosclerosis in diabetics is frequently combined with neuropathy. The result is a greater frequency of complications which demand amputation.

Many investigations have suggested that the thickening of the capillary basement membrane may contribute to the skin changes. In a study of the small vessels of the great toe the average thickness of the basement membrane in diabetics was 1330 nm and in the non-diabetics 590 nm (Banson & Lacy 1964). In spite of this change in the basement membrane, there is no evidence that microangiopathy in vessels other than those of the glomerulus and retina, play a part in the production of the late complications of diabetes.

Combined lesions

Neuropathic skin changes may be complicated by sepsis and ischaemia. A proper appreciation of the relative role played by each complication in the production of the lesion influences the treatment and affects the prognosis. In a typical case the patient is elderly, presenting with an obviously inflamed but painless lesion. The area of destruction may be large, hidden in that part of the foot least easily seen. The single symptom leading to consultation may have been the discharge of offensive pus or gangrene appearing in one of five equally clawed toes. The diagnosis is made on clinical observations.

The history may reveal the painlessness or relative painlessness of the lesion. It may record previous sensory symptoms such as 'burning' pain or 'walking on cotton wool'.

Inspection reveals the shape of the foot, the skin texture and the position of the toes. The skin colour is noted, together with the presence or absence of hairs. The latter are a reliable index of an adequate blood supply.

Examination records the range of movement suggestive of Charcot-like changes. The nature and site of any localized swelling or obvious abscess is noted. A neurological survey completes the clinical examination, both motor and sensory changes being carefully observed (Fig. 9.5).

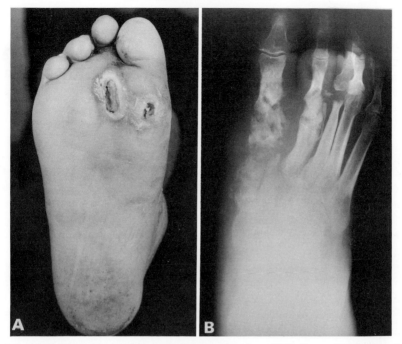

Fig. 9.5   (a) Hidden lesion in the foot of a 60 year-old patient. (b) Radiograph of the same foot.

SPECIAL INVESTIGATIONS

Radiography

Attention should be directed to the following aspects.

Skeletal changes

Neuropathic   In the absence of sepsis there is often an attenuated appearance of the metatarsal shafts with a tendency to lack of differentiation between cortex and medulla. Hypertrophic and atrophic joint destruction may be apparent. Neuropathic changes are most frequently seen in the talonavicular portion of the midtarsal joint, though any joint of the foot may be affected.

Septic   Sepsis is usually exogenous, entering through the base of an ulcer. Involucrum formation does not occur. Rarefaction of the affected area, usually near a joint, rapidly proceeds to disorganization and the formation of sequestra.

Other changes   Degenerative changes due to long-standing congenital deformity or osteoarthritis may complicate the radiographic appearance.

Soft tissue changes   Infection can be seen as soft tissue swelling, a break in the outline or subcutaneous air suggesting ulceration. Oedema is shown as patchy areas of different density due to separation of fat by oedema fluid (Fig. 9.6).

Vascular changes   Calcification of major vessels is not an uncommon finding in the elderly. It is of little value in prognosis in the individual case, but is to be noted as an unfavourable sign.

Doppler scanning

The Doppler ultrasound flowmeter is an invaluable tool. In a busy clinic a small portable machine will readily demonstrate those with increased, normal or reduced arterial flow. A valuable measurement is the ratio of the systolic blood pressure at the ankle to that recorded in the antecubital fossa. In the normal subject it is approximately one, but it may fall considerably where there is peripheral vascular disease. Wagner and Buggs (1978) have called it the ischaemic index. They have used it to predict healing of surgical procedures and in selection of amputation levels in ischaemic limbs. Elective surgery and amputations, including Syme's procedure, healed in 93.3% when the ischaemic index was above 0.45 in the diabetic patient. In the non-diabetic patient healing will occur at an index 0.35.

Arteriography

This is of limited value and should be reserved for cases with clinical evidence of major vessel disease. It should not be undertaken unless surgery is seriously contemplated. The investigation itself is not without major complications.

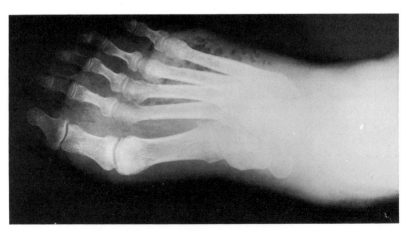

Fig. 9.6   Air in the soft tissues associated with infection of the head of the second metatarsal and a perforating ulcer of the sole.

The diagnosis can usually be made on clinical grounds. With experience and regular examination it is possible to differentiate between the predominantly neuropathic infected lesion and the predominantly ischaemic infected lesion. To offer repeated limited amputation in the latter case can result in the early and unnecessary loss of a limb.

TREATMENT

The orthopaedic surgeon with his experience in joint deformities, degenerative disease and bone sepsis, and trained to pay more attention to function than structure, is ideally suited to take part in the management of the 'diabetic foot'.

The nature of the diabetic condition and its wide range of complications render total care by a specialist of one discipline impossible. The diabetic needs care throughout his lifetime. With combined care many of the complications can be diminished and surgery can be carried out safely with every confidence of a successful outcome.

Joint consultation in relation to foot problems is essential in any diabetic clinic. The attendance of a chiropodist, interested and experienced in the problems, greatly reduces the incidence of gross pathological states.

Treatment may be divided into prophylactic, conservative and operative measures.

Prophylactic

The effects of neuropathy can be delayed for many years by a simple regime of foot care. The patient must be made aware of the risks involved and informed of the principles of prophylaxis. These may be summarized:

1   The feet should be inspected daily for accidental damage, using a suitably placed mirror if necessary. The inspection can be combined with a simple regime of cleanliness of the feet, socks and stockings and footwear. Damaged areas should be cleansed with a mild antiseptic and lightly dressed. Inflammation should be reported to a doctor immediately.

2   Socks should be well fitting and made of wool for softness, and regularly washed. Shoes should be of the correct size and shape with soft and pliable uppers. Great care should be taken when buying new shoes. All shoes should be inspected regularly for foreign objects, nail points, etc.

3   Extremes of temperature should be avoided. The feet should not be allowed to remain wet, especially in winter months. Proximity to fires, radiators and hot water bottles is dangerous.

4   Walking barefoot can result in accidental damage, particularly outside the home.

5   The nails should be cut transversely at the centre. Corns and calluses should not be treated except by a chiropodist. This advice should be emphasized to those patients who have failing vision.

6   Smoking causes vasoconstriction. Alcohol may aggravate neuropathy.

7   A patient who cannot care for his feet should seek the regular aid of a chiropodist.

Subacute neuropathy, particularly of the sensory type, improves with good diabetic control, though there is no evidence that insulin is of exceptional value in this regard. A period of rest in hospital with controlled nutrition and analgesia is sometimes necessary. There is no objective evidence to support the use of vitamin B therapy (Collens *et al* 1950) but subjectively many patients are improved with a course of intravenous Parenterovite (10 injections of 10 ml at twice weekly intervals).

The prophylaxis of ischaemia is unrewarding. The patient with intermittent claudication can be taught to anticipate the onset of symptoms and advised to walk more slowly. A change to more sedentary employment may be necessary. It must be remembered that claudication of sudden onset may improve with time as a collateral circulation develops. Chemical and physical methods of vasodilatation are disappointing. Sympathectomy is of no value.

Conservative

Mobile claw toes may be corrected by the application of a metatarsal pad, preferably on an insole. The correction makes the foot longer and shoe length must therefore be carefully checked (Fig. 9.7).

The deformity eventually becomes fixed as the neuropathy progresses, the metatarsal pad then becomes no more than a space-occupying lesion. Any such appliance should be presented to the patient with an explanation of its purpose and its potential dangers.

Proper fitting footwear is necessary for any diabetic with neuropathic changes. This is best supplied by a surgical fitter. Moulded cork insoles are preferred. For the patient with neuropathic ulceration, thought must be given to the accommodation of dressings and in such cases Plastazote insoles are better than cork. In acute phases of infection, with associated inflammation and oedema, cheaper forms of ready made footwear into which a moulded Plastazote insole can be placed are available (see Chapter 14).

Pressure sores can easily develop when the patient is put to bed. Pressure on the heels must be avoided. Extensive neuropathic sores can be healed by elevation in well-padded slings and springs suspended from a beam, with a toe strap to prevent equinus deformity. The spring tension should be such that the heels are just off the mattress so that the patient can sit up and move comfortably in bed.

The small, solitary purely neuropathic sore will usually heal without operation. The patient need not lose time from work, though treatment may continue for many months. Any purulent discharge is examined bacteriologically and the appropriate antibiotic prescribed. Radiographs are taken to exclude any underlying bone sepsis, which carries a poor prognosis. Correct attention is paid to the footwear. Those who cannot be fitted with commercial shoes require purpose-

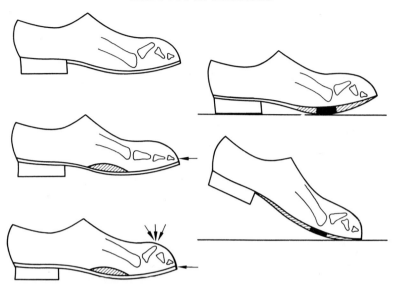

Fig. 9.7 The effect of a metatarsal insole contrasted with that of a rocker bar on the sole. (From Oakley *et al.* 1968.)

built moulded shoes, if only for the period of treatment. The moulding should be taken in the presence of such padding as is needed to relieve pressure on the affected area and of any dressings. A regime of regular cleansing with gentle removal of necrotic material from the ulcer edges is instituted. Non-adherent dressings should be used. The value of local antibiotic sprays and powders (e.g. Cicatrin) to hasten ulcer closure is disputed. Healing is inevitably slow, which renders the assessment of such application difficult.

In the ischaemic foot, rest pain is a common problem. In patients unsuitable for arterial surgery it can be controlled for a time with analgesics and sedatives. The pain is generally worse at night when the limb is at rest, warm and subject to passive vasodilatation. A bed cradle with the coverings adjusted to enable cool air to circulate, so that the limb is effectively 'out of bed' will bring some relief. It is unwise to persist with conservative measures once the pain is no longer controlled by simple analgesics. Amputation should then be advised. Long standing preoperative pain may result in addiction to narcotic agents and is a common cause of 'phantom limb'.

The conservative management of cases of infection in the presence of ischaemia may lead to disaster. Carefully repeated examination can avoid the tragedy of a high amputation which carries a high mortality if it is carried out as an emergency.

Operative treatment

General principles

1   Urgent surgery is seldom indicated. Adequate control of the diabetes, improvement in the general condition of the patient and the administration of the
appropriate antibiotic improves the chance of a successful outcome. A few days
preparation may lead to a planned procedure more limited than originally
contemplated.

2   Pressure sores on unaffected areas must be avoided by appropriate nursing
measures in the wards and in the operating theatre.

3   A tourniquet is to be avoided because of the frequent association with some
degree of ischaemia. The damage caused by a tourniquet can lead to the failure of a
planned procedure even in the apparently neuropathic limb.

4   Sutures should not be used as a routine. The incision should be designed to
allow the skin edges to fall together without tension. They may be gently apposed
by sterile adhesive paper strips and the occasional stitch or by the application of a
petroleum jelly gauze dressing. Suture can result in infection being retained
beneath the flaps, or gangrene due to tissue tension with resulting delay or failure
in healing.

   All amputations in diabetic patients should be treated as if they were old
wounds with the risk of infection ever present.

   The problems of operative surgery in diabetic patients fall broadly into four
groups:

Young deformed foot

If possible deformity should be corrected before neuropathy or ischaemia develop.
Sadly it is still the deformed foot in the diabetic that leads to early major
amputation. The patient is often not referred until serious sepsis has occurred,
when corrective surgery is no longer possible because of bone or joint damage.

Ischaemic foot

The purely ischaemic foot is rare in the diabetic. The indications for major arterial
surgery are the same as in the non-diabetic. In this group of patients major
reconstructive surgery is thought to be less successful since obliterative disease
may be more common below the knee. Many failures are due to poor selection and
the lack of recognition of severe coexistent neuropathy, which is associated with a
grave risk of infection.

   Once rest pain persistently prevents sleep, amputation becomes inevitable.
Mid-thigh amputations carry a higher mortality than through-knee or below-knee
procedures (Martin *et al* 1967). The level selected must depend on the degree of
ischaemia. A long stump is obviously better for the bilateral amputee.

Predominantly ischaemic infected foot

If the lesion is confined to one toe, local amputation offers a one in three chance of saving the foot. However, 90% will come to major amputation within a year. The remainder may have a useful limb for up to five years. There is no question of limited amputation in patients with more than one toe involved.

Predominantly neuropathic infected foot

It is here that limited amputation has a major part to play in the management of the diabetic foot.

A common presentation is a perforating ulcer on the metatarsal head, with x-ray changes of joint destruction and sequestrum formation. The foot is generally swollen with widespread cellulitis, though the circulation is often intact.

If a lesion is confined to a single toe then it can be removed through a dorsal racquet incision (Fig. 9.8). The involvement of several toes is best treated by several incisions avoiding the need for suture of a large plantar flap. All toes may be removed in this fashion if necessary. In the latter case a prosthesis is required, either worn next to the skin or built into the shoe. Any sock must fit the stump exactly.

If infection has spread to a metatarsal bone, then the whole 'ray' must be removed in such a way as to allow the skin edges to fall together. The removal of one or two rays is compatible with function. In the case of the great toe the Faraboeuf operation has been found satisfactory (Fig. 9.9).

The midtarsal and Syme operations have little to offer in the diabetic foot. The

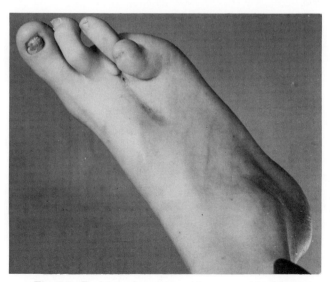

Fig. 9.8   Excision of a ray through a racquet incision.

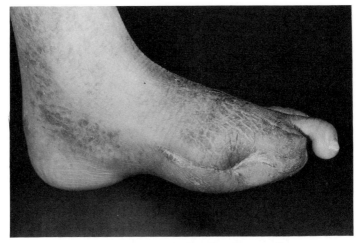

Fig. 9.9   End result of a Faraboeuf amputation.

former requires a large posterior flap with sutures, and drifts inevitably into equinus. The latter reduces the weight-bearing area and further neuropathic sores with loss of the heel pad soon occur.

In the neuropathic foot with multiple bone involvement, local drainage procedures and limited amputation procedures can still be considered. With appropriate footwear and regular dressings, an unhealed neuropathic sore does not prevent a reasonably active life. The most surprising results can be achieved by thorough surgical toilet.

Should such limited procedures fail and infection persist, below-knee amputation will result in a sound, useful limb. Many techniques are available, all of which have their firm supporters. The essence of success lies in careful preparation of the patient and selection of the technique with which the surgeon is familiar. The limb fitter naturally prefers a scar away from the end of the stump. The surgeon must balance the risk of obtaining an ideal scar against the risk to the patient. Planned surgery will result in the lowest amputation possible and avoid the risk to life inherent in mid-thigh procedures.

The most successful technique is that of Burgess (Burgess & Zettl 1969). This procedure will produce a sound stump suitable for early fitting. Flaps must be handled with great care and the use of crushing instruments (even toothed forceps on skin edges) should be minimal. However, if skin sensation is reduced in the field of the long posterior flap, then equal flaps may have to be used. (Fig. 9.10).

There is no point in removing an infected foot if neuropathic skin from the back of the calf is placed on the end of the stump! In diabetes, because of the varying oedema of the limb, stumps are often a different size at different times of the day.

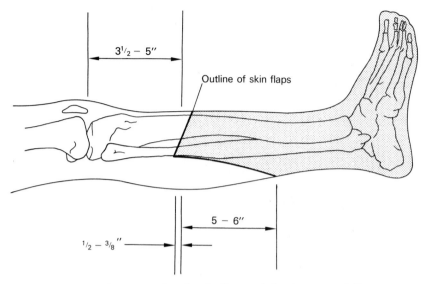

Fig. 9.10   The correct flaps for the Burgess below-knee amputation.

However expertly the patella-bearing socket is made, the stump may well be end-bearing from time to time. A neuropathic stump is almost as dangerous as a neuropathic foot.

SUMMARY

In the management of the complications of diabetes as they affect the foot, a combination of disciplines will provide the best care for the patient. Regular combined clinics with the diabetic physician will detect the development of complications. Prompt advice and skilled chiropody will maintain mobility and identify the patients at risk.

Once ulceration or gangrene has developed the success of treatment depends on the efficiency of the local blood supply. Local amputation is often successful, but if it fails, below-knee amputation, where conditions allow, has been shown to be a safe and reliable procedure.

Surgery should be delayed until the patient has been brought to his maximum state of fitness. Surgery is then safe and the incidence of postoperative complications reduced. In nearly all cases the changes are bilateral and the sound limb must be carefully protected. With treatment based on these principles the quality of life for the diabetic with lesions of the feet, though never enviable, need seldom be considered desperate.

REFERENCES

BANSON B.B. & LACEY P.E. (1964) Diabetic microangiopathy in human toes; with emphasis on the ultrastructural change in dermal capillaries. *American Journal of Pathology* **45**, 41.

BURGESS E.M. & ZETTL J. (1969) Amputation below the knee. *Artificial Limbs* **13**, 1–12.

CHOPRA J.S. & HURWITZ L.J. (1969) A comparative study of peripheral nerve conduction in diabetes and non-diabetic chronic occlusive peripheral vascular disease. *Brain* **92**, 83–96.

COLBY A.O. (1965) Neurologic disorders of diabetes mellitus. *Diabetes* **14**, 424–9.

COLLEGE OF GENERAL PRACTITIONERS (1962) A diabetes survey: Report of a Working Party. *British medical Journal* **1**, 1497–1503.

COLLENS W.S., RABINER A.M., ZILINSKY J.D., BOAS L.C. & GREENWALD J.J. (1950) The treatment of peripheral neuropathy in diabetes mellitus. *American Journal of the Medical Sciences* **219**, 482–7.

ELLENBERG M. (1966) Diabetic neurogenic vesical dysfunction. *Archives of Internal Medicine* **117**, 348–54.

MARTIN P., RENWICK S. & THOMAS E.M. (1967) Gritti-Stokes amputation in atherosclerosis: A review of 237 cases. *British medical Journal* **3**, 837–8.

MULDER D.W., LAMBERT E.H., BASTRON J.A. & SPRAGUE R.G. (1961) The neuropathies associated with diabetes mellitus. A clinical and electromyographic study of 103 unselected diabetic patients. *Neurology* **11**, 275–84.

OAKLEY W. (1954) Diabetes in surgery. *Annals of the Royal College of Surgeons* **15**, 108–19.

OAKLEY W.G., PYKE D.A. & TAYLOR K.W. (1968) *Clinical Diabetes and its Biochemical Basis*, p. 524. Blackwell Scientific Publications, Oxford.

RACKOW F. (1968) *Clinical Diabetes and its Biochemical Basis*, p. 542. Blackwell Scientific Publications, Oxford.

STRANDNESS D.E., PRIEST R.E. & GIBBONS G.E. (1964) Combined clinical and pathological study of diabetic and non-diabetic peripheral arterial disease. *Diabetes* **13**, 366–72.

THOMAS P.K. & LASCELLES R.G. (1966) The pathology of diabetic neuropathy. *Quarterly Journal of Medicine* **35**, 489–509.

WAGNER F.W. & BUGGS H. (1978) Use of Doppler ultrasound in determining healing levels in diabetic dysvascular lower extremity problems. In Bergan J.J. & Yao J.S.T. (eds.), *Gangrene and Severe Ischaemia of Lower Extremities*. Grune & Stratton, New York.

10

Common Neurological Disorders Affecting the Foot

L. KLENERMAN & J.A. FIXSEN

This chapter deals with problems affecting the feet as a result of a generalized neurological disorder. Mention has already been made of pes cavus (see Chapter 5) and the diabetic foot is mentioned in Chapter 9. Probably the commonest disease of this type is leprosy, which affects 12–15 million of the population of the world, although there are only about one thousand sufferers in Great Britain.

CEREBRAL PALSY

The majority of patients present to the paediatrician or the neurologist. The aim of surgical treatment is to improve function and prevent disability and deformity. The timing of an operation may be difficult. It is usually undertaken when a deformity remains or increases despite adequate conservative treatment. The neurological diagnosis should be established if possible before considering any surgery. Operative treatment for an undiagnosed progressive disorder may result in great disappointment for both patient and surgeon if the progressive nature of the condition is not fully understood at the time. Surgery is largely confined to the spastic type of cerebral palsy, and is rarely indicated in the athetoid and ataxic types.

In the hemiplegic, an equinus deformity that has persisted despite adequate physiotherapy should be corrected if it is causing a functional disability (Fig. 10.1). Serial plasters can be useful when the foot is still passively correctible, particularly in the younger patient. These plasters can be applied with or without anaesthetic. They need to be changed at 2–3 week intervals and should be retained for 6–8 weeks. Below-knee plasters are usually adequate unless the child develops significant knee flexion spasm, when an above-knee plaster may be necessary.

Elongation of the tendo-Achilles is required if conservative methods fail. As pointed out by Fixsen (1979), there are many papers extolling the virtues of elongating either the tendo-Achilles, the gastrocnemius or both. He recommends the slide elongation technique of White (1943) as the technique of choice. In this operation, the medial half of the tendon is divided proximally and the anterior half distally. The tendon can then be elongated by sliding the fibres apart. The tendon

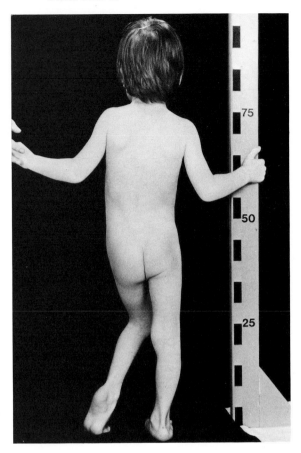

Fig. 10.1 Posterior
view of child with right
hemiplegia with severe
equinus foot.

does not have to be sutured and the patient can get up, walking within 48 hours in a
below-knee plaster. The plaster is usually retained for 4 weeks.

Varus and valgus deformities may also develop in the hemiplegic foot. It is
essential to correct the equinus deformity first before considering tendon transfer
or any other treatment for the varus deformity. An overactive or paralysed tibialis
posterior tendon is the chief reason for varus or valgus deformity (Bennet *et al*
1980). Elongation of the tendon at or above the ankle is a simple procedure which is
unlikely to cause overcorrection. Lateral transfer of the tibialis posterior tendon
should be used cautiously. Very careful pre-operative assessment is necessary to
avoid converting a varus deformity into a valgus one. It is important not to transfer
the tendon too far laterally. Valgus deformity of the foot is more common in
diplegia than in hemiplegia (Figs. 10.2 a & b). The classic operation of extra-articular subtalar fusion described by Grice (1952) remains a very satisfactory procedure
for controlling the deformity. It can be performed from the age of 4–6 years
upwards, once the bones of the hindfoot have reached a reasonable size. The

modified technique described by Dennyson and Fulford (1976), in which a screw is used to provide control of the subtalar joint while awaiting bony fusion from the iliac or tibial graft is very satisfactory. In the pronated and everted foot at or near maturity, triple arthrodesis may be used to provide a reasonably shaped foot which will accept normal footwear. Triple arthrodesis for a valgus foot is always a rather difficult operation. The technique of inlay-grafting described by Williams and Menelaus (1977) is very attractive, but is only suitable for valgus feet where the removal of bony wedges is unnecessary.

In spastic diplegia the tendo-Achilles may appear to be tight because the patient walks with his heels off the ground. However, this is often secondary to flexion at the hip and knee. If the tendon is lengthened, the patient sinks to the ground, adopting the so-called 'crouch' position. It is essential in this situation to deal with the proximal deformities at the hip and knee before considering tendo-Achilles lengthening. Similarly in the valgus foot the tendo-Achilles often appears tight. However, lengthening of the tendo-Achilles in these feet with so-called 'valgus ab-equino' is rarely successful, as the feet already have a hypermobile subtalar joint, and lengthening of the tendo-Achilles does not improve the valgus. In this situation it is better to stabilize the subtalar joint by Grice arthrodesis, and then consider lengthening the tendo-Achilles.

SPINAL DYSRAPHISM

As pointed out by James and Lassmann (1972), spinal dysraphism is a term revived by Lichenstein (1940), referring to all forms of developmental abnormality occurring in the midline of the back. It includes all forms of spina bifida occulta, aperta, anterior and posterior. Where there has been herniation of the meninges outside the vertebral canal, with or without neural content, the diagnosis is 'aperta'; where there is no such herniation, the case is classed as one of 'occulta'.

Myelomeningocele

In this lesion the neural tube is closed and covered by a membrane centrally and skin peripherally, but the spinal cord and/or the nerve roots are outside the vertebral canal. It occurs mainly in the thoracic and lumbar region.

The initial enthusiasm regarding the orthopaedic future of children with myelomeningocele has proved unfounded (Frank & Fixsen 1980). The concept that a myelomeningocele produced a lower motor neuron lesion to be treated like poliomyelitis was too simple. Stark and Baker (1967) showed that the majority of patients have complex neurological lesions and distal reflex movements. If this is not recognized and surgery is based simply on the presence or absence of muscle activity, it is likely to fail. Foot deformities have to be assessed in relation to the whole of the lower limbs. Conservative means of correction using strapping should be used, if possible, during the first year to eighteen months, until the general

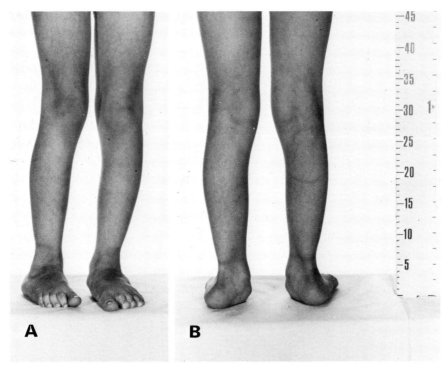

Fig. 10.2 Severe valgus feet in child with spastic diplegia (A) posterior view, (B) anterior view.

prognosis for the child is known. Care must be taken with the management of the skin when using these methods. The aim is to achieve a plantigrade foot in those children who are going to remain reasonable standers and walkers. Any excessive pressure that is not taken on the weight-bearing skin of the sole of the foot produces recurrent pressure sores. Often simple tenotomy of an overactive muscle is better than a complex tendon transfer, particularly in those cases with reflex muscle action. Again, great care must be taken with plaster application to prevent skin problems which can ruin an otherwise successful procedure.

Spina bifida occulta

The clinical importance of spina bifida occulta lies in the extrinsic anomalies which bind down the spinal cord or its nerve roots and prevent them from changing their position within the vertebral canal to accommodate for growth of the vertebral column. If the spinal cord is tethered it will suffer a traction force during vertebral growth. It can accommodate this to some degree by increasing its own rate of growth, but when this compensatory action is exceeded the traction force will cause failure of neuronal conduction and ischaemia, due to failure of blood supply or venous congestion with possible thrombosis. The fat and fibrous tissue which so commonly occur in association with abnormal development of embryonic tissues further complicates matters by increasing in bulk and causing pressure. These factors all combine to produce changes in the lower limbs, and affect control of the bladder and bowel.

Clinical presentation

Occult forms of spinal dysraphism are not uncommonly evident at birth. In some the spinal cord is affected *in utero*, in which case the infant may be incontinent and have a foot deformity at birth. More commonly the foot deformity is a severe calcaneovalgus, but forms of talipes equinovarus occur; these may be unilateral or bilateral and the two feet may have opposite deformities, i.e. one calcaneovalgus and the other equinovarus. These are the foot deformities so commonly seen in cases of spina bifida aperta and, while not always present at birth, in spina bifida occulta they may develop during the course of growth, so that the pattern of neurological deficit in the growing child is that of spina bifida aperta, but over an extended time-scale.

Examination of the spine will reveal one of five principal cutaneous manifestations (James & Lassman 1972): a lumbosacral lipoma, hypertrichosis, pigmented naevi, dermal dimples or dermal sinuses (Fig. 10.3).

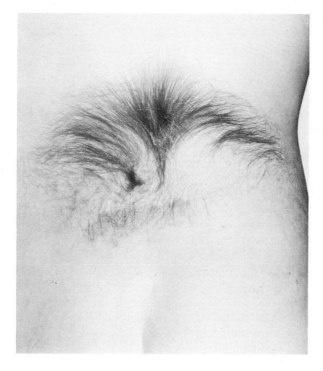

Fig. 10.3 Hairy patch over lumbar spine in spinal dysraphism.

The most common symptom is a peculiarity of gait, which may occur at any age from 1–16 years. The complaint may be of distortion of one shoe or of poor posture associated with a short leg or because one foot is smaller than the other. Pain is not a feature, but occasionally there is a complaint of metatarsalgia resulting from a protective gait. The gait is often as if there is a verruca beneath the great toe resulting in an elevation of the first metatarsal, while the great toe remains flexed. A cavovarus deformity may develop, which is usually unilateral and not unlike the deformity seen in late cases of poliomyelitis or cases of relapsed club foot. There is often shortening of one leg or foot.

As in all progressive neurological conditions the reflexes may be normal at the outset but later become exaggerated and finally disappear. Sensory changes are difficult to assess in children unless they are old enough to co-operate.

Treatment

The treatment depends on early recognition of the condition and the extent of the underlying neurological problem. If the neurological condition is progressive, myelography and neurosurgical intervention will be needed. The treatment of the foot or feet will depend on the nature of the deformity which is present, and all efforts are directed at producing a plantigrade foot.

HEMIPLEGIA

Hemiplegia in the adult, which may be either the result of intracranial injury or disease, produces stereotyped patterns of deformity in the lower extremity. Two basic patterns of either flexor or extensor synergy may be observed (Tracy 1976). Flexor synergy is characterized by hip flexion, knee flexion and ankle dorsiflexion during the swing phase of gait. However, extensor synergy, which is characterized by hip extension, plantar flexion and heel inversion with curling of the toes during the swing phase, is more amenable to orthopaedic treatment. It is possible to balance the foot of a patient with extensor predominance by means of orthoses or surgical techniques and to considerably improve their gait.

In order to achieve stability, some form of appliance is required. A below-knee walking plaster is cheap and readily applied and useful for short term use. Nevertheless, a double below-knee iron with square ankle sockets provides more satisfactory stabilization. The appropriate surgical procedures have to be selected for each individual patient. No single operation will answer all problems. The extensor pattern of muscle spasm often places the foot in an extreme equinovarus deformity and this can only be relieved by lengthening of the tendo-Achilles. Spastic toe flexors are frequently a cause of major disability to the active, mildly involved patient. Tenotomy of the flexor tendons at the bases of the toes should control this problem. The varus component of the foot deformity during stance results from the combined influence of the spastic gastrocnemius–soleus, toe flexors, tibialis posterior and tibialis anterior muscles. The tibialis anterior is active in the reflex flexor patterns of gait and continues its influence in the extensor pattern of the stance phase by holding the foot in an unbalanced position and accentuates the varus pull of the tibialis posterior. Mooney and his co-workers (1967) have described a useful procedure for the patient with extensor synergy, which includes lengthening the tendo-Achilles, lengthening of the tibialis posterior at the ankle, section of the flexors of all five toes at the bases of the toes and transfer of one half of the distal portion of the tibialis anterior tendon to the lateral cuneiform. The split tibialis anterior tendon transfer results in an inverted Y-shaped insertion which allows the foot to dorsiflex in a neutral position of inversion–eversion.

ANTERIOR POLIOMYELITIS

This is a rare condition in Great Britain nowadays. The effects of paralysis of the muscles around the ankle and foot are varied and deformities result, depending on the muscles involved. Equinus or fixed plantarflexion arises when the dorsiflexors of the ankle and foot are weak and the calf muscles have remained strong. The tendency to equinus is aggravated by gravity. Calcaneus or a fixed dorsiflexion deformity arises when the triceps surae is weak or paralysed and the dorsiflexor muscles have remained strong. Weight is borne on the posterior surface of the heel (the so-called 'pistol-grip heel') and at the same time the foot becomes cavus. Valgus or fixed eversion is probably the commonest deformity to be seen as the tibialis muscles are the most frequent to be paralysed in poliomyelitis (Sharrard 1957), and the position of the foot may be further displaced by weight-bearing. Varus (or fixed inversion) is less common and is a result of weak peroneal and active tibialis muscles. Deformity due to muscle imbalance is aggravated by growth as the weak muscles are further stretched and weaked as the bone grows.

Techniques of correction of the deformities produced by poliomyelitis have been well documented in the literature (see list of recommended reading). In the growing child it may be possible to prevent deformity by transfer of an overacting tendon. Weakness of muscles may be supplemented by external supports in the form of orthoses. Once the foot is skeletally mature, residual deformity can be corrected by formal triple arthrodesis.

LEPROSY

This ancient disease still affects 12–15 million people (White & Feagin 1972). Leprosy has remained definitely endemic only in Africa, India, Burma, South China, Japan, Central and South America, Mexico, the West Indies, the Malaysian Archipelago and many of the Pacific Islands (Riordan 1960). There are two main forms, the lepromatous and the tuberculoid.

Lepromatous leprosy is generally considered to be the progressive or malignant form of the disease. It is characterized by nodules throughout the skin, considerable thickening of the involved skin and widespread involvement throughout the body. *Mycobacterium leprae* can be demonstrated in practically all the tissues of the body but true pathological lesions are found only in the skin, the mucous membranes of the respiratory tract, the testicles, the anterior chambers of the eyes and the nerves. In contrast, tuberculoid leprosy is generally thought to be the self-limiting form of the disease, because the host has reacted defensively and sometimes successfully against the bacillus. The disease is restricted to one or more areas of the body and in some instances there is eventual destruction of the bacilli and eradication of the infection (Riordan 1960).

It has been found that anaesthetic feet without deformity or muscle imbalance produce significantly higher pressures than normal feet during barefoot walking on a flat surface (Bauman *et al* 1963). Loss of toes or function of the toes resulted in high, sharp pressure peaks under the anterior end of the foot during push-off, and in deformed feet these pressures are concentrated on one or two small areas. In anaesthetic feet the prevention of trophic ulceration depends on the even distribution of pressure over the sole of the foot. Carefully placed arch supports or metatarsal bars effectively re-distribute plantar pressure. For shortened, deformed feet, a shoe with a rigid sole supported by a rocker near the centre of the foot effectively reduces pressures under the forefoot.

There seem to be two distinct modes of destruction of the foot, once pain sensibility has been lost (Harris & Brand 1966). The first is a slow erosion and shortening associated with perforating ulcers under the distal weight-bearing end of the foot. The second is a proximal disintegration of the tarsus in which mechanical forces often determine the onset and progress of the condition, and once the tarsus has begun to disintegrate it is difficult to halt the rapid destruction of the foot. Routine palpation of anaesthetic feet will reveal patches of warmth localized to bones and joints which are at risk. Patients with insensitive feet need to realize that their feet will only last them a lifetime provided that their activities are severely curtailed and that running, jumping or walking on rough, uneven ground may set in train a process of calamitous destruction. A penetrating ulcer should be treated as a potential destroyer of the foot. To obtain healing the only effective treatment, other than bed rest, is immobilization in a plaster boot, preferably non-weight bearing or if not, with a rocker sole. A useful prophylactic or reconstructive procedure is transfer of the tibialis posterior tendon through the interosseous membrane for the patient with a drop foot.

TRAUMATIC PARAPLEGIA

Although surgery of the foot is relatively infrequent in patients who have damaged spinal cords, it has a place. Surprisingly, ingrown toe nails are often a source of trouble, and overlooked because there is little or no associated pain. Serious pyrexia may result with increase in spasm. Formal ablation of the nail bed may be required.

Claw toes may be a problem with incomplete cord lesions. Interphalangeal fusions are sometimes indicated, but often tenotomy of the flexor tendons at the bases of the toes is sufficient.

Equino-varus deformities may result in pressure sores over the lateral malleolus or on the dorsum of the foot, because of difficulty with resting the feet on the footplate of a wheelchair. Lengthening of the tendo-Achilles or transfer of an overacting tibialis anterior tendon may be needed for incomplete lesions of the cord. Occasionally, bony correction by means of a wedge tarsectomy or triple arthrodesis will be indicated.

Pressure sores may occur on the heels, malleoli or at the base of the fifth metatarsal. To produce healing, it is often necessary to resect bone to allow the soft tissues to fall together. A penetrating heel sore can be especially troublesome and may require excision of the whole calcaneum.

ACKNOWLEDGEMENT

The editor would like to acknowledge the invaluable help of Mr T. McSweeney FRCS and Mr D.K. Evans FRCS in providing information for the section on traumatic paraplegia.

REFERENCES

BAUMAY J.H., GIRLING J.P. & BRAND P.W. (1963) Plantar pressures and trophic ulceration. *Journal of Bone and Joint Surgery* **45B**, 652–73.

BENNET G.C., JONES D. & LANG M. (1981) Varus and valgus deformities of the feet in cerebral palsy. *Journal of Bone and Joint Surgery* (in press).

DENNYSON W.G. & FULFORD G.E. (1976) Subtalar arthrodesis cancellous grafts and metallic internal fixation. *Journal of Bone and Joint Surgery* **58B**, 507–10.

FIXSEN J.A. (1979) Surgical treatment of the lower limbs in cerebral palsy. *Journal of the Royal Society of Medicine* **72**, 761–5.

FRANK J.D. & FIXSEN J.A. (1980) Spina bifida. *British Journal of Hospital Medicine* 422–37.

GRICE D.S. (1952) An extra-articular arthrodesis of the subastragalar joint for the correction of paralytic feet in children. *Journal of Bone and Joint Surgery* **34A**, 927–40.

HARRIS J.R. & BRAND P.W. (1966) Patterns of disintegration of the tarsus in the anaesthetic foot. *Journal of Bone and Joint Surgery* **48B**, 4–16.

JAMES C.C.M. & LASSMAN L.P. (1972) *Spina Bifida Occulta*. Butterworths, London.

MOONEY V., PERRY J. & NOCKEL V.L. (1967) Surgical and non-surgical orthopaedic care of stroke. *Journal of Bone and Joint Surgery* **49A**, 989–1003.

RIORDAN D.C. (1960) The hand in leprosy. *Journal of Bone and Joint Surgery* **42A**, 661–90.

SHARRARD W.J.W. (1957) Muscle paralysis in poliomyelitis. *British Journal of Surgery* **44**, 471–80.

STARK G.D. & BAKER G. (1967) Developmental Medicine and Child. *Neurology* **9**, 732–44.

TRACY H.W. (1976) Operative treatment of the plantar-flexed inverted foot in adult hemiplegia. *Journal of Bone and Joint Surgery* **58A**, 1142–5.

WHITE A.A. & FEAGIN J.A. (1972) The management of the foot in leprosy. *Clinical Orthopaedics* **85,** 115–21.

WILLIAMS P.F. & MENELAUS M.B. (1977) Triple arthrodesis by inlay grafting—a method suitable for the undeformed or valgus foot. *Journal of Bone and Joint Surgery* **59B,** 333–6.

Further reading

SHARRARD W.J. (1967) Paralytic deformity in the lower limb. *Journal of Bone and Joint Surgery* **49B,** 731–47.

SEDDON H.J. (1954) Poliomyelitis, Part II. Treatment of Poliomyelitis. In *British Surgical Practice, Surgical Progress* p. 162 *et seq.* Butterworths, London.

11

Fractures of the Foot

D.W. WILSON

Fractures of the toes and metatarsals are common and present few problems in treatment. Apart from those of the calcaneum, injuries of the hindfoot and midfoot are uncommon and any one surgeon is unlikely to have a wide experience of them all. While a considerable amount has been written about fractures of the calcaneum and talus, other regions of the foot are less well documented.

Opinions concerning the mechanisms producing and the management of major injuries are diverse. This chapter attempts a collection and synthesis of these diverse views and draws heavily on the work of others. It will be easier to understand the text and the diagrams if they are viewed together with the corresponding dried bones.

PRINCIPLES

In the management of major injuries of the foot, especially of the midfoot and the hindfoot, certain principles should be emphasized.

Diagnosis

While injuries of the forefoot and toes seldom cause diagnostic difficulty, those of the midfoot and the hindfoot may be missed or wrongly assessed. A full set of radiographs is essential. It does the patient no service to omit comparison views of the sound foot because of anxieties about radiation dosages.

The skin and infection

The prompt handling of any primary wound or secondary skin necrosis is of the greatest importance. Once deep infection is established in the tarsal bones or joints, it is difficult to eradicate without extensive and destructive surgery.

Soft-tissue injury

A severe sprain of an important region of the foot (e.g. the midtarsus or the tarsometatarsal joints) is a relatively major insult and merits the correct treatment. It must not be dismissed as a minor matter. A normal radiological appearance should not outweigh the clinical assessment of the severity of the injury.

The shape of the foot

It is important to restore the foot to as normal a shape as possible, even if joint mobility cannot be achieved, and the relative lengths of the medial (talonaviculo-cuneiform) and the lateral (calcaneocuboid) columns of the foot should be restored. Abnormal bony prominences on the plantar surface of the foot must be avoided.

It may be worthwhile undertaking operative correction of an injury solely to prevent residual deformity. This is well illustrated in the calcaneum, the navicular, the cuboid and the tarsometatarsal region of the foot. 'Normal foot function is dependent upon maintenance of the proper weight-bearing lines of the foot. . . . Bony displacement which alters the weight-bearing lines or disturbs the arch must be corrected.' (P. Wilson 1933.)

Joints

Retention of only a trace of motion may not be useful, especially if it represents an unsound fibrous ankylosis and is painful. Movement is not likely to be regained fully if joint surfaces remain notably incongruous. In these circumstances open reduction may be indicated. Conversely, a stable ankylosis in a good position may be painless and yield an acceptable result.

While a period of immobilization is of benefit to achieve soft-tissue healing, it is illogical to prolong it if joint motion is the aim. In these circumstances, internal fixation of a fracture may allow earlier mobilization of the foot than might be permissible in a conservative regimen.

Complications

It is important to adopt methods of treatment which anticipate and avoid or eliminate complications such as mal-union, delayed union or non-union, avascular necrosis and secondary soft-tissue problems, such as tendon entrapment. This principle is especially important for injuries of the talus.

The ruined foot

The foot presenting in a state of complete disorganization after very severe trauma (Fig. 11.1) is best managed by early definitive amputation at the lowest level compatible with good function and satisfactory prosthetic fitting.

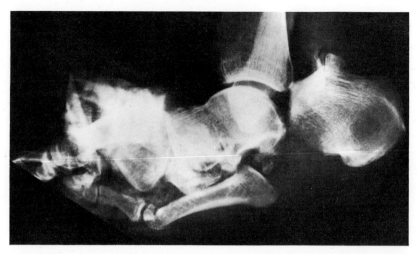

Fig. 11.1   The ruined foot of a man who fell five stories. The forefoot was reduced to a jumble of bones. The heel pad could be salvaged and treatment was by Chopart amputation, replacing the calcaneum below the talus.

CALCANEUM

Anatomy and radiological appearance

The calcaneum is an irregularly cuboidal bone whose gross appearance is well described in anatomy texts.

On the upper and lateral part of the middle of the bone there is a strong, angled strut of cortex, supporting the lateral process of the talus. The bend in this strut forms the so-called 'crucial angle' across which primary fracture lines commonly pass. Radiologically, on lateral views with the foot in a neutral posture, the cortical strut is seen along the upper surface of the bone, partly concealed by the oval shadow of the sustentaculum tali. On eversion the sustentacular shadow moves downward and no longer overlies the cortical strut.

The radiological projections needed to assess injuries of the calcaneum are set out in Table 11.1. On strictly mediolateral views fracture lines may not be easy to see (Fig. 11.2).

The appearance of the axial projection depends on the angle of the x-ray beam in relation to the foot. With the beam at less vertical angles the calcaneum appears elongated and vice versa.

Classification

A classification is suggested and is set out in Table 11.2. It is based on the classifications of Essex–Lopresti (1952) and Allan (1955).

Table 11.1. Radiological examination of the fractured calcaneum.

View	Position of patient & comments	
Lateral	The ankle lies with its lateral side on the plate. A pad is placed. under the knee	
Axial	Patient supine, the heels are separated by a small pad, but the great toes are together. Maximum dorsiflexion is maintained with a sling. The plate lies under the heels	45° 55°
Oblique lateral view of the talocalcaneal joint (Anthonsen)	Method (a); Anthonsen (1943), Allan (1955) Patient on injured side, lateral side of dorsiflexed foot on the plate	25°
	Method (b); Clark (1973) Patient on injured side, lateral side of dorsiflexed foot on the plate. Leg is rolled a further 40° forward, bringing the patella to the couch and raising heel from plate with a pad	20°

	Ray centre point	Direction of central ray	View obtained
	2 cm below the medial malleolus	Vertical (directly mediolaterally)	
	In the midline of the foot, 5 cm above the plate	40–45° from vertical in a headward direction, 55° for the elongated view	
	Just below the tip of the medial malleolus	25° toward the foot end of the couch and 30° forward along the foot toward the toes	
	At the tip of the medial malleolus	20° toward the foot end of the couch	

Table continued overleaf

Table 11.1. (cont.)

View	Position of patient & comments	
Oblique lateral	Patient supine, foot rotated 45° externally This view shows posterior sub-talar joint	
Oblique medial	Patient supine, foot rotated 45° internally Useful if axial views are un-satisfactory or difficult to obtain	
Over-everted oblique of the foot (Greenwood)*	Position as for oblique foot views, but with increased eversion until the sole is 45° to the plate This view shows anterosuperior process of the calcaneum and anterior facet of subtalar joint	

* I am indebted to Mrs Eileen Greenwood DCR, Superintendent Radiographer at the Royal Free Hospital, London, for help with this table and for the over-everted oblique view of the foot.

	Ray centre point	Direction of central ray	View obtained
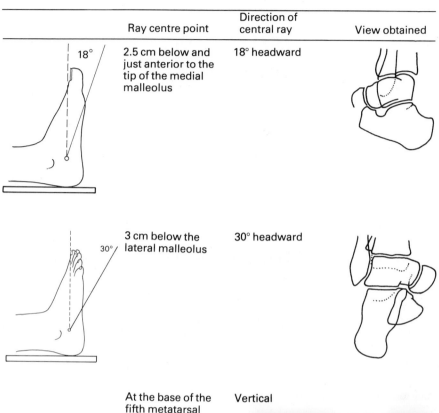	2.5 cm below and just anterior to the tip of the medial malleolus	18° headward	
	3 cm below the lateral malleolus	30° headward	
	At the base of the fifth metatarsal	Vertical	

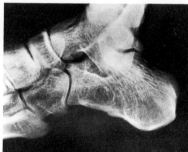

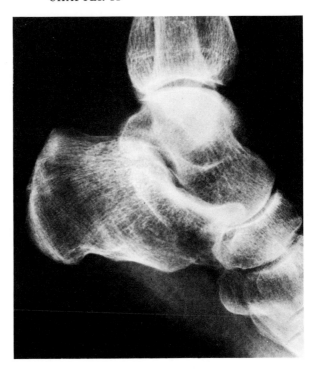

Fig. 11.2 Same case
as Fig. 11.25. True
lateral projection. The
fracture is very
difficult to see.

The incidence of the various types of fracture is shown in Table 11.3. Three-quarters of all calcaneal fractures involve the central regions of the bone and the subtalar joint, and half are displaced.

Fractures of the posterior end (tuberosity) of the calcaneum

Posterosuperior avulsion fractures

These fractures were described by Lowy (1969) within four groups, corresponding to Group 1 of Bohler (1958) (Figs. 11.3–11.9). He drew attention to the variable extent of the attachment of the tendo-Achilles to the posterior surface of the calcaneum. In the majority the tendon was inserted into the middle part of the bulge on the posterior surface of the bone, but in 20% was higher than this.

In genuine beak fractures (Fig. 11.3) a triangular portion of the posterosuperior part of the bone is hinged upward on its anterior end. Only the deeper part of the tendon is attached to it and the tendon remains functionally intact. Conversely, in false beak fractures, all the effective tendon is included with the triangular fragment, due either to a high insertion (Fig. 11.5) or to degeneration and easy rupture of the remaining superficial fibres (Fig. 11.7). Lowy (1969) noted that radiographs could not distinguish the genuine from the false beak fracture. This distinction could only be made by clinical tests of the continuity of calf muscle

Table 11.2 Classification of fractures of the calcaneum.

Region	Name	Comments and equivalent in other classifications
Fractures not involving the subtalar joint		
	Posterosuperior avulsion	
	(a) Beak types	Essex-Lopresti: beak fracture
		Watson-Jones: horizontal fracture tuberosity
		Bohler: groups 1a to 1c
	(b) Avulsion type	Lowy: beak & avulsion fractures
	Posteromedial process	Fractures of the medial plantar process—
		Essex-Lopresti: avulsion of medial border
		Warrick & Bremner: vertical fracture of tuberosity
		Watson-Jones: vertical fracture of tuberosity
		Bohler: group 2
Posterior end of calcaneum (tuberosity)	Posterior primary (horizontal)	Horizontal fracture in the tuberosity
		Devas: horizontal compression fracture of tuberosity
	Posterior primary (vertical)	Vertical and oblique fracture across the tuberosity—
		Essex-Lopresti: vertical fracture of tuberosity
		Allan: primary fracture behind posterior facet
		Bohler: group 4
		Devas: vertical compression fracture of tuberosity
Anterior end of calcaneum	Anterosuperior	Fracture of the anteromediosuperior process—
		Dachtler: anterosuperior beak fracture
		Watson-Jones: fracture of the anterior end
		Bohler: group 3b
	Anterior comminuted	Watson-Jones: crush fracture of calcaneocuboid joint
		Dewar & Evans: } mid-tarsal fracture dislocation
		Main & Jowett: }

Table 11.2 (*Cont.*)

Fractures involving the body of the calcaneum and the subtalar joint

Region	Name	Comments and equivalent in other classifications
Primary fractures of the body	Undisplaced central primary	Undisplaced oblique fissure anterior to facet— Allan: primary fracture anterior to facet Undisplaced oblique fissure through the facet— Essex-Lopresti: undisplaced fracture Allan: primary fracture through the facet Souer & Remy: stage 1 fracture
	Sustentaculum tali	Essex-Lopresti: fracture of sustentaculum tali Bohler: group 3a
	Displaced central primary	Oblique fracture through the facet with displacement of the lateral fragment— Allan: secondary compression of part of subtalar joint Watson-Jones: fracture with displacement of lateral half of joint Bohler: group 5
Secondary fractures of the body	Trapdoor central secondary	Palmer: type 1 Essex-Lopresti: joint depression type Allan: secondary compression of all of subtalar joint Bohler: group 5 Soeur & Remy: semilunar stage 2
	Seesaw central secondary	Morestin: bascule (seesaw) Palmer: type 2 Essex-Lopresti: tongue type Allan: tongue type Soeur & Remy: comet-shaped stage 2

Table 11.2 (*Cont.*)

Region	Name	Comments and equivalent in other classifications
Secondary fractures of the body (*Cont.*)	Additional central secondary	With additional fracture lines in the body of the calcaneum— Allan: tertiary fracture lines Bohler: group 8 Soeur & Remy: stage 2 with additional fracture lines
Comminuted fractures of the body	Central comminuted	Without dislocation of the subtalar joint— Essex-Lopresti: type from below Bohler: group 6 Soeur & Remy: stage 3 With dislocation of the subtalar joint— Essex-Lopresti: type from behind forward Bohler: group 7
Posterior end of calcaneum	Stress	Hullinger: insufficiency fracture Leabhart: stress fracture Devas: compression stress fracture

Table 11.3 Incidence of the types of fracture of the calcaneum. (All figures are percentages unless otherwise indicated.)

	Essex-Lopresti 1952	Warrick & Bremner 1953	Allan 1955	Bohler 1958	Lance et al 1963	Soeur & Remy 1975	Aggregate
Number of cases:	230	300	81	250	199	112	117
Posterosuperior avulsion		1		$\frac{1}{2}$			
Posteromedial process	17		17	$15\frac{1}{2}$	$9\frac{1}{2}$		1
Posterior primary		$10\frac{1}{2}$				17	
Anterosuperior			2	4*			
Anterior comminuted	8	$13\frac{1}{2}$			$23\frac{1}{2}$		1
Totals (%)	25	25	19	20	33	17	2
Undisplaced central primary							
Anterior to facet	$15\frac{1}{4}$ ($20\frac{1}{2}$)	$16\frac{1}{2}$ (22)		27 (34)	18 (27)	(36)	2
Through facet		9 (12)	5 (6)				
Sustentaculum tali	$\frac{1}{2}$ ($\frac{1}{7}$)	$\frac{1}{2}$ ($\frac{1}{2}$)		*	4 (6)		
Displaced central primary		$35\frac{1}{4}$ ($47\frac{1}{2}$)	54 (67)				
Central secondary				33			
Trapdoor	33 (44)			($41\frac{1}{2}$)	$23\frac{1}{2}$ (35)	(62)†	4
Seesaw	20 ($26\frac{1}{2}$)	$13\frac{1}{2}$ (18)	8 (10)		$7\frac{1}{2}$ (11)		
Additional				11 (13)			
Central comminuted							
Without dislocation	$3\frac{1}{2}$ (5)		14 (17)	3 (4)	13 ($19\frac{1}{2}$)	(2)	
With dislocation	$2\frac{1}{4}$ ($3\frac{1}{4}$)			6 ($7\frac{1}{2}$)	1 ($1\frac{1}{2}$)		
Totals (%)	75	75	81	80	67	83	

* Includes 3c. Sustentaculum tali
† Quoted ratio trapdoor:seesaw = 5:1
Figures in brackets are percentage incidence within the group of central fractures which involve the subtalar joint.

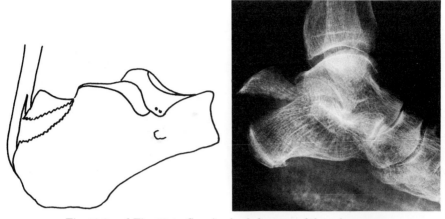

Fig. 11.3 and Fig. 11.4 Genuine beak fracture of the calcaneum.

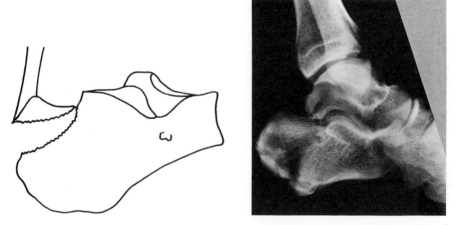

Fig. 11.5 and Fig. 11.6 False beak fracture of the calcaneum, showing a high insertion of the tendo-Achilles (*left*).

function. Although it is possible to treat true beak fractures by closed manipulation, if tests of calf continuity are abnormal or equivocal, open exploration to replace the fragment and to secure it with a screw is indicated. Rarely, the triangular fragment extends forward far enough to encroach upon the posterior subtalar joint facet (Fig. 11.8).

In the avulsion type of fracture the whole attachment of the tendo-Achilles is lifted as an oval plaque of bone, which comes to lie above and parallel to its bed (Fig. 11.9). Open reduction and fixation with a screw is essential.

All posterosuperior avulsion fractures should be immobilized in a below-knee cast in some equinus for 6 weeks after reduction.

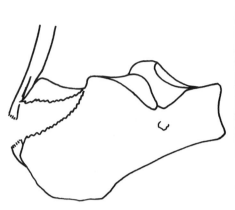
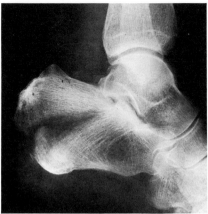

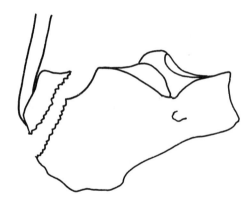

Fig. 11.7 (*Above left*) False beak fracture of the calcaneum, showing rupture of the remaining part of the tendo-Achilles.

Fig. 11.8 (*Above right*) Beak-type fracture in which the elevated bone includes part of the posterior subtalar joint facet.

Fig. 11.9 (*Right*) Avulsion type fracture of the calcaneum, showing the entire attachment of the tendo-Achilles lifted from its bed.

Posteromedial process

Bohler (1958) attributed fracture of the medial (plantar) process of the posterior part of the calcaneum to direct shearing when the heel impacted on the ground. However, Essex-Lopresti (1952) regarded it as an avulsion fracture caused by force transmitted along the plantar fascia.

The fracture is best seen in the axial projection radiograph (Figs. 11.10–11.12). Rest in a below knee cast for 4–6 weeks is adequate treatment.

Posterior primary fractures

Horizontal fracture was considered by Devas (1961) to be due to direct compression

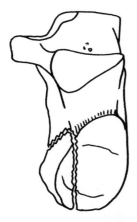

Fig. 11.10 (*Left*) Fracture of the medial (plantar) process of the calcaneum. Compare with Fig. 11.11.

Fig. 11.11 (*Below left*) Axial view of fracture of the medial process.

Fig. 11.12 (*Below right*) Same as Fig. 11.11. Lateral view.

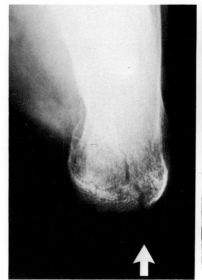

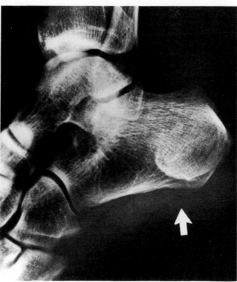

infracture against the ground (Fig. 11.16). He contrasted this and also vertical compression fracture, due to trauma, with the oblique stress (fatigue) fracture (see p. 232).

The injury is not included in other classifications.

Vertical fracture of the posterior part of the calcaneum runs obliquely forward across the bone. Bohler (1958) postulated that this fracture occurred when the heel alone impacted against a projecting step.

Allan (1955) included this injury with the primary fracture lines and considered that it differed only in its position behind the facet (Figs. 11.13, 11.14).

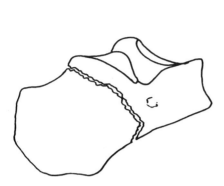
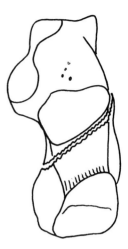

Fig. 11.13 (*Left*) Primary vertical fracture in the tuberosity of the calcaneum. The vertical fracture plane crosses the heel from posteromedial to anterolateral.

Fig. 11.14 (*Right*) Same as Fig. 11.13. Superior view.

Devas (1961) recorded a case of this type which he attributed to the compression of the tuberosity of the combined tensions in the tendo-Achilles and the plantar fascia (Fig. 11.15).

Fractures of the anterior end of the calcaneum

Anterosuperior

Fractures of the anteromediosuperior process of the calcaneum were described by Dachtler (1931) and attributed to hyperdorsiflexion forces, typically inflicted when a heavy, low-loading truck ran up the heel from behind, forcing the leg forward on the fixed foot. These injuries accounted for 58% of fractures of the anterior end of the calcaneum in his series of 26 cases.

A triangular fragment is elevated from the front of the top of the calcaneum at the junction of the calcaneocuboid joint and the anterior subtalar joint (Warrick & Bremner 1953) (Figs. 11.17, 11.18). Occasionally (7%), the fragment is large and extends into the region below the talus. It is best seen on superoinferior or over-everted oblique radiographs of the foot and does not appear on ankle radiographs.

The physical sign typical of these injuries is tenderness on the dorsilateral foot 3 cm anterior to and slightly below the lower end of the lateral malleolus, with swelling and bruising. Too-early mobilization after these injuries leads to prolonged discomfort (Bohler 1958; Dachtler 1931) and a period of rest in a below-knee cast is recommended.

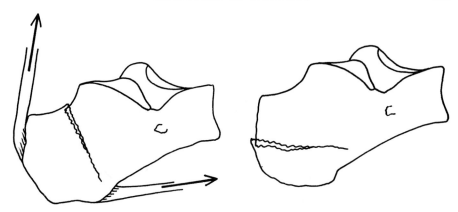

Fig. 11.15 (*Left*) Primary vertical compression fracture of the calcaneum. The forces acting in the tendo-Achilles and the plantar fascia set up a resultant force which compresses the tuberosity.

Fig. 11.16 (*Right*) Primary horizontal compression fracture of tuberosity (Devas 1961).

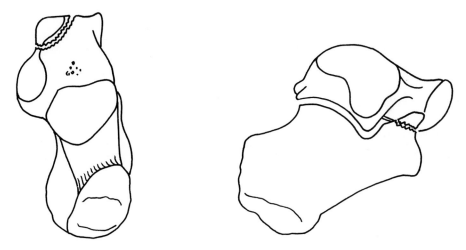

Fig. 11.17 (*Left*) Anterosuperior fracture of the calcaneum. Superior view.

Fig. 11.18 (*Right*) Same as Fig. 11.17. Lateral view.

The remaining 42% of fractures in Dachtler's series were typical inversion and adduction sprain fractures with shards avulsed from the region of the calcaneo-cuboid joint. Among the sites described were the anteroinferior border of the calcaneum (11%) and the lateral and superior borders (19%).

Anterior comminuted

Comminuted fractures of the anterior end of the calcaneum at the calcaneocuboid joint, without fractures in the remainder of the bone, represent part of a midtarsal injury (see p. 274). Comminution of the anterior end also occurs as an additional fracture in combination with other fractures of the bone (see p. 230).

Central fractures

Fractures of the central region (body) of the calcaneum involve the posterior facet of the subtalar joint and the sustentaculum tali (the middle subtalar facet). They are best considered as a sequence of increasing damage to the bone, in which the causative violence may stop at any time leaving the injury in an intermediate stage. These injuries are caused by falls from a height (commonly 2–5 metres) and are rarely due to vertical compression alone (2% in the series of Soeur & Remy 1974; Fig. 11.19).

Undisplaced central primary fracture

When the calcaneum impacts against the ground, it rotates into eversion (Figs. 11.20, 11.21). It is then compressed by the talus, which continues to descend under the body's weight. The wedge-shaped lateral process of the talus impacts into the crucial angle of the top, outer border of the calcaneum and it is immediately below this spot that the anterior end of the primary fracture line emerges through the lateral cortex (Figs. 11.22, 11.23).

This primary fracture line runs obliquely across the bone from proximomedial to distolateral (Figs. 11.24–11.26). It commonly crosses the posterior facet of the subtalar joint near to the root of the sustentaculum tali (Fig. 11.27, middle fracture line). A variable amount of the articular surface of the posterior facet remains attached to the sustentaculum tali.

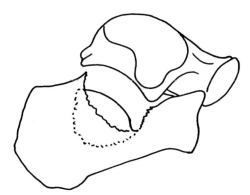

Fig. 11.19 Vertical depression of the posterior subtalar facet. Compare with Fig. 11.38.

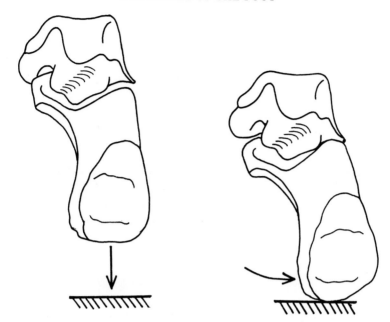

Fig. 11.20 (*Left*) The falling calcaneum in neutral posture before impact. Posterior view.

Fig. 11.21 (*Right*) The calcaneum everting on impact. Posterior view.

Fracture of the sustentaculum tali

At the same time or a little after the main fracture is occurring, the head of the talus descends upon the middle facet of the subtalar joint. The talus shears the shelf-like sustentaculum tali off the medial side of the body of the calcaneum.

After this initial depression, and when the violence has ceased, the sustentacular fracture tends to relocate itself in relation to the talus, rather than in relation to the rest of the calcaneum (see p. 224).

Commonly this injury is added to the central primary fracture, but rarely it may occur in isolation (Figs. 11.28–11.31). Some of the posterior subtalar facet remains attached to the sustentaculum tali (Essex-Lopresti 1952).

Displaced central primary fracture

Continuing violence either displaces the lateral half of the calcaneum downward or laterally at the primary fracture line (Figs. 11.32–11.36), the mechanism stressed by Warrick and Bremner (1953) and Allan (1955), or displaced secondary fracture lines appear (Figs. 11.37, 11.42), the concept of Essex-Lopresti (1952) and Soeur and Remy (1975) (see Table 11.3).

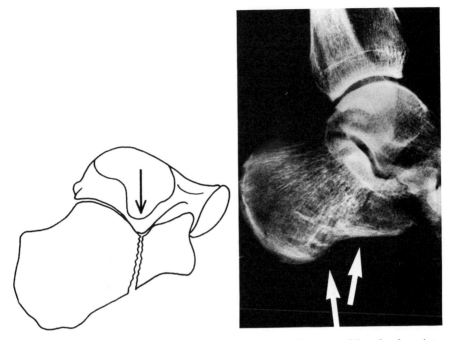

Fig. 11.22   (*Left*) Eversion of the calcaneum brings the lateral process of the talus down into the crucial angle.

Fig. 11.23   (*Right*) Undisplaced, primary central fracture of the calcaneum. Lateral view.

Central secondary fractures

As an alternative to pure displacement of the primary fracture, the primary fissure opens inferiorly, the tuberosity becomes elevated and further fracture lines appear. These separate the posterior subtalar facet from the rest of the lateral half of the calcaneum. Other fracture lines may appear in the lateral wall and the anterior end of the bone (Essex-Lopresti 1952; Soeur & Remy 1975).

Further compression and eversion depress the posterior subtalar facet into the cancellous interior of the body of the calcaneum. There are two ways in which this may happen.

The trapdoor fracture   The more common of these two is the joint depression type of Essex-Lopresti (1952) or the semilunar type of Soeur and Remy (1975). The posterior subtalar facet alone becomes separated from the lateral fragment by a transverse fracture line just behind it (Fig. 11.37). The facet is then rotated downward like a trapdoor on a transverse, posterior hinge (Figs. 11.38–11.41). The trapdoor descends inside the lateral cortex of the body of the calcaneum, crushing the cancellous interior as it does so.

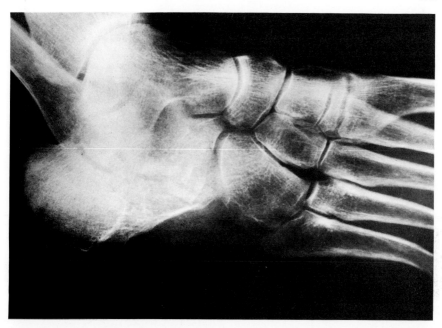

Fig. 11.24   Primary oblique fracture line across the calcaneum behind the posterior subtalar facet. Compare with Fig. 11.2.

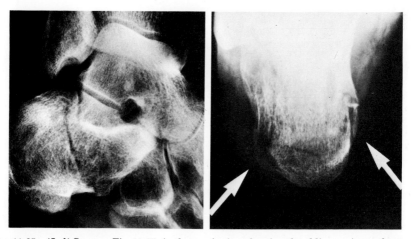

Fig. 11.25   (*Left*) Same as Fig. 11.25. Anthonsen's view showing the oblique primary fracture line. Compare with Fig. 11.2.

Fig. 11.26   (*Right*) Same as Fig. 11.23. Axial view.

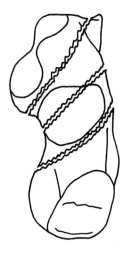

Fig. 11.27 The typical primary fracture lines in the central part of the calcaneum as described by Allan (1955). The posterior fracture has been described with fractures of the tuberosity. The middle fracture is the typical primary fracture described by Essex-Lopresti (1952) and Soeur and Remy (1975). It crosses the posterior facet, leaving a small portion attached to the sustentaculum tali. The anterior fracture line corresponds to the anterior splits described by Soeur and Remy (1975) (See Fig. 11.48) or to a sustentacular fracture.

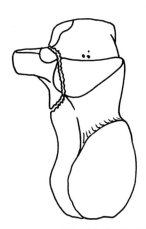

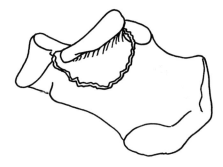

Fig. 11.28   (*Left*) Fracture of the sustentaculum tali. Axial view.

Fig. 11.29   (*Right*) Same as Fig. 11.28. Medial view.

The seesaw fracture   Less commonly the fractures delimiting the fragment containing the posterior subtalar facet extend backward along the upper surface of the tuberosity to its posterior margin (Fig. 11.42). The long, plank-like fragment then tilts like a seesaw (Morestin 1902), upward posteriorly and downward anteriorly, inside the lateral wall of the bone (Figs. 11.43–11.46). This is the tongue fracture of Essex-Lopresti (1952) or the comet-shaped fracture of Soeur and Remy (1955).

The trapdoor or seesaw fragment includes whichever part of the posterior subtalar facet has not been retained on the sustentacular fragment (Fig. 11.46). At the moment of greatest compression, the sustentacular fragment is depressed as much as the lateral fragment. However, when the violence ceases and the foot is no

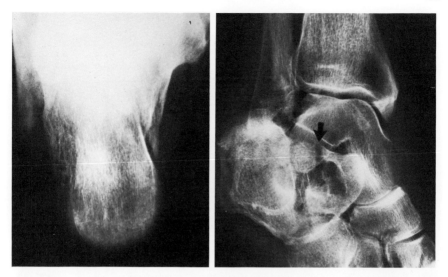

Fig. 11.30   (*Left*) Fracture of the sustentaculum tali. Axial view, compare with Fig. 11.28.

Fig. 11.31   (*Right*) Oblique view showing separation of the sustentaculum tali.

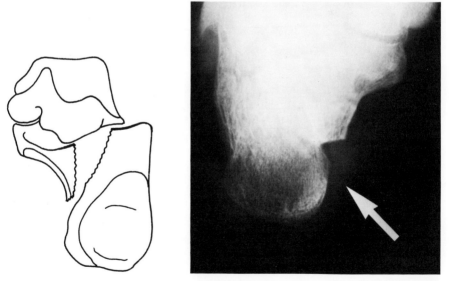

Fig. 11.32   (*Left*) Displaced primary central fracture of the calcaneum, with lateral displacement of the lateral half of the bone.

Fig. 11.33   (*Right*) Displaced primary central fracture of the calcaneum.

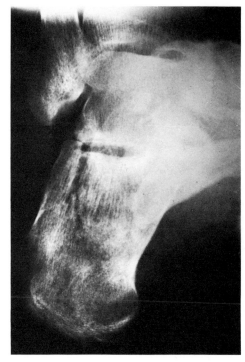 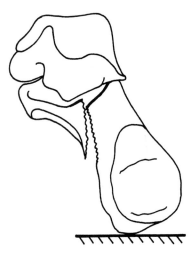

Fig. 11.34   (*Left*) Displaced primary central fracture of the calcaneum.

Fig. 11.35   (*Right*) Displaced primary central fracture of the calcaneum, with depression of the lateral half of the bone.

longer bearing weight, the elasticity of the medial ligamentous attachments pulls the sustentaculum tali back into its normal relation to the talus. The lateral fragment of the calcaneum has no comparable ligamentous attachment and remains jammed within the body of the bone, producing a step deformity in the upper contour of the posterior subtalar facet.

If the sustentaculum tali has chanced to remain intact, the posterior subtalar facet may still be depressed in any of the above ways by continuing eversion of the calcaneum.

Additional central secondary fracture lines

Additional fracture lines involving the lateral wall of the bone and its anterior end are common.

When the posterior subtalar facet is depressed within the body of the calcaneum, the lateral wall is ballooned outward (Fig. 11.47). Soeur and Remy (1975) record three common additional fractures: a triangular plate, with its base

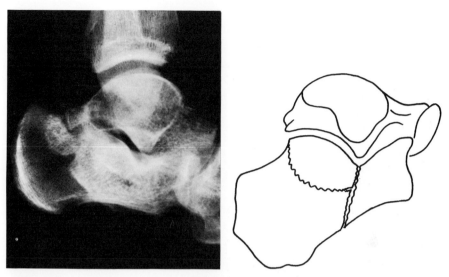

Fig. 11.36 (*Left*) Same as Fig. 11.33. Lateral view.

Fig. 11.37 (*Right*) Secondary fracture lines appearing just behind the posterior facet.

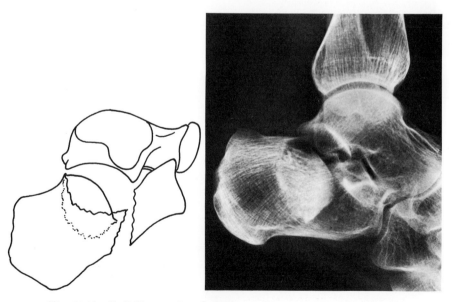

Fig. 11.38 (*Left*) The trapdoor fracture.

Fig. 11.39 (*Right*) Trapdoor secondary central fracture of the calcaneum.

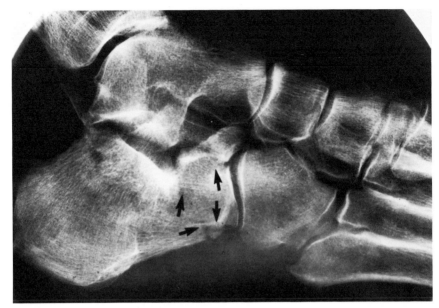

Fig. 11.40 Trapdoor fracture, sustentacular fracture and anterior fracture of the calcaneum.

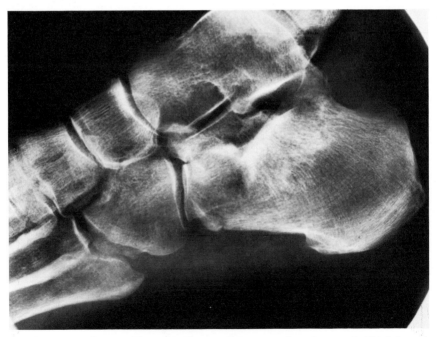

Fig. 11.41 Same as Fig. 11.40. Fracture lines enter the calcaneocuboid joint.

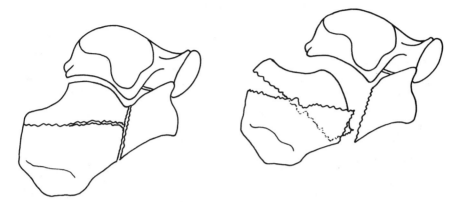

Fig. 11.42 (*Left*) Secondary fracture lines appearing and extending back to the rear of the calcaneum.

Fig. 11.43 (*Right*) The seesaw fracture of Morestin (1902).

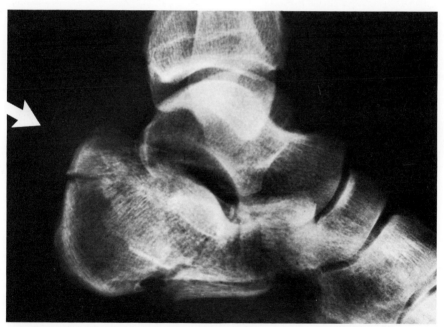

Fig. 11.44 Slightly atypical seesaw central secondary fracture of the calcaneum. The plank of the seesaw is broken near its hinge. Note the additional fracture lines separating the triangular plate from the lateral wall, compare Fig. 11.48.

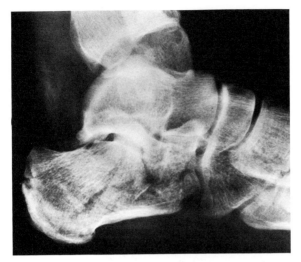 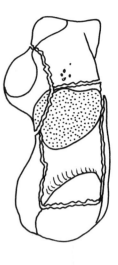

Fig. 11.45 (*Left*) A relatively undisplaced seesaw fracture. Note the additional fracture lines in the anterior end of the bone, compare Fig. 11.48.

Fig. 11.46 (*Right*) The plank of the seesaw. Superior view.

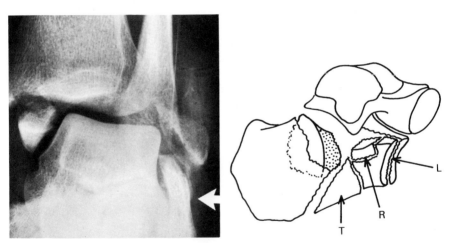

Fig. 11.47 (*Left*) Same as Fig. 11.45. Note the lateral displacement of the lateral wall of the calcaneum and the associated ankle injury.

Fig. 11.48 (*Right*) The additional fracture lines of Soeur and Remy (1975).

inferior, split off from the lateral wall (Fig. 11.48 'T'; & Fig. 11.44); a rod-shaped fragment from the edge of the sinus tarsi (Fig. 11.48 'R'); and a longitudinal split in the anterior end of the bone into the calcaneocuboid joint (Fig. 11.48 'L' & Figs. 11.45, 11.49). Less commonly these additional fracture lines may complicate a

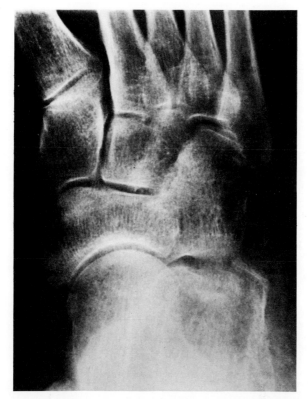

Fig. 11.49 Same as Fig. 11.25. A fracture line runs obliquely forward into the lateral edge of the calcaneocuboid joint. Note also the minor avulsion of the tuberosity of navicular.

simple undisplaced primary fissure, especially the longitudinal split into the calcaneocuboid joint.

Central comminuted fracture

As a final, but uncommon, stage the calcaneum is extensively comminuted, with the posterior subtalar facet buried near the plantar cortex, surrounded by crushed fragments.

FRACTURES OF THE CALCANEUM IN CHILDREN

While these injuries are uncommon in children, Matteri and Frymoyer (1973) described typical fissures in three children aged 16, 27 and 30 months, forming about 6% of a series of injuries. They pointed out the difficulties of radiological diagnosis (Fig. 11.50), the importance of the axial view (Fig. 11.51) and that the fracture may be misdiagnosed as a sprain.

The characteristic clinical picture which they described was of a child refusing to bear weight on the heel, walking with the limb joints in semiflexion and the foot in equinus, and with tenderness on lateral compression of the heel. Disability is minimal compared with the adult and the children do well either with a period of rest or in a plaster cast.

Thomas (1969) described injuries in five children aged 6–12 years. Four of the five had slight depression of the posterior subtalar joint, probably of the trapdoor type, but only two had trivial limitation of subtalar joint motion at follow-up. He ascribed the good results in children to their ability to mould the shape of the talar facet to fit the altered calcaneal facet. He devised a radiological angle measurement to illustrate this moulding (Figs. 11.52–11.55). He described the inverse relationship of his angle measurement to the classical one of Bohler (1931).

STRESS FRACTURES

Stress fractures of the calcaneum were described by Hullinger (1944) and Leabhart (1959) in two series of Army recruits. The classical clinical picture is of painful diffuse swelling of the hindfoot and occasionally of the calcaneal bursa, after unaccustomed activity. There is tenderness on both sides of the heel, but no

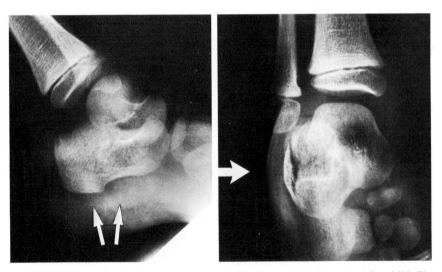

Fig. 11.50 (*Left*) Undisplaced primary central fracture of the calcaneum of a child. The fracture is not easy to see.

Fig. 11.51 (*Right*) Same as Fig. 11.50. Oblique medial projection shows the split in the lateral wall.

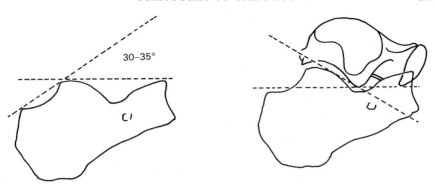

Fig. 11.52 (*Left*) The traditional 'tuber-joint angle' of Bohler (1931) on the lateral radiograph.

Fig. 11.53 (*Right*) The normal 'talar facet angle' of Thomas (1969), between a tangent to the highest point of the posterior facet and a second line joining the lowest points of the head and posterior facet of the talus on the lateral radiograph.

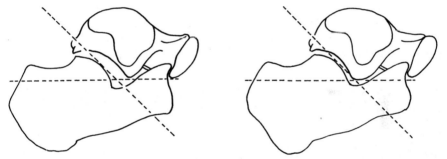

Fig. 11.54 (*Left*) The 'talar facet angle' is increased if the posterior facet of the calcaneum is depressed.

Fig. 11.55 (*Right*) The 'talar facet angle' remains abnormal, but the joint is no longer incongruous, due to increased convexity of the talar facet with remodelling in the child.

bruising, no pain on tiptoe and no pain on passive dorsiflexion of the ankle. The symptoms settle quickly with rest, but recur if activity is resumed prematurely. Radiographs are slow to show changes, which may not appear until the fifth week.

The cortex of the bone remains intact and the fracture is revealed as a haze of endosteal callus within the cancellous bone (Fig. 11.56). The fracture is almost always in posterior part of the bone (the tuberosity). Hullinger (1944) recorded only two patients with stress fractures in the anterior end of the calcaneum in a series of 53 patients. Fracture lines may be multiple (Devas 1961).

The line of the callus is transverse to the axis of the tuberosity and approximately parallel to the posterior cortex. The cause of the lesion is not the

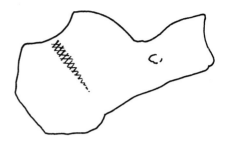

Fig. 11.56 Stress fracture of the calcaneum. A haze of callus forms within the cancellous bone. The cortex remains intact.

repetitive impact of the heel on the ground, but repeated compression stresses along the axis of the tuberosity, due to the resultant force from the tensions in the plantar fascia and the tendo-Achilles (Devas 1961) (Fig. 11.15). Treatment is by rest, followed by graduated return to activity with a sponge heel pad in the shoe (Devas 1961).

THE MANAGEMENT OF DISPLACED FRACTURES OF THE CALCANEUM

Sources of residual disability

After fractures of the central part of the bone involving the subtalar joint disability may arise from various sources which were well summarized by McLaughlin (1963). They include:

Deformity Broadening of the heel and especially bulging of the lateral wall (see below). Fixed valgus posture of the heel. Elevation of the back end of the calcaneum with flat foot and calf muscle weakness due to relative lengthening.

Persistent swelling

Stiffness Fibrous ankylosis or osteoarthritic changes in the damaged subtalar joint. Periarticular fibrosis around any of the hindfoot or midfoot joints.

Pain From the subtalar joint, more severe if there is osteoarthritis or unstable ankylosis, less severe if extensive damage leads to a firm fibrous ankylosis. From the peroneal tendons in the presence of sheath stenosis due to bony encroachment. From calcaneofibular abutment due to bulging of the lateral wall (Evans 1968; Isbister 1974) (Fig. 11.47). Tenderness under the heel from plantar fasciitis or from bony spicules.

Factors influencing the end result

The classification of the original injury

Fractures not involving the posterior subtalar joint and undisplaced fractures almost invariably yield satisfactory results. In the series of extra-articular fractures of Lance *et al* (1963), all but three of 74 cases were satisfactory and in a similar group from Essex-Lopresti (1952) 93% of the 47 cases had either no or only trivial residua. Considering undisplaced fractures involving the posterior subtalar joint, Lance *et al* (1963) quoted 70% as satisfactory and Essex-Lopresti noted that four of each five recovered well. In injuries affecting the subtalar joint, results vary with the severity of the joint damage. Lance *et al* (1963) noted 60% of good results after conservative treatment of trapdoor type displaced central fractures, but the group contained a number of cases without serious incongruity of the joint. In contrast, their cases with the seesaw type of fracture were more severely damaged and were less favourable. Central comminuted and open fractures each carried a 66% risk of a poor result.

Deformity

Lance *et al* (1963) noted that mild broadening and slight valgus of the heel might be compatible with a good result (in 86%). However, poor results were to be expected in patients with marked deformity (61–67% poor) or lateral displacement of the lateral wall of the calcaneum (88% poor).

Too early weight-bearing

In the series of Lance *et al* (1963), 14 patients had a significant increase in the displacement of the fracture after weight-bearing prior to bony healing, converting a mild into a severe injury with deterioration in the quality of the result. This problem did not occur after the eighth week.

Stiffness

Failure to regain subtalar joint motion at least to a half of the normal range lead to an unsatisfactory result in 75% (Lance *et al* 1963). The occurrence of stiffness either in the ankle or in the tarsus gave dissatisfaction in 65%.

Conversely, all cases with more than half range of subtalar movement did well, as did 75% of those with normal ankle and tarsal mobility.

Age and sex

In the series of 173 cases of Essex-Lopresti (1952), the results of the same operative procedure for displaced fractures were only half as good in patients over the age of fifty years, compared with their younger fellows. Lance *et al* (1963) agreed with this principle, but thought the selected critical age to be too low. They also noted generally better results in women, with 75% satisfactory.

Atrophy of the heel pad

All patients with this phenomenon did badly (Lance *et al* 1963).

Certain treatment methods

In general, traction through a pin in the heel gave poor results (Lance *et al* 1963) and unsuccessful attempts at open reduction produced a 70% rate of disability as judged by return to work (Essex-Lopresti 1952).

Length of follow-up

Most authors are agreed that improvement ceases after a period of time of the order of 18 months (Essex-Lopresti 1952) to 2 years (Nade & Monahan 1972).

Methods of treatment

The possible methods of treatment of displaced fractures of the calcaneum and their results are summarized in Tables 11.4 & 11.5. While each of the methods has its enthusiasts, an admixture of conservative and operative methods might seem logical. No one method can reasonably be expected to suit all cases of calcaneal fracture.

There seems to be a general feeling against primary subtalar joint arthrodesis (Roberts 1968; Evans 1968) although more recently Noble and McQuillan (1979) found over 94% of 47 patients had an excellent, good or satisfactory result.

Conservative methods

Most authors advocate the treatment of favourable groups of fracture (extra-articular and undisplaced central fissures and sustentacular fractures) by entirely conservative means. Whether this is by immobilization in a plaster cast or by a regimen of early mobilization seems to be a matter of individual preference. Anterosuperior fractures need a period of rest in a plaster cast (Dachtler 1931). When considering displaced central fractures, the reasoned attitude of Lance *et al* (1963) has much to commend it. They would select for treatment by early mobilization the following groups:

1   Those in whom reasonable alignment of the posterior subtalar facet is preserved.

2   Those without gross clinical deformity and without displacement of the lateral wall of the bone.

Table 11.4 Methods of treatment of displaced fractures of the calcaneum.

Method	Proponents
Plaster cast	
Early mobilization by exercises	Barnard & Odegard (1955) Lance *et al* (1963)
Closed reduction methods	
Spike methods	Westhues (1934) Essex-Lopresti (1952) Aaron (1974)
Traction methods	Bohler (1958) Harris (1963)
Manipulation	Herman (1937) Aitken (1963)
Open reduction	Morestin (1902) Palmer (1948) Essex-Lopresti (1952) Maxfield & McDermott (1955) McReynolds (1972) Soeur & Remy (1975) Fisk (1981)
Primary subtalar arthrodesis	Dick (1953) Noble & McQuillan (1979)
Late subtalar arthrodesis	Gallie (1943) Kalamchi & Evans (1977)

3   Patients in the older age groups, for whom operative reduction is less suited.
4   As a special group, those with the grossest comminution, where a firm fibrous ankylosis of the ruined subtalar joint offers the optimum result obtainable short of formal late arthrodesis.

The conservative regimen of Lance *et al* (1963) is representative. The injured extremity is elevated and wrapped in elastic bandages over wool wadding. The patient is instructed to move all the joints within the limits imposed by pain. After a few days, when swelling is reduced, the patient progresses to walking with crutches, but all weight-bearing is prohibited. Dependency of the limb for too long at one time should be avoided at this stage. At the end of the one or two weeks the radiological assessment and the clinical examination are repeated. If the original assessment is maintained, the patient is instructed in the exercise programme and allowed home.

Close out-patient supervision should follow until weight-bearing may begin (say at 6–8 weeks in linear fractures and 10–12 weeks for the more severe types). The transition from non-weight-bearing to full weight-bearing should be gradual

Table 11.5 Results of treatment of displaced fracture of the calcaneum. (All figures are percentages unless otherwise indicated.)

Method	Author	No. of cases	Results			Subtalar motion			Disability	
			Good	Fair	Poor	50% or more	Under 50%	Ankylosis	None	Notable
Early mobilization	Lance et al (1963)	205	60–87 (in suitable cases)							
	Nade & Monahan (1972)	93	0–40 (in unfavourable cases)							57
Closed reduction by manipulation	Herman (1937)	152	73	14	13					
	Aitken (1963)		75	15	10					
Open reduction & grafts	Allan (1955)	12	92		8	67	33			
	Maxfield & McDermott (1955)	19	69	26	5					
	Fisk (1981)	126	90			50	25	25		
Open reduction & Kirschner wires	Soeur & Remy (1975)	45				45	29	26	5 (Slight = 95)	
Open reduction & staple	McReynolds (1972)	29	76			50				

Recovery time

				Within 9 month	At work within		With no disability
					6 month	12 month	
Spike & POP	Essex-Lopresti (1952)	138	Successful redn. under age 50 years	80	80		80
			Successful redn. over age 50 years	40	40		40
			Unsuccessful redn.		20	30	

over 2 weeks. The patient can usually resume reasonable work about a month after recommencing weight-bearing.

Reduction methods

Reduction by forcible manipulation might well yield good results by producing enough additional trauma to the calcaneum to result in firm, painless fibrous ankylosis (McLaughlin 1963). Reduction by classical traction methods produced poor results in the series of Lance *et al* (1963) and of Harris (1963). Following Westhues (1934), Essex-Lopresti (1952) favoured reduction of the seesaw type of fracture by closed reduction with a slender spike introduced from behind into the fragment itself. With the patient prone and the knee flexed to a right angle the spike is introduced in the long axis of the seesaw fragment, inclining slightly outward in the axial view. Radiological control of the manoeuvre is necessary. Lifting the foot and leg upward by the spike and the dorsum of the foot at the head of the talus (not by the toes) reduces the displacement (Figs. 11.57, 11.58). Direct manual pressure replaces the lateral wall of the bone. Redisplacement is prevented by enclosing the foot and the spike in a plaster slipper which maintains a constant relation of the spike (and hence of the seesaw fragment) to the sole of the foot (and hence to the rest of the calcaneum). However, the slipper permits exercises for the joints. The patient is mobilized using crutches and taking no weight on the foot for 8–10 weeks. The spike is removed at four weeks and a below-knee cast is substituted for the slipper. This method seems little used in current practice and has been replaced by open reduction and internal fixation. For the trapdoor type of fracture Essex-Lopresti (1952) favoured open reduction, but he used a similar, but stouter, spike without bone grafts to maintain reduction. Soeur and Remy (1975) advocated open reduction through a lateral approach for both trapdoor and seesaw types of fracture, with multiple Kirschner wires to secure the reduction and no bone grafts

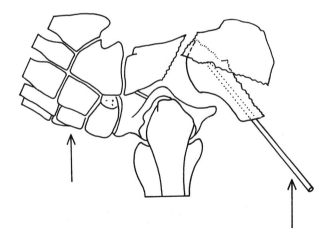

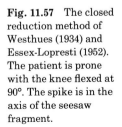

Fig. 11.57 The closed reduction method of Westhues (1934) and Essex-Lopresti (1952). The patient is prone with the knee flexed at 90°. The spike is in the axis of the seesaw fragment.

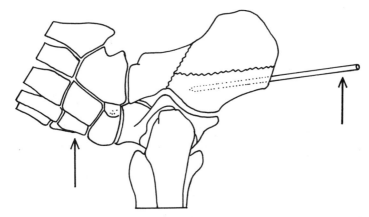

Fig. 11.58 Same as Fig. 11.57. Lifting the foot by the talus and the spike reduces the seesaw fracture. Manual compression is then needed to replace the bulging lateral wall of the bone.

(Fig. 11.59). Their aftercare called for immobilization in a plaster cast for 12 weeks, with four weeks in bed with the foot elevated followed by weight-bearing in the plaster. The wires were removed some time after the third month from operation.

Palmer (1948) advocated open reduction, but used cancellous bone grafts from the ilium to prop up the reduced fragment. Again, he recommended immobilization

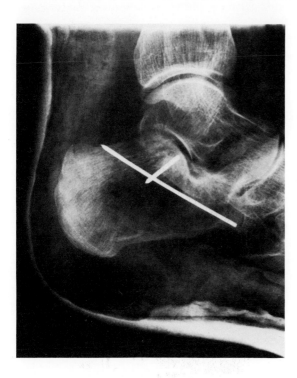

Fig. 11.59 Same as Fig. 11.39 after open reduction by the method of Soeur and Remy (1975).

in plaster for 12 weeks. Fisk (1981), in a series of 126 cases of depressed fractures of the posterior subtalar joint, favoured open reduction through a lateral incision and the insertion of an iliac bone graft. His recommended postoperative regimen differed from the above in that he continued immobilization for only 2–3 weeks to achieve sound wound healing and thereafter began mobilization. This approach seems more logical than one of prolonged rigid immobilization and is in accord with common practice after open reduction of the similar injury of plateau fracture of the knee. Fisk (1981) permits weight-bearing at six weeks. He claimed that osteoarthritis did not occur and that the subtalar joint remained mobile unless there was gross comminution or unless the calaneocuboid joint was involved in the fracture. He held that, even if there was too much comminution for hope of restoration of subtalar motion, correction of the height of the calcaneum and of valgus deformity and the production of a normal foot shape were important gains.

McReynolds (1972) described a method of open reduction from the medial side and of internal fixation with staples. It is probable that it is immaterial which method of fixation is employed (spike, wires, staples or bone block) provided that it remains secure. Certainly filling of the cavity within the crushed cancellous bone of the calcaneum is not essential to union and grafts are used for their mechanical properties.

With firm internal fixation and in accord with the view of Fisk (1981) it seems logical to propose non-weight-bearing exercises out of the plaster cast as soon as wound healing is assured. Weight-bearing would seem more safely deferred until the eighth week (Lance et al 1963).

The advantages of reduction methods, especially accurate open reduction, are that the shape of the foot is restored, including the anatomy of the subtalar joint, the heel size and shape and the contour of the lateral wall. This offers hope of restoration of the critical half range of joint motion and prevents the peroneal entrapment and calcaneofibular abutment problem. Performed through a lateral incision, the operation is less daunting than at first might seem.

Late operative procedures

These are principally indicated for persistent pain. Isbister (1974) clearly stated that lateral heel pain at the tip of the lateral malleolus and beginning when weight-bearing was commenced, was frequently due to bulging of the lateral wall of the calcaneum and abutment against the fibula, with perhaps also entrapment of the peronei. He pointed out that triple arthrodesis, by shortening the heel as the joints were excised, made the abutment worse. He suggested excision of the distal non-articular one centimetre of the tip of the lateral malleolus in these cases, reserving triple or subtalar fusion for those not relieved by the preliminary operation.

Triple or subtalar arthrodesis is the salvage procedure of choice in subtalar osteoarthritis, which typically produces a more diffuse pain felt on both sides of the heel and worse on eversion and inversion strains or on rough terrain. The posterior method of Gallie (1943) is the most suitable. Gallie obtained firm fusion in all but 6% of patients at three months from operation.

TALUS AND PERITALAR INJURIES

Classification

No fundamental change in classification is proposed and the scheme of Table 11.6 is a mixture from many authors. A terminology similar to that of carpal injuries is used. The incidence of the types of injuries is shown in Table 11.7.

Fractures

Avulsion fractures and fractures of the processes

Fracture of the lateral process of the talus This may occur in three degrees (Hawkins 1965): a single fracture involving only the posterior talocalcaneal joint (Fig. 11.60), a single fracture extending into both talocalcaneal and talofibular joints (Figs. 11.61, 11.62) and a comminuted fracture affecting an extensive part of the lateral process (Fig. 11.63). These fractures are caused by shearing forces and direct compression by the posterior subtalar facet of the calcaneum in forced dorsiflexion of the inverted foot (Hawkins 1965; Mukherjee *et al* 1974), probably combined with external rotation of the leg (Dimon 1961; Figs. 11.64, 11.65).

The injury is not due to avulsion of the attachments of the lateral ligaments, which do not insert into the lateral process, but more anteriorly (Fig. 11.69). Nor are they caused by impaction against the lateral malleolus during eversion, for they are not seen in association with abduction fracture of the lateral malleolus (Dimon 1961). However, they are seen combined with adduction (vertical) fractures of the medial malleolus (Hawkins 1965).

Clinically, they are characterized by swelling in the region of the lateral malleolus and tenderness just anterior to its tip.

Radiologically, they may not appear on lateral views, except for the type illustrated in Fig. 11.60, which shows against the sinus tarsi. They are better seen in oblique radiographs taken with the foot in 45° of internal rotation and 30° of plantarflexion. On anteroposterior views they may present a slight step in the articular surface of the talus below the lateral malleolus, but they do not appear in the mortise of the ankle joint (contrast avulsion fractures, see p. 247). Definitive treatment should be undertaken early (Mukherjee *et al* 1974). The optimum is the replacement of large pieces with a small screw (Dimon 1961) and the excision of small fragments. Conservative treatment offers a satisfactory solution in only half of the cases (Table 11.8).

Fracture of the posterior process of the talus This was said by Pennal (1963) to be due to compression between tibia and calcaneum in extreme plantarflexion. How-

Table 11.6 Classification of talar and peritalar injuries.

Name	Described by
Fractures	
Avulsion fractures	Dimon (1961); Hawkins (1964);
Fractures of the processes	Bigelow (1974); Mukherjee *et al* (1974)
Fractures of the head	
Fractures of the body:	
Transcorporeal	Dunn (1966)
Osteochondral	Marks (1952); Nisbet (1954);
	Berndt & Harty (1959); Rosenberg (1963);
	Mukherjee & Young (1973): stages 1–4
Transcervical fractures	Hawkins (1970): stage 1
	Canale & Kelly (1978): stage 1
Fracture–dislocations	
Dislocations of the subtalar joint	
Transcervical peritalar	Hawkins (1970): stage 2
dislocation of the tarsus	Canale & Kelly (1978): stage 2
Transcorporeal peritalar	Coltart (1952); Kenwright & Taylor (1970)
dislocation of the tarsus	
Dislocations of the (body of the) talus	
Transcervical dislocation	Detenbeck & Kelly (1969);
of the talus	Hawkins (1970): stage 3
	Canale & Kelly (1978): stage 3
Transcervical total	Canale & Kelly (1978): stage 4
dislocation of the talus	
Dislocations	
Peritalar dislocation of the tarsus	Penhallow (1937); Leitner (1955): stage 1
Dislocation of the talus	Mitchell (1936); Newcomb (1948);
	Leitner (1955): stage 3
	Detenbeck & Kelly (1969)

Note Coltart (1952), Mindell *et al* (1963), Kenwright & Taylor (1970) and Wilson (1976) include all the serious injuries listed above in their classifications.

ever, Ombredanne (1902) produced the injury experimentally most frequently (in 10 of 22 specimens, 45%) by a forced movement of dorsiflexion, internal rotation and adduction of the foot. The irregular outline of the fractured bone and the usual tilting of the fragment should distinguish it from the common congenitally separate os trigonum (os intermedium). As the posterior tubercle forms the lateral wall of the groove for the tendon of flexor hallucis longus and represents the posterior lip of the subtalar joint (Fig. 11.66), residual displacement may cause disability (compare the lateral process above). Early excision of the fragment is indicated.

Table 11.7 Incidence of the types of talar and peritalar injuries. (All figures are percentages unless otherwise indicated.)

	Miller & Baker (1939)	Coltart (1952)	Larson et al (1961)	Mindell et al (1963)	Pennal (1963)	Dunn et al (1966)	Detenbeck & Kelly (1969)	Hawkins (1970)	Kenwright & Taylor (1970)	Peterson et al (1977)	Canale & Kelly (1978)	Aggregate
Number of cases	28	217	20	40	98	34	9	57	48	46	71	668
Avulsion fractures and fractures of the processes	11	26			$22\frac{1}{2}$							12
Fractures of the head	11	3	5		6	9			4			3
Fractures of the body:												
Transcorporeal	39	7	30	$7\frac{1}{2}$	11	9			$8\frac{1}{2}$			8
Osteochondral		*			*	14						$\frac{1}{2}$
Transcervical fractures	7	17	35	20	$17\frac{1}{2}$	9		$10\frac{1}{2}$	$6\frac{1}{2}$	28	21	17
Dislocations of the subtalar joint:												
Transcervical peritalar dislocation of the tarsus		$17\frac{1}{2}$	25	$27\frac{1}{2}$	10	59		42	29	48	$42\frac{1}{2}$	26
Transcorporeal peritalar dislocation of the tarsus	7	3		$17\frac{1}{2}$					4			$2\frac{1}{2}$
Dislocations of the (body of the) talus:												
Transcervical dislocation of the talus	25	$14\frac{1}{2}$		†	$14\frac{1}{2}$		67	$47\frac{1}{2}$	$8\frac{1}{2}$	24	$32\frac{1}{2}$	$18\frac{1}{2}$
Transcervical total dislocation of the talus											4	$\frac{1}{2}$
Peritalar dislocation of the tarsus	8	8	5	20	$15\frac{1}{2}$	33			$35\frac{1}{2}$			9
Dislocation of the talus	4	4	5	$7\frac{1}{2}$	3	33			4			3

Note All but 17 of 685 cases ($2\frac{1}{2}\%$) in the literature quoted above may be classified in the above scheme.
* Osteochondral fractures included with avulsion and processes.
† Transcervical dislocation of the talus included with transcervical peritalar dislocation of the tarsus.

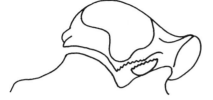
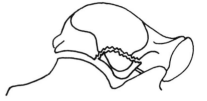

Fig. 11.60 (*Left*) Fracture of the lateral process of the talus, involving only the talocalcaneal joint surface.

Fig. 11.61 (*Right*) Fracture of the lateral process of the talus, involving both the talocalcaneal and the talofibular joints.

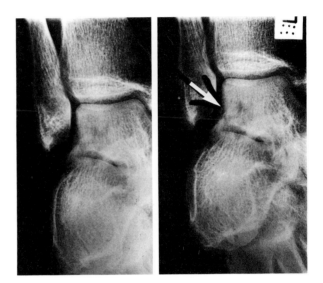

Fig. 11.62 Fracture of the lateral process of the talus.

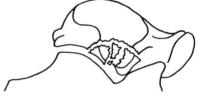

Fig. 11.63 Comminuted fracture of the lateral process of the talus.

Avulsion fractures of the talus These may occur near any of the joints, but are commonest on the top of the neck (Figs. 11.67, 11.69) at the attachment of the upper part of the anterior talofibular ligament or of the dorsal talonavicular ligament and on the medial surface of the body of the talus below and behind the tip of the medial malleolus (Fig. 11.68), at the attachment of the posterior talotibial liga-

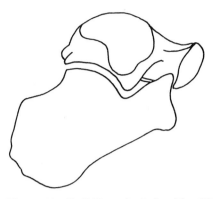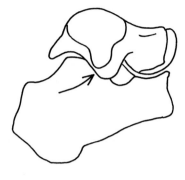

Fig. 11.64 (*Left*) Normal relationship of the posterior facet of the calcaneum to the lateral process of the talus.

Fig. 11.65 (*Right*) Same as Fig. 11.64, but in inversion, with the talus riding higher (more posteriorly) on the calcaneal facet. The edge of the calcaneal facet is applied to the articular surface of the talus which overhangs it. Forced dorsiflexion of the foot and external rotation of the leg will drive the calcaneum into the lateral process of the talus.

ment. Occasionally this medial shard is large enough to include the medial wall of the groove for the tendon of flexor hallucis longus and to block ankle motion (Coltart 1952) and then needs excision.

On the lateral aspect avulsion fractures are seen at the lower attachment of the anterior talofibular ligament just in front of the lateral malleolar articular surface of the talus (Fig. 11.69). These small fragments should be distinguished from the fracture of the lateral process of the talus. They appear on anteroposterior radiographs in the talofibular joint space (Fig. 11.70). Small extrasynovial avulsion fragments may be managed conservatively as for sprains, but larger intrasynovial pieces should be excised.

Fractures of the head of the talus

The head of the talus is fractured by longitudinal compression (Pennal 1963) and involves usually the medial and dorsal parts of the head. Three varieties have been

Table 11.8 Results of treatment of fractures of the lateral process of the talus.

	Number of cases	Method of treatment	Percentage satisfactory
Hawkins (1965)	13	Conservative	54
Mukherjee *et al* (1974)	13	Conservative	0
		Early operation	75
		Late operation	33

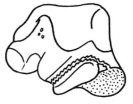

Fig. 11.66   Fracture of the posterior
process of the talus.

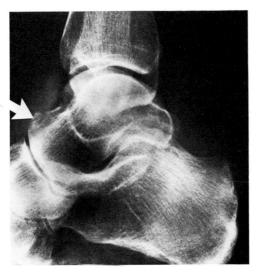

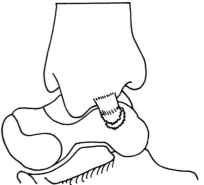

Fig. 11.67   (*Left*) Avulsion fracture of the upper surface of the neck of the talus.

Fig. 11.68   (*Right*) Avulsion fractures on the medial side of the talus.

noted: several undisplaced fissures may radiate through the head (Coltart 1952), or
a substantial piece of the head may be displaced either with (Coltart 1952) or
without dislocation of the triple joint complex (Kenwright & Taylor 1970; Figs.
11.71–11.73).

　　While undisplaced fractures can be treated by immobilization in a plaster cast
for 6 weeks (Dunn *et al* 1966), those with displacement should be replaced or excised
by operation to restore surface alignment in the talonavicular and triple joints
(Kenwright & Taylor 1970).

Transcorporeal fractures of the talus

Fractures of the talus present in two forms: transverse or oblique fissures (Morrison 1937; Coltart 1952; Dunn *et al* 1966) may be undisplaced or associated with
dislocation of the subtalar joint (Figs. 11.74–11.76), while comminution of the
whole body is seen after falls from a height (Pennal 1963; Fig. 11.77). 'Horizontal'

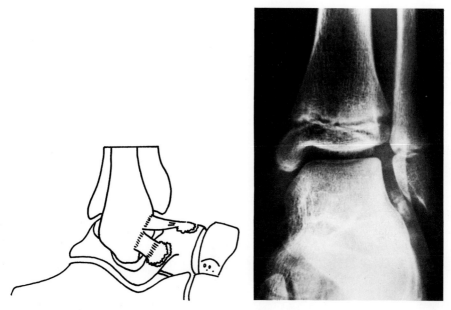

Fig. 11.69   (*Left*) Avulsion fractures on the lateral side of the talus.

Fig. 11.70   (*Right*) Avulsion fracture of the lateral side of the talus by the anterior talofibular ligament. The piece was excised.

fracture of the talus represents only the anteroposterior radiological view of a transcervical fracture with dislocation of the subtalar joint.

Undisplaced fractures may be managed by immobilization in a plaster cast for 6 weeks or more, but those associated with displacement and dislocation of the subtalar joint should be reduced and fixed internally as for fractures of the neck (see p. 260). Avascular necrosis of the body is a real risk (Coltart 1952; Table 11.9). Comminuted fractures which are unsalvagable are best treated by excision of the fragments and tibiocalcaneal fusion at about the fourth week. Most authors condemn astragalectomy (talectomy) alone.

Osteochondral fractures   Osteochondral fractures of the dome of the body of the talus were described by Berndt and Harty (1959), together with experimental work on their aetiology.

These injuries are uncommon, forming 0·8% of ankle fractures and dislocations (Mukherjee 1973), 0·09% of all fractures (Berndt & Harty 1973) or 8% of talar and navicular injuries (Marks 1952; Table 11.10).

They occur as two types and in two sites (Fig. 11.78). Lateral osteochondral fractures are elevated by leverage against the lateral malleolus during inversion strains with the ankle in dorsiflexion (Figs. 11.79–11.84), and usually present as

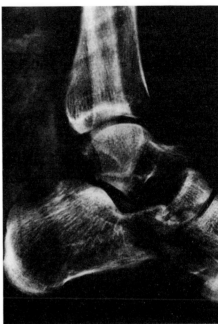

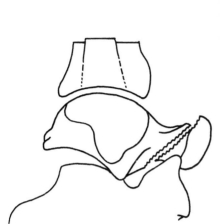

Fig. 11.71 (*Above left*) Fracture of
the head of the talus with
subluxation of the subtalar joint.

Fig. 11.72 (*Above right*) Fracture of
the head of the talus with
subluxation of the subtalar joint.

Fig. 11.73 Fracture of the head of
the talus with displacement of the
fragment, while the subtalar joint
remains intact.

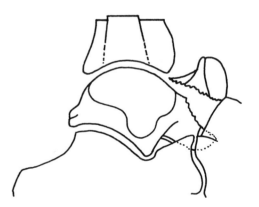

acute, symptomatic injuries (Rosenberg 1964). Medial osteochondral fractures are
rarely displaced, are caused by the compression and shearing impact of the tibia
and its medial malleolus on the posterior and medial margin of the talus during
strains combining inversion of the foot, plantarflexion of the ankle and external
rotation of the leg (Figs. 11.85–11.88). The compression fracture of the trabeculae
may not become visible on radiographs until absorption takes place. The fractures
are often asymptomatic and only half of the patients give a history of trauma.

In the acute stage, lateral osteochondral fractures present in a fashion similar
to sprains of the ankle, and indeed ligament damage is associated. Tenderness is

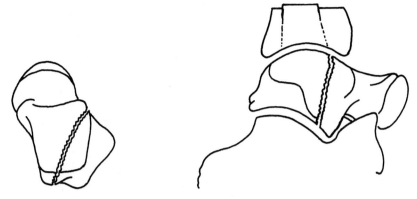

Fig. 11.74 (*Left*) Oblique, undisplaced transcorporeal fracture of the talus. Superior view.

Fig. 11.75 (*Right*) Same as Fig. 11.74. Lateral view.

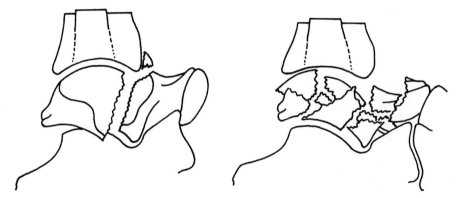

Fig. 11.76 (*Left*) Displaced transcorporeal fracture of the talus, with dislocation of the subtalar joint.

Fig. 11.77 (*Right*) Comminuted transcorporeal fracture of the talus.

anterior. In chronic cases symptoms are those of an ankle arthropathy or of locking.

A complete set of ankle radiographs is necessary to visualize all lesions. Anteroposterior views both in neutral position and in plantarflexion to show medial lesions and in neutral position combined with 10° of internal rotation to show lateral ones. Lateral views allow assessment of the size and the site of the lesion.

Berndt and Harty (1959) reported the results of the treatment of a large series of cases from the literature, which made it obvious that conservative management

Table 11.9. Incidence of avascular necrosis in talar and peritalar injuries. (All figures are percentage unless otherwise indicated.)

	Coltart (1952)	Larson *et al* (1961)	Mindell *et al* (1963)	Dunn *et al* (1966)	Hawkins (1970)	Kenwright & Taylor (1970)	Peterson *et al* (1977)	Canale & Kelly (1978)	Aggregate
Number of cases	130	20	38	31	57	44	46	67	433
Fractures of the head		0				0			0
Transcorporeal fractures	0	83				25			8
Transcervical fractures	0	57	20	0	0	0	0	13	$8\frac{1}{2}$
Dislocations of the subtalar joint									
Transcervical peritalar dislocation of the tarsus	$31\frac{1}{2}$	60	55	80	42	$36\frac{1}{2}$	$13\frac{1}{2}$	50	43
Transcorporeal peritalar dislocation of the tarsus	83		50	50		50			59
Dislocations of the talus									
Transcervical dislocation of the talus	93				91	75	27	84	67
Transcervical total dislocation of the talus								50	50
Peritalar dislocation of the tarsus	0	} 27				0			} 11
Dislocation of the talus	50	100				0			
Overall incidence of avascular necrosis	25	65	37	$64\frac{1}{2}$	72	20	13	51	$35\frac{1}{2}$

Table 11.10 Incidence of the two types of osteochondral fracture of the talus. (All figures are percentages unless otherwise indicated.)

	Berndt & Harty (1959)	Rosenberg (1965)
Number of cases	214 from the literature	38
Lateral osteochondral fractures	44	26
Medial osteochondral fractures	56	74

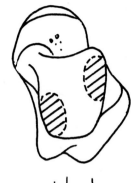

Fig. 11.78 The anterolateral and the posteromedial sites on the dome of the talus where osteochondral fractures occur.

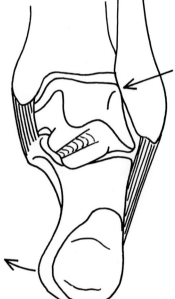

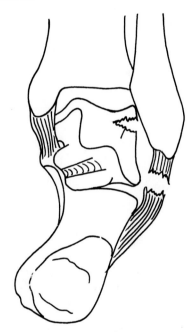

Fig. 11.79 (*Left*) Impact of the lateral edge of the talus on the fibular malleolus during inversion in ankle dorsiflexion.

Fig. 11.80 (*Right*) The osteochondral shard hinges upward as the calcaneofibular ligament ruptures.

was inappropriate. These lesions should be removed if small, and replaced and fixed internally if very large (Table 11.11).

Transcervical fractures of the talus

Fractures of the neck of the talus account for about 17% of talar injuries (Table 11.7), which themselves form about 6% of foot and ankle trauma (Coltart 1952). Thus transcervical fractures make up about 1% of foot injuries.

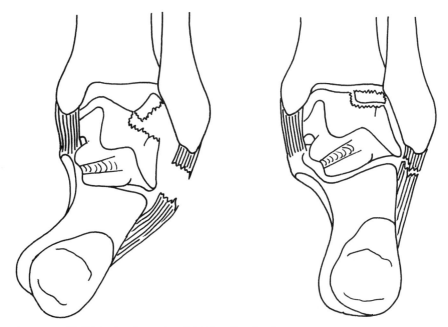

Fig. 11.81   (*Left*) Further inversion detatches the shard.

Fig. 11.82   (*Right*) Return of the foot to neutral leaves the shard loose in the joint or inverted in its bed.

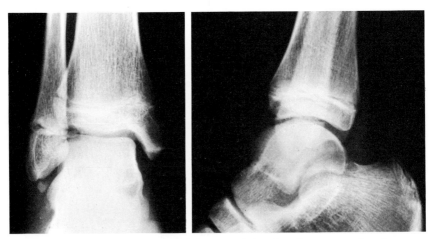

Fig. 11.83   (*Left*) Osteochondral fracture of the talus. Anteroposterior view.

Fig. 11.84   (*Right*) Same as Fig. 11.83. Lateral view.

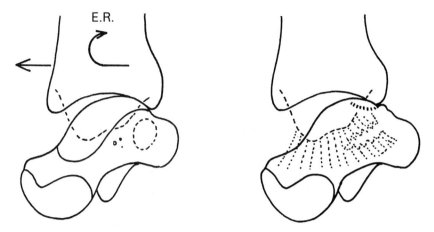

Fig. 11.85 (*Left*) With the foot in inversion and plantarflexion, external rotation of the leg impacts the posterior lip of the tibia tangentially against the posteromedial edge of the dome of the talus.

Fig. 11.86 (*Right*) Rupture of the posterior part of the deltoid ligament allows the tibia to plough into the surface of the talus.

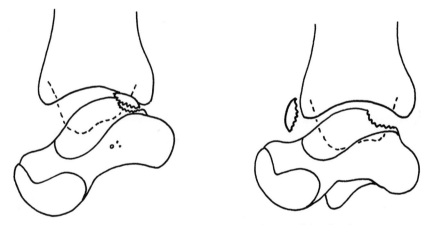

Fig. 11.87 (*Left*) Progression completes the detatchment of the shard.

Fig. 11.88 (*Right*) Return of the foot to neutral leaves the shard loose in the joint.

Aetiology Classical theory holds that these fractures are caused by acute dorsi-flexion of the ankle, breaking the neck of the talus against the anterior lip of the tibia (Coltart 1952; Pennal 1963; Hawkins 1970). This theory is almost certainly incorrect.

The talus is the most robust of the tarsal bones. Forcible dorsiflexion of the ankle combined with compression causes a fracture of the *tibia* by the talus!

Table 11.11. Results of treatment of osteochondral fractures of the talus. (From Berndt & Harty 1959.)

Treatment	Number of cases	Results				Requiring some secondary operation (%)
		Good		Fair & poor		
		No.	(%)	No.	(%)	
Conservative	154	26	17	128	83	33
Operative	72	47	84	9	16	3

Burwell & Charnley (1965), when discussing pronation–dorsiflexion injuries of the ankle joint, state ' . . . pressure from the upper surface of the talus causes fracture of the anterior part of the tibial articular surface'.

In cases of transcervical fracture of the talus, Schrock (1952) and Peterson *et al* (1977) noted that one did not see the minor impact damage to the lip of the tibia which might have been expected. Ombredanne (1902) could produce only one transcervical fracture of the talus in 42 specimens subjected to forced dorsiflexion, although he did produce other talar injuries (Table 11.12). Peterson & Romanus (1976) carried out experimental work on cadaveric feet to determine the mechanism of this fracture. They simulated the localized rudder bar–foot pedal impact body so commonly involved with a heavy pendulum, arranged to strike the sole of the dorsiflexed foot at a point just distal to the level of the anterior margin of the tibia (Fig. 11.89). A variety of injuries was obtained, including fracture of the distal tibia, but no transcervical fracture of the talus (Table 11.12). Obviously force was not concentrated in the neck of the talus and some additional mechanism was involved. The shod cadaveric foot was fixed so that the ankle joint could not move, by stressing the forefoot and the heel with turnbuckles applied to an ordinary shoe (Fig. 11.90). In these circumstances the localized blow produced transcervical fracture in 6 of 9 consecutive tests (67%), and the three failures were explicable by errors of technique. Contact with the lip of the tibia did not occur. The necessary ankle rigidity is provided in an accident situation by the tendency of the victim to extend the legs and to press down with the feet in involuntary bracing motions just before the impact, the calf muscles acting in the same manner as the turnbuckle of the experiment.

The factors necessary may be summarized as:

1   The accident involve high kinetic energies, e.g. a car or aeroplane crash (Table 11.13).

2   The victim be in a state of emergency reaction, i.e. rigidly extended limb with the joints fixed by muscular action.

3   The arch of the foot be poised on a small impact body, e.g. the pedal of the car or the rudder bar of an aircraft.

Table 11.12 Experimental fractures.

	Peterson & Romanus (1976)	Ombredanne (1902)			Totals
	Forced dorsiflexion alone	Forced d'flexion alone	D'flexion + internal rotation + adduction	D'flexion + external rotation + abduction	
Fractures					
TALUS					
Transcervical	1				1
Transcorporeal				1	1
Inner face of talus	1			1	2
POSTERIOR TUBERCLE					
Inner lip		3	6	6	15
Outer lip		2	4	1	7
MALLEOLI					
Medial	2	4	1	10	17
Lateral	8	4	2	3	17
Tibia: Distal end shaft	7				7
Calcaneum	6				6
Joint injuries					
Ligament rupture or avulsion		2	1	3	6
Ankle subluxation	3				3
Subtalar subluxation		1			1
Totals					
Number of injuries	26	18	14	25	83
Number of feet	20	13	9	20	62

Fracture-dislocations

Transcervical peritalar dislocation of the tarsus

Once fracture of the neck of the talus has occurred (Figs. 11.91–11.93) and the momentary involuntary tension in the tendo-Achilles is released by inhibition by pain (Peterson & Romanus 1976), dorsiflexion can take place with secondary displacements. With impaction of the body of the talus in the ankle mortise (Pennal 1963) and with rupture of the posterior talocalcaneal ligament, the calcaneum, the talar head and the foot slide forward and sideways into inversion (Coltart 1952) producing transcervical peritalar dislocation of the tarsus (Figs. 11.94–11.95). In

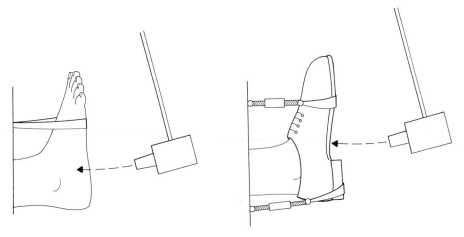

Fig. 11.89   (*Left*) The initial experiment of Peterson & Romanus (1976).

Fig. 11.90   (*Right*) The later experiment in which fixation of the foot by pretensioning the heel and forefoot allowed the pendulum to produce transcervical fracture of the talus.

these circumstances the talus becomes plantarflexed relative to the dorsiflexing foot, with its fractured surface resting on the calcaneum (Pennal 1963).

Transcervical dislocation of the talus

Alternatively, with continuing dorsiflexion, the ankle and the subtalar joints gape posteriorly and the posterior ligaments joining to tibia, fibula and calcaneum all rupture. The body of the talus is forced backward, swinging on the deltoid ligament (Pennal 1963) and following the curve of the posterior subtalar articular facet of the calcaneum. It is so directed that its underside faces downward and outward,

Table 11.13   Incidence of road accidents and aviation crashes in all types of transcervical injury of the talus.

Author & date	Number of cases	Road accidents No.	(%)	Aviation crashes No.	(%)
Detenbeck & Kelly (1969)	9	6	67	1	11
Hawkins (1970)	55	33	60	5	9
Kenwright & Taylor (1970)	58	25	43	3	5
Peterson *et al* (1977)	46	26	57	0	0
Overall totals	168	90	54	9	5

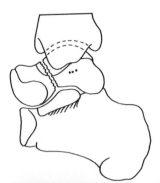

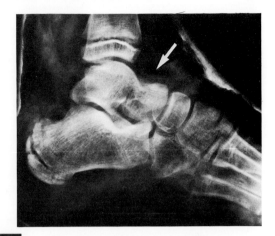

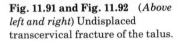

Fig. 11.91 and Fig. 11.92 (*Above left and right*) Undisplaced transcervical fracture of the talus.

Fig. 11.93 Slightly displaced transcervical fracture of the talus. Note the gap at the fracture line and the associated ankle and tibial injuries.

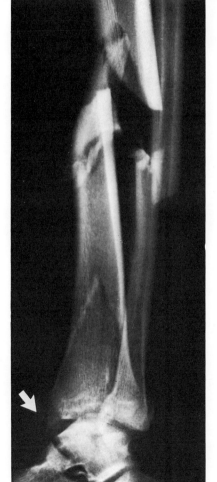

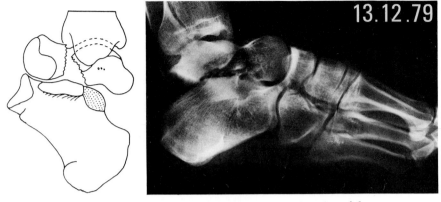

Fig. 11.94 and Fig. 11.95   Transcervical peritalar dislocation of the tarsus.

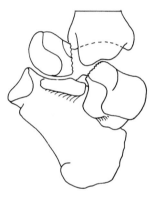

Fig. 11.96   Transcervical
dislocation of the talus. Note how
the body of the talus escapes
posteromedially from the
tibiocalcaneal gap, being guided
there by the shape of the posterior
facet of the calcaneum and the
deltoid ligament.

and the fractured surface of its neck upward and outward. When the foot is
released and springs back to a neutral position, the talar body remains jammed
behind the sustentaculum tali in the position of established transcervical dislocation of the talus (Fig. 11.96). This is more easily understood by reference to the
dried, disarticulated skeleton of the foot.

The management of fractures and fracture–dislocations of the talus   Undisplaced
transcervical fracture of the talus may be treated by immobilization in a plaster
cast until union is complete. While some transcervical peritalar dislocations,
reduced early and accurately, may be treated in a similar fashion, a plaster cast in
the equinus posture is necessary. If attempts are made to bring up the foot into a
neutral position, redisplacement at the level of the neck may occur.

   To avoid the undesirable equinus posture, to prevent redisplacement, and in
cases where accurate reduction has not been obtained, open reduction with internal fixation should be undertaken. A screw is easily inserted through a nonarticu-

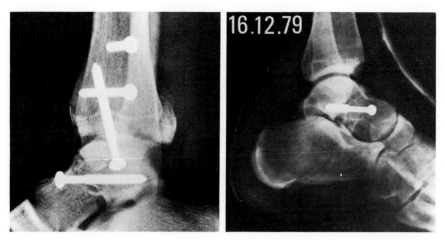

Fig. 11.97 (*Left*) Same as Fig. 11.93 after open reduction and internal fixation of all three injuries.

Fig. 11.98 (*Right*) Same as Fig. 11.95 after open reduction and internal fixation with a screw.

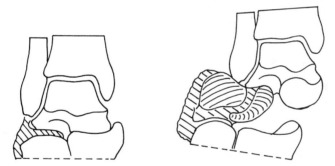

Fig. 11.99 (*Left*) Diagrammatic anterior view of the normal disposition of the ankle and triple joints. This forms the starting point of the two series of Leitner (1955). It is recommended that the diagrams be followed with the disarticulated dried bones to hand.

Fig. 11.100 (*Right*) Lateral peritalar dislocation of the tarsus. The talocalcaneal and talonavicular joints are dislocated, but the calcaneocuboid joint is intact. The foot is markedly displaced to the lateral side, but only slightly everted (pronated).

lar area (Figs. 11.97, 11.98) or stout Kirschner wires may be used (McKeever 1963; Pennal 1963). Transcervical dislocation of the talus should be managed by immediate reduction. Although Pennal (1963) described a technique of reduction by strong dorsiflexion of the foot, distraction and eversion of the calcaneum with a Steinman pin in the heel and direct pressure over the displaced body of the bone, it is likely that open reduction will be needed. If so, internal fixation of the fracture should be added. Avascular necrosis of the body may well follow (Hawkins 1970; Table 11.9). Hawkin's sign (see p. 270) is useful in diagnosis.

To avoid collapse of the avascular bone, weight-bearing should be prohibited for many months. A patellar-bearing calliper may be a useful way of avoiding prolonged use of crutches. This complication is discussed on p. 270.

Transcorporeal dislocation of the tarsus is rare ($2\frac{1}{2}\%$ of talar injuries) and is managed on principles similar to those for the transcervical injury. Risks of avascular necrosis are greater and the prospects of a satisfactory outcome are less than with the transcervical injury.

Transcervical total dislocation of the talus is described only by Canale and Kelly (1978) as their stage 4 injury. All three cases were compound injuries, presumably amenable to open reduction, and all did badly.

Disclocations

Dislocations around the talus were described by Leitner (1955), who postulated that dislocation of the triple joint was the first stage of a total dislocation of the talus. The sequence which he described may be summarized as follows:

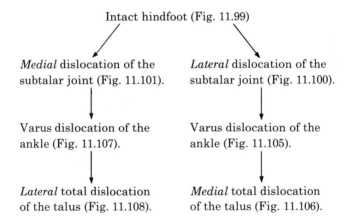

Intact hindfoot (Fig. 11.99)

Medial dislocation of the subtalar joint (Fig. 11.101).

Lateral dislocation of the subtalar joint (Fig. 11.100).

Varus dislocation of the ankle (Fig. 11.107).

Varus dislocation of the ankle (Fig. 11.105).

Lateral total dislocation of the talus (Fig. 11.108).

Medial total dislocation of the talus (Fig. 11.106).

Peritalar dislocation of the tarsus

The dislocation may occur to either side, but is more common to the lateral side with forcible movements of plantarflexion and eversion. In lateral peritalar dislocation the foot is displaced laterally and moderately everted, but not usually abducted (so in only one-fifth of cases, Leitner 1955) (Fig. 11.100). In medial peritalar dislocation, due to plantarflexion and inversion, the foot lies in strong inversion (Figs. 11.101–11.104). These simple dislocations are easily reduced by closed methods and remain stable. A period of rest in a plaster cast followed by physiotherapy to remobilize the joints is appropriate. Avascular necrosis seldom occurs and results are usually satisfactory (Tables 11.9, 11.14).

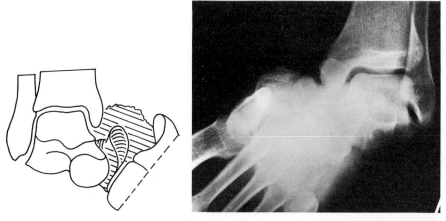

Fig. 11.101 (*Left*) Medial peritalar dislocation of the tarsus. The same joints are dislocated as in Fig. 11.100 but to the opposite side. The foot is strongly inverted (supinated), indicated by the dotted line.

Fig. 11.102 (*Right*) Medial peritalar dislocation of the tarsus.

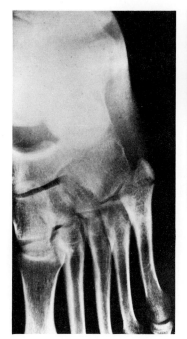

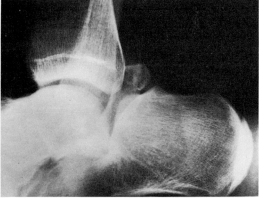

Fig. 11.103 (*Left*) Posteromedial and plantarward peritalar dislocation of the tarsus. Note the avulsion of the styloid of the fifth metatarsal.

Fig. 11.104 (*Right*) Same as Fig. 11.103. Note the avulsion of the posterior process of the talus.

A rare form of plantar peritalar dislocation of the triple joint was described by Main and Jowett (1975) as an extension of plantar mid-tarsal dislocation if the interosseous talocalcaneal ligament becomes torn.

Dislocation of the talus

Leitner (1955) studied 42 cases of peritalar dislocation and found six cases (14%) of simultaneous ankle joint instability, unsuspected until varus strain radiographs of the ankle were taken. He postulated that there was no special type of injury which led to total dislocation of the talus, but that this injury was due to continuation of the same forces which had produced the preliminary peritalar dislocation. He pointed out that it was unlikely that the ankle should dislocate first, as Coltart (1952) thought, as then the talus would have no tendency to separate from the tarsus.

He demonstrated that, after either type of peritalar dislocation, and regardless of the final position into which the talus dislocated, the talus quitted the ankle joint always by a movement of inversion (supination, varus). In cadaveric experiments he found that the medial malleolus and the calcaneum acted as obstacles to eversion (pronation, valgus) dislocation of the bone when the subtalar joint was dislocated medially. He envisaged the steps of the injury as in Figs. 11.105–11.108 (see captions for details).

Dislocation of the talus is a severe injury and, if not compound from the beginning, may well become so due to skin necrosis. Even if reduction can be obtained, avascular necrosis is highly likely. No less than 7 of 9 cases of Coltart (1952) were treated by astragalectomy and of the two which were not, one became avascular. Of the three cases of Pennal (1963) one was reduced, but developed avascular necrosis with a poor result, one was treated with primary tibiocalcaneal fusion and the third suffered amputation for recurrent infection.

It is difficult to be dogmatic about the best advice in so rare an injury. Probably the optimum management is early tibiocalcaneal fusion. The results of the treatment of talar injuries are summarized in Table 11.14.

The blood supply of the talus

Extra-osseous

The extra-osseous blood supply of the talus is derived from the three main foot arteries: the anterior tibial (dorsalis pedis), the posterior tibial and the peroneal (through its perforating branch).

On the medial side (Fig. 11.109) the artery of the tarsal canal is a large, constant branch of the posterior tibial artery (present in 13 of 14 (93%) dissections by Haliburton 1958), which enters the tarsal canal between talus and calcaneum and which anastomoses with the artery of the tarsal sinus. From the artery of the tarsal canal a large deltoid branch enters the medial side of the body of the talus

Table 11.14 Results of treatment of talar and peritalar injuries. (All figures are percentage unless otherwise indicated.)

	Miller & Baker (1939)	Mindell et al (1963)	Hawkins (1970)	Kenwright & Taylor (1970)	Mukherjee et al (1974)	Peterson et al (1977)	Canale & Kelly (1978)	Aggregate
				Percentage of results which were satisfactory				
Number of cases	27	40	43	44	12	36	71	273
Avulsion fractures and fracture of the processes	100							67
Fracture of the head	33			100	58			60
Fractures of the body								
Transcorporeal	40	*		50				43
Osteochondral								
Transcervical fractures	100	82	100	100		75	93	87
Dislocations of the subtalar joint								
Transcervical peritalar dislocation of tarsus		64	44	73		$31\frac{1}{2}$	57	52
Transcorporeal peritalar dislocation of tarsus	0	29		0				18
Dislocations of the talus								
Transcervical dislocation of talus	29	50	15	75		$55\frac{1}{2}$	48	38
Transcervical total dislocation of talus							0	0
Peritalar dislocation of tarsus		73		$87\frac{1}{2}$				} 83
Dislocation of talus		†		100				
Overall satisfactory results	44	60	37	77		47	59	$56\frac{1}{2}$

* Transcorporeal fractures included with transcervical fractures.
† Dislocation of talus included with peritalar dislocation of tarsus.

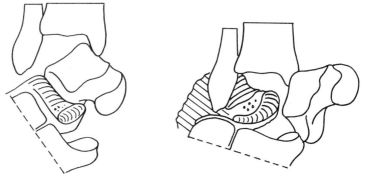

Fig. 11.105 (*Left*) Progression of the lateral peritalar dislocation to include adduction (supination) subluxation of the ankle joint. Note that the foot is now more strongly everted. As the foot everts the sustentaculum tali engages against the lateral process of the talus and rolls it out of the ankle mortise into adduction (varus).

Fig. 11.106 (*Right*) Medial dislocation of the talus. The injuries shown in Fig. 11.100 and Fig. 11.105 form the earlier stages of this. As the foot swings back from its position of extreme eversion, it pushes the subluxated talus medially. The talus lies anteromedial to the ankle with its trochlea facing laterally.

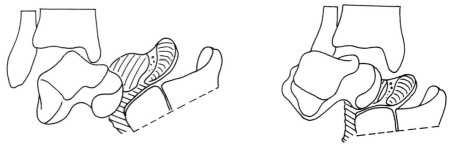

Fig. 11.107 (*Left*) Progression of the medial peritalar dislocation to include adduction (supination) subluxation of the ankle joint. The foot is less strongly inverted and more markedly displaced medially.

Fig. 11.108 (*Right*) Lateral dislocation of the talus. The injuries shown in Fig. 11.101 and Fig. 11.107 form the earlier stages of this. As the foot returns under the leg, the subluxated talus is pushed laterally. The talus lies anterolateral to the ankle with its trochlea facing laterally, its head medially, and its calcaneal surface backward.

just below the medial malleolus (present in 20 of 30 dissections by Mulfinger & Trueta 1970).

From the posterior tibial artery itself, branches supply the posterior tuberosity of the talus. From the medial tarsal branch of the doralis pedis artery, and from this vessel itself, twigs enter the head and neck of the talus and anastomose with the deltoid artery.

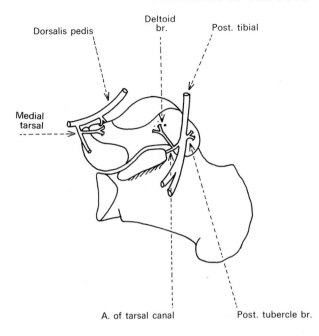

Dorsalis pedis

Deltoid br.

Post. tibial

Medial tarsal

A. of tarsal canal

Post. tubercle br.

Fig. 11.109 The medial side of the talus with its blood vessels.

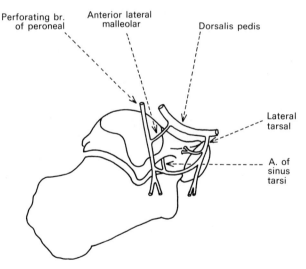

Perforating br. of peroneal

Anterior lateral malleolar

Dorsalis pedis

Lateral tarsal

A. of sinus tarsi

Fig. 11.110 The lateral side of the talus with its blood vessels.

On the lateral side (Fig. 11.110) the artery of the tarsal sinus arises from the anastomotic vessel linking the perforating peroneal artery to the lateral tarsal artery (Mulfinger & Trueta 1970; Peterson *et al* 1974) or from the anterior lateral malleolar artery (anterior tibial artery) or from the perforating peroneal artery itself (Haliburton 1958). Branches from the lateral tarsal artery enter the head and the anterolateral side of the body of the talus.

Superiorly, tributaries from the dorsalis pedis artery or its medial tarsal branch enter the top of the neck of the bone.

Intra-osseous

The intra-osseous vessels of the talus 'form a richly interconnected system of branches' and 'interconnection of the interosseous vessels is distributed in a way which gives no impression of segmental delineation based on the source from which the anastomotic vessels arise' (Peterson *et al* 1974). The main supply into the body of the bone is derived from the artery of the tarsal canal by a vessel entering the roof of the canal (Haliburton *et al* 1958) and via the deltoid branch (Mulfinger & Trueta 1970). The main supply of the head is from the artery of the tarsal sinus or via the anterolateral surface of the neck. Haliburton (1958) feels that the importance of branches entering the superior surface of the neck has been exaggerated.

Peterson *et al* (1974) pointed out many ligamentous vessels linking the talus with the intra-osseous networks of the tibia and the navicular.

A study of the vessels in relation to experimentally-produced fractures of the neck of the talus in eleven feet, was carried out by Peterson & Goldie (1975). In undisplaced transcervical fracture all the main vessels remained intact, but the intra-osseous network was always destroyed at the fracture line. In displaced transcervical fracture the arteries of the tarsal canal and of the tarsal sinus disintegrated at the fracture site and in all specimens their ascending twigs were torn. Similarly, in displaced fractures, the descending branches from the dorsalis pedis artery were ruptured, although the main artery escaped damage.

In five cases with little or no displacement of the transcervical fracture, there was no disturbance of the interosseous capsular vessels. In one case with great displacement, the anterior but not the posterior capsular vessels were ruptured. Hawkins (1970) considered that of three routes by which blood might reach the talus, one was lost each time the injury advanced from group 1 to group 3 in his classification (Table 11.9).

Potential problems and treatment after injuries of the talus

These were well documented by McKeever (1963), Dunn *et al* (1966) and Canale and Kelly (1978), and include: primary skin injury or pressure necrosis, infection (following skin problems or postoperatively); inadequate reduction or redisplacement during treatment; mal-union, either dorsal or varus, following poor or unstable reduction; delayed or non- union, avascular necrosis; osteoarthritis of the subtalar or ankle joints.

The skin

A quarter of all major talar injuries are open and this proportion is higher when there is dislocation of the talus (Table 11.15). Similarly, in displaced but closed

Table 11.15 Compound injuries of the talus.

Author & date	Type of injury	Number of cases	Compound cases No.	Compound cases (%)	Incidence of infection No.	Incidence of infection (%)
Detenbeck & Kelly (1969)	Dislocation of the talus	9	7	78	7	78
Kenwright & Taylor (1970)	Major injuries	58	13	22	2	$3\frac{1}{2}$
Birt & Townsend (1976)	Major fractures	22	4	18	0	0
Canale & Kelly (1978)	Transcervical dislocations	71	17	24	5	7
Overall totals		160	41	26	14	9

injuries, the projecting bone may so stretch the intact skin that necrosis rapidly ensues. Such severe injuries as these produce extensive ecchymosis and oedema, adding to skin tension. Prompt reduction of the lesion is essential. If necrosis does occur the skin should be replaced at once by flap repair (e.g. the gracilis musculocutaneous flap of Orticochea 1972) with the assistance of the plastic surgeon, or cover obtained by local muscle pedicle techniques (e.g. the abductor hallucis transfer of Ger 1971). Delay is likely to result in infection.

Infection

Once the injured and possibly avascular talus becomes infected, any conservative surgery is doomed to failure (McKeever 1963). Radical treatment is needed.

Astragalectomy gives poor results as a definitive procedure (Detenbeck & Kelly 1969; Canale & Kelly 1978). Coltart (1952) reported 25 astragalectomies among 166 cases of talar injury and only 6 of 22 reviewed gave a good result (27%), and those only because they had developed a firm tibiocalcaneal ankylosis.

The best final treatment probably is formal tibiocalcaneal fusion after preliminary astragalectomy to clear the infection.

Inadequate reduction, redisplacement, mal-union and delayed union

Dunn *et al* (1966) pointed out the need for complete radiological assessment of the quality of the reduction of talar fractures. This may include comparison views of the opposite foot. He found tomograms useful in assessing union. On anteroposterior views angulation of the neck may be detected. On lateral projections rotatory deformity may be revealed as distortion of the characteristic shape of the talus, with the head and neck appearing broader.

Dunn *et al* (1966) point out that, if a portion of the interosseous talocalcaneal ligament in the sinus tarsi remains intact and retains its anterior attachment to the head, it will maintain the head in correct alignment on the calcaneum. If the entire ligament is torn the distal talar fragment is able to rotate and closed reduction is made more difficult.

McKeever (1963) showed that redisplacement of transcervical fractures may occur easily in plaster casts and resulted in dorsal mal-union, which restricts dorsiflexion at the ankle joint. Both he and Dunn *et al* (1966) favoured internal fixation to prevent this problem and to obviate prolonged external fixation in equinus. Pennal (1963) noticed that associated malleolar fractures may impair the stability of transcervical fractures of the talus and recommended internal fixation of both injuries (Fig. 11.97). Canale and Kelly (1978) reported 18 cases of dorsal mal-union from 71 cases (25%) of all types of transcervical fracture, in eleven of whom treatment had been conservative. Some relief of the limitation of ankle dorsiflexion was gained in three cases by excision of the prominence on the top of the neck of the talus. They also reported 14 cases of varus mal-union with prominence of the fibula and some rotatory deformity. Five of these cases suffered painful secondary osteoarthritis in the subtalar joint.

Mindell *et al* (1963) found that the average time to union in transcervical fracture of the talus was five months. Delay in union was noted in association with comminution or a gap at the fracture line and with avascular necrosis. Kenwright and Taylor (1970) noted four cases of delayed union in transcervical peritalar dislocation of the tarsus ($7\frac{1}{2}$%) and Hawkins (1970) three cases among 27 of his group 3 injuries (11%).

Avascular necrosis

The classical radiological sign of this complication, relative density of the body of the talus, is slow to appear. Hawkins (1970) popularized a relatively early and favourable sign of the *absence* of avascular necrosis. This sign appeared positive on radiographs taken 6–8 weeks after injury as a zone of subchondral osteoporosis in the dome of the talus on anteroposterior views. This was presumed to be the ordinary disuse porosis able to take place because of preservation of a blood supply.

Canale and Kelly (1978) showed that of 23 cases of transcervical fracture with Hawkins sign positive within 12 weeks of injury, only one (4%) developed avascular necrosis. Conversely, of 26 cases with the sign negative, 20 (77%) suffered the complication. In those likely to develop the complication, the incidence rises with the severity of the initial injury (Table 11.9). Revascularization proceeds over a period of two or three years (McKeever 1963). Treatment of the complication is controversial and results discouraging (Table 11.16). Conservative measures include prolonged non-weight-bearing with crutches, immobilization in plaster casts or in a brace and therapeutic inactivity (Table 11.17).

Astragalectomy while possible is not favoured, so that practical surgical

Table 11.16 Results of treatment of talar and peritalar injuries in cases with avascular necrosis.

	Percentage of results which were satisfactory			
	Hawkins (1970)		Canale & Kelly (1978)	
	No. of cases	% satisfactory	No. of cases	% satisfactory
Transcervical fractures			2	100
Transcervical peritalar dislocation of the tarsus	6	0	21	48
Transcervical dislocation of the talus	18	17		
Overall satisfactory results	24	$12\frac{1}{2}$	23	52

treatment includes only various fusions. Ankle or subtalar arthrodesis or both (Miller & Baker 1939; Schrock 1952), fusion of the talar head to the tibia (Blair 1943; Morris *et al* 1971) (Fig. 11.111) and tibiocalcaneal fusion (Coltart 1952; Detenbeck & Kelly 1969) have been suggested. Certainly early subtalar arthrodesis does not hasten revascularization (Pennal 1963; Morris *et al* 1971). Probably the best alternatives are the Blair operation and tibiocalcaneal fusion.

Morris *et al* (1971) performed ten modified Blair operations, eight for fracture-dislocation and two for avascular necrosis, resulting in satisfaction in all, with solid talotibial fusion in all, a 10–20° range of residual hinge motion and about a half range of inversion–eversion movement, in a foot of near normal, unshortened appearance. They advocate the operation for established avascular necrosis in transcervical fracture (Hawkins group 1) or in transcervical peritalar dislocation of the tarsus (Hawkins group 2) and as a delayed primary treatment (at 4–6 weeks after primary excision of the body) in transcervical dislocation of the talus (Hawkins group 3).

Table 11.17 Results of conservative treatment for avascular necrosis of the talus. (From Canale & Kelly 1978)

Treatment	Number of cases	Percentage satisfactory
No special treatment (full weight-bearing)	8	25
Brace or cast (partial weight-bearing)	6	33
Prolonged non-weight-bearing	9	89

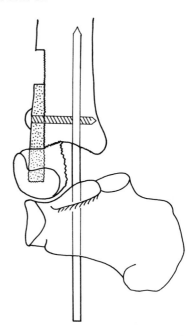

Fig. 11.111 The Morris (1971)
modification of the Blair (1943)
talotibial fusion operation.

Osteoarthritis

Degenerative arthritis in the peritalar joints presents as limitation of movement
and typical radiological signs (Fig. 11.112), with or without pain. Canale & Kelly
(1978) found some evidence of this in about half of their series of 71 cases. As
predisposing factors they noted the severity and type of the initial injury, fracture
of the dome of the talus, mal-union, associated ankle injuries (Fig. 11.113) and
avascular necrosis. If symptoms are severe arthrodesis of the affected joint or
joints is indicated.

THE MIDTARSUS

Injuries of the midtarsus include fractures of cuboid and navicular and sprains,
instability and dislocations of the talonavicular and calcaneocuboid joints. Also
included is comminuted fracture of the anterior end of the calcaneum. The best
classification of these injuries is that of Main and Jowett (1975), who divide them
into five groups by the type and direction of the causative violence (Table 11.18).
The relative incidence of the types is displayed in Table 11.19.

Sprains

Sprains of the midtarsal joint caused by forced inversion and plantarflexion of the

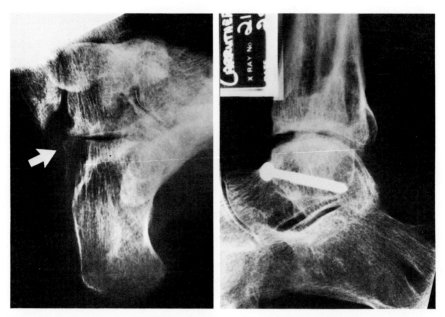

Fig. 11.112 (*Left*) Osteoarthritis of the subtalar joint secondary to fracture of the head of talus with subluxation of the subtalar joint.

Fig. 11.113 (*Right*) Same as Fig. 11.93. 2 years 9 months later the transcervical fracture is united, but there are osteoarthritic changes in the ankle joint. There is no evidence of avascular necrosis.

foot, avulse fragments from the lateral margins of the calcaneum or cuboid or from the top of the talus or navicular (attachment of the dorsal talonavicular ligament). Conversely, sprains due to forcible eversion after low falls give rise to avulsion fractures of the navicular tuberosity or of flakes from the dorsum of the talus or navicular together with impaction fractures of the lateral margins of calcaneum or cuboid or both. Sprains due to laterally directed force are potentially more serious than those caused by medially directed ones. Care must be taken to avoid misdiagnosis of lateral fracture–dislocation as a sprain.

Forcible plantarflexion of the midfoot commonly involves the tarsometatarsal region (see p. 283), but strain may fall on the midtarsal joint, with fragments avulsed from the dorsum of talus and navicular or the front of the calcaneum. Longitudinal and crushing forces do not produce this type of injury.

Midtarsal sprains produce considerable reaction in the foot with bruising and oedema out of proportion to the radiological appearance. It is advisable to rest the foot in a plaster cast for 3–4 weeks before remobilizing the patient. As with fractures of the front of the calcaneum (Dachtler 1931), too early unsupported use of the foot may precipitate prolonged disability. A temporary valgus insole may increase foot comfort during rehabilitation.

Table 11.18   Classification of midtarsal injuries. (From Main and Jowett 1975)

Direction of or type of force	Type of injury
Medially directed	Inversion sprains
	Avulsion fractures
	Medial dislocation
	Medial swivel dislocation
Laterally directed	Eversion sprains
	Avulsion fractures
	Avulsion of the navicular tuberosity
	Lateral fracture–dislocation
	Lateral swivel dislocation
Longitudinal	Fracture of the navicular
	Fracture–dislocation of the navicular
Plantarward	Sprains
	Avulsion fractures
	Plantar dislocation
Crushing	No constant pattern of fracture
Isolated dislocation	Medial dislocation of navicular
	Inferomedial dislocation of cuboid
Stress fracture	Vertical stress fracture of navicular

Fracture–dislocations of the midtarsal joint

Corresponding to the directions of violence producing the sprains, more severe strain will produce dislocation of the midtarsal joint, perhaps accompanied by fractures of the adjacent bones.

In medial midtarsal dislocation the foot is displaced inward, while the hindfoot bones remain in their normal relationship to each other and to the tibia (Figs. 11.114, 11.115, 11.118). Reduction and immobilization in a plaster cast for 4–6 weeks followed by rehabilitation is satisfactory management. In lateral midtarsal dislocation there is usually a notable fracture component, with lateral dislocation of the talonavicular joint and collapse of the lateral column of the foot due to comminution either of the cuboid or of the front end of the calcaneum (Main & Jowett 1975; Dewar & Evans 1968; Hermel & Gershon-Cohen 1953). The navicular tuberosity is frequently avulsed (Figs. 11.116, 11.117).

Dewar and Evans (1968) noted that this injury was frequently missed if the dislocation had reduced spontaneously. Instability of the whole midtarsus may be demonstrated by abduction strain radiographs under anaesthesia. Both Main and Jowett (1975) and Dewar and Evans (1968) advocate stabilization of the lateral column of the foot by primary arthrodesis of the calcaneocuboid joint and by replacement and internal fixation of the navicular tuberosity.

With plantarflexion violence applied to the foot, dislocation at the midtarsal joint is uncommon. For the injury to occur the interosseous talocalcaneal ligament

Table 11.19 Incidence of the types of midtarsal injury. (All figures are percentages unless otherwise indicated.)

	P.Wilson (1933)	Eichenoltz & Levine (1964)	Main & Jowett (1975)	Nine other authors	Aggregate
Number of cases	20	66	71	33	190
Medial					
Sprains	5		$15\frac{1}{2}$		$6\frac{1}{2}$
Dislocation			4		$1\frac{1}{2}$
Swivel			10		$3\frac{1}{2}$
Lateral					
Sprains		47	10		20
Fracture–dislocation	15		$5\frac{1}{2}$	52	$12\frac{1}{2}$
Swivel			$1\frac{1}{2}$		$\frac{1}{2}$
Fracture of tuberosity of navicular		24			$8\frac{1}{2}$
Longitudinal					
Navicular	80	29	7	3	$11\frac{1}{2}$
Fracture–dislocation of navicular			34	21	27
Plantar					
Sprains			3		1
Dislocation			4	3	2
Crush			$5\frac{1}{2}$	6	3
Dislocation of cuboid				3	$\frac{1}{2}$
Dislocation of navicular				6	1
Stress fracture				6	1

Note The other authors included in the above are; Berman (1924); Penhallow (1937); Day (1947); Hermel & Gershon-Cohen (1953); Dewar & Evans (1968); Drummond & Hastings (1969); Eftekhar *et al* (1969); Kenwright & Taylor (1970); Towne *et al* (1970).

must remain intact, or a dislocation of the triple joint occurs instead. Reduction and treatment on the above lines is adequate.

Swivel dislocations

Swivel injuries are uncommon and form about 4% of midtarsal trauma (Main & Jowett 1975), which itself accounts for about $\frac{1}{2}$% of all fractures and dislocations (Wilson 1933). The lesion presents as a pure dislocation of the talonavicular joint with the calcaneocuboid joint intact and the interosseous talocalcaneal ligament

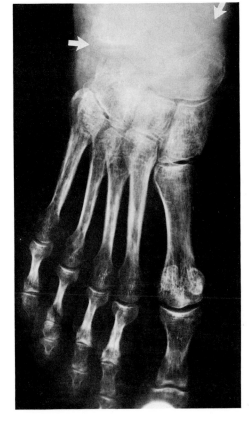

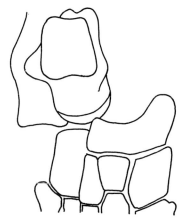

Fig. 11.114   (*Left*) Lateral dislocation of the midtarsal joint.

Fig. 11.115   (*Right*) Fracture–dislocation of the midtarsal joint associated with crush fracture of the navicular and the head of the talus.

unruptured. The subtalar joint is slewed sideways, medially or laterally, without corresponding inversion or eversion. This contrasts with full subtalar dislocation (see p. 262) in which the interosseous talocalcaneal ligament is torn and the calcaneum displaced from the talus.

Radiologically the swivel dislocation is revealed when both oblique and lateral projections of the bones appear on the same plate (Figs. 11.119, 11.120). Swivel dislocation is more common to the medial side than to the lateral side (Fig. 11.121). Lateral swivel dislocation may be associated with impact fractures of the cuboid (the 'nutcracker fracture' of Hermel & Gershon-Cohen 1953).

These injuries should be managed by prompt reduction followed by the usual rehabilitation.

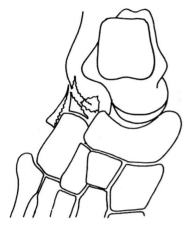

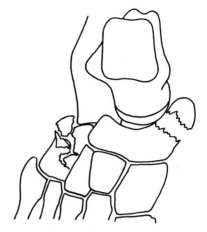

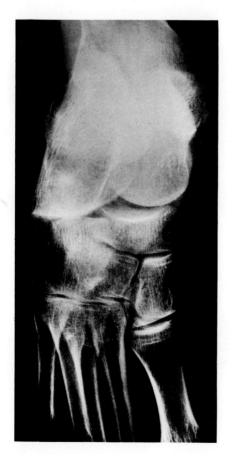

Fig. 11.116 (*Above left*) Lateral fracture–dislocation of the midtarsal joint. Note the comminution of the anterior end of the calcaneum.

Fig. 11.117 (*Above right*) Lateral fracture–dislocation of the midtarsal joint. Note the avulsion of the navicular tuberosity and the comminution of the cuboid.

Fig. 11.118 Medial dislocation of the midtarsal joint.

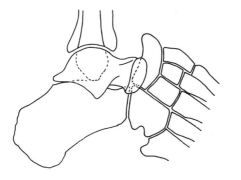
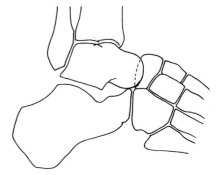

Fig. 11.119 (*Above left*) Medial
swivel dislocation of the midtarsal
joint. Note on the diagram the
mixture of oblique forefoot and
calcaneal alignment with true lateral
ankle and talar position.

Fig. 11.120 (*Above right*) Medial
swivel dislocation of the midtarsal
joint. Note on the diagram the
mixture of oblique ankle and talar
alignment with true lateral forefoot
and calcaneal position.

Fig. 11.121   Lateral swivel
dislocation of the midtarsal joint.
The talonavicular joint is dislocated,
but both the calcaneocuboid joint
and the inerosseous talocalcaneal
ligament remain intact. The
calcaneum swivels sideways under
the talus.

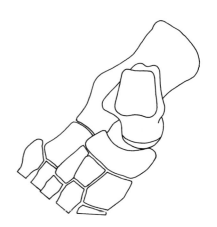

Fracture of the navicular tuberosity

This fracture may occur as an isolated injury (Main & Jowett 1975; Eichenholtz &
Levine 1964) and the tuberosity probably is pulled away by the plantar calcaneonavicular ligament rather than by tibialis posterior. Care is necessary to exclude
the more serious injury of midtarsal fracture–dislocation. If it is of any size, the
fragment should be reattached by open operation.

Fracture of the navicular

Main & Jowett (1975) divided the navicular into zones (Fig. 11.122) with one zone
corresponding to each cuneiform and the fourth to the tuberosity.

Longitudinally-directed forces of moderate severity, transmitted from the plantarflexed forefoot by the metatarsal-cuneiform rays, shear the navicular at the junctions of the zones (typically between zones A and B or zones B and C). Longitudinal, undisplaced fissures with the fracture plane vertical are produced (Figs. 11.123, 11.124). Simple immobilization until the fracture is united (6–8 weeks) followed by rehabilitation is satisfactory treatment.

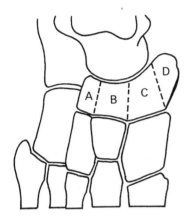

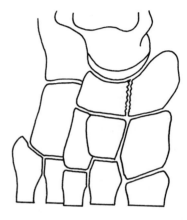

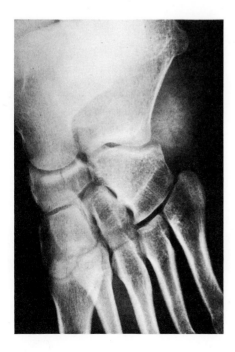

Fig. 11.122 (*Above left*) The navicular zones of Main & Jowett (1975).

Fig. 11.123 (*Above right*) Undisplaced fracture of the navicular. The fissure corresponds to the junction of zones B and C.

Fig. 11.124 Undisplaced fracture of the navicular. The fissure corresponds to the junction of zones A and B.

Fracture-dislocations of the navicular

More severe longitudinal violence produces extensive injury, the exact nature of which depends on the main direction of the thrust, which ray transmits it and the degree of plantarflexion of the foot at the moment of injury.

Force transmitted up the second ray crushes zone B, displacing medially the remainder of the bone (Fig. 11.125). Violence ascending the lateral rays pushes the forefoot medially crushing zone A and shifting zones B to D inward. There may be associated impact fracture of the talar head or medial subluxation of the calcaneo-cuboid joint (Fig. 11.115).

With lesser degrees of plantarflexion of the foot, violence is transmitted more evenly up the rays and falls more to the plantar side of the navicular. The lower margins of the central zones are crushed and their dorsal, largely intact portions are extruded dorsally (Fig. 11.126)). The results of the treatment of these injuries correlate with the severity of the initial trauma, the quality of reduction and the degree of residual joint incongruity. An attempt to reconstruct the bones and joints by open reduction and internal fixation should be made, although this is not easy. If reasonable alignment can be achieved and if the medial column of the foot can be brought to its proper length, an acceptable result can be obtained (Eftekhar *et al* 1969). Fusion should be reserved as a salvage procedure. If it proves necessary, Main and Jowett recommend triple arthrodesis rather than isolated talonaviculo-cuneiform fusion.

Crush fractures

As in the tarsometatarsal region, crushing of the midfoot produces no constant pattern of fractures. Bones are crushed and the joints sprung open. The injuries are commonly compound. Treatment follows basic principles for the management of soft-tissue trauma rather than specific manoeuvres for the bony splintering.

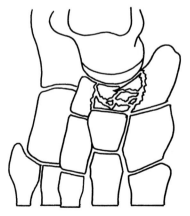

Fig. 11.125   Fracture–dislocation of the navicular. Zone B is crushed and zones C and D are displaced medially. The first and second rays are displaced proximally.

Isolated dislocations

Isolated dislocation either of cuboid (Figs. 11.127, 11.128; Drummond & Hastings 1969; Penhallow 1937) or of navicular (Fig. 11.129; Day 1947; Berman 1924) are rare and usually occur in reports of single cases. Stable reduction, by operation and internal fixation with Kirschner wires if necessary, should be obtained, followed by aftercare similar to that for the injuries already described.

Stress fracture of the navicular

Stress fractures of the navicular are uncommon. Two cases were reported by Towne *et al* (1970), presenting as pain and swelling of the foot after prolonged physical activity. The vertical fissure in the tarsal navicular was delayed in its appearance and difficult to see on plain radiographs, although easier to see on tomograms.

Towne *et al* (1970) distinguish the stress fracture from the congenital bipartite

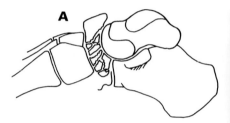

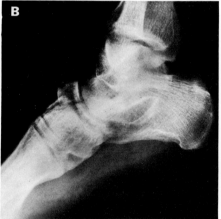

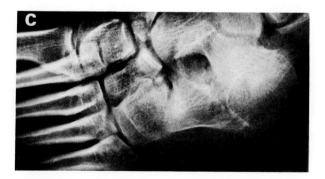

Fig. 11.126 (A) Fracture–dislocation of the navicular. The plantar part of the bone is crushed and the dorsal part is displaced dorsally out of the talocuneiform gap. (B) Fracture–dislocation of the navicular. Compare with (A). (C) Fracture–dislocation of the navicular. Compare with (A).

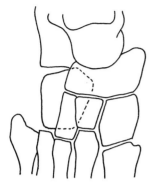

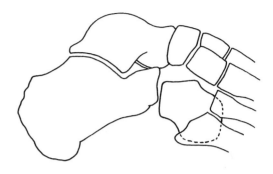

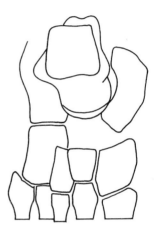

Fig. 11.127   (*Above left*) Isolated
inferomedial dislocation of the
cuboid. Dorsiplantar view.

Fig. 11.128   (*Above right*) Same as
Fig. 11.127. Lateral view.

Fig. 11.129   Isolated medial
dislocation of the navicular.

navicular by the radiological appearance. On anteroposterior views, the congenital anomaly shows as a comma-shaped, bent navicular and on the lateral view as a cleft from proximoplantar to distodorsal, separating a triangular block on the dorsal side of the bone.

Results of treatment of midtarsal injuries

Results are set out in Table 11.20. which is a condensation of the figures of Main and Jowett (1975).

CUNEIFORMS

While the cuneiform bones may be splintered as part of a general crushing injury, little is recorded of any type of injury specific to this region.

Therefore these bones have been included with the adjacent regions, where

Table 11.20   Results of treatment of midtarsal injuries. (From Main & Jowett 1975.)

	Managed by conservative methods		Managed by operative methods		Totals	
	No.	% satisfactory	No.	% satisfactory	No.	% satisfactory
Sprains						
Medial	11	100				
Lateral	7	71			20	90
Plantar	2	100				
Dislocations & fracture dislocations						
Medial	3	33				
Lateral	4	0			10	30
Plantar	3	67				
Swivel						
Medial	4	25	3	67	8	50
Lateral	1	100				
Undisplaced fracture of navicular	5	100			5	100
Displaced fracture–dislocation of navicular	21	29	3	0	24	25
Crush fractures	3	33	1	0	4	25

injuries often involve a longitudinal segment comprising metatarsal, cuneiform (or cuboid) and navicular (Huet & Lecoeur 1946; Holstein & Joldersma 1950; Wilson 1972; Main & Jowett 1975).

THE TARSOMETATARSAL REGION

On a basis of clinical experience and cadaveric experimental work, injuries of the tarsometatarsal region were classified into five types (Table 11.21; Wilson 1972). These injuries are caused by forcible forefoot rotation (Jeffreys 1963) with the foot in a position of full plantarflexion, or by plantarflexion alone (Novotny 1953). The injury may take a variety of forms, including dislocation or fracture–dislocation of the metatarsal base, fracture of the extreme proximal end of the metatarsal or fracture or fracture–dislocation of the adjacent cuneiform or cuboid. There is no fundamental difference between these variations on the basic theme and the same principle of treatment may be applied to all. Separation of the first and second

Table 11.21   Classification of tarsometatarsal injuries.

Direction of violence	Name	Detail of displacement
Plantarflexion and forefoot eversion (pronation)	Stage 1 = P1	Medial dislocation of the first metatarsal alone
	Stage 2 = P2	Medial dislocation of the first metatarsal and dorsilateral dislocation of the four lesser metatarsals
Plantarflexion and forefoot inversion (supination)	Stage 1 = S1	Dorsilateral dislocation of up to four lesser metatarsals
	Stage 2 = S2	Dorsilateral dislocation of all five metatarsals
Plantarflexion alone	PF	*Either* Dorsal subluxation of the base of the second metatarsal, *or* Coronal fracture–dislocation of the base of the first metatarsal

Note   In P1, P2 and S1 injuries there will be diastasis of the first and the second metatarsals. This has no especial significance

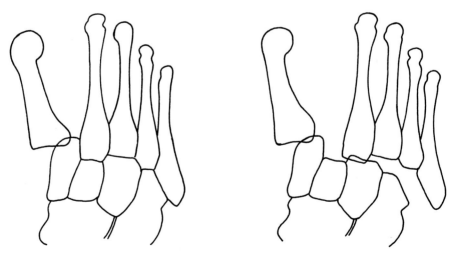

Fig. 11.130   (*Left*) P1 type tarsometatarsal dislocation.

Fig. 11.131   (*Right*) P2 type tarsometatarsal dislocation.

metatarsals (diastasis) was stressed by Quenu and Kuss (1909) and Ashhurst (1926), but experiment showed that it was merely a result of the sequence in which the components of the injury took place (Table 11.22; Figs. 11.130–11.131). The relative incidence of the types of injury is set out in Table 11.22.

Experimental work   Fixing the hindfoot and forcing the forefoot into plantar-flexion and inversion, produced dorsilateral dislocation of the four lesser metatarsals, beginning laterally and progressing medially (Figs. 11.132, 11.134). Little displacement of the lateral three bones was seen until after the second had given way. With further force dorsilateral dislocation of the first metatarsal was added (Figs. 11.133, 11.135). In agreement with this finding, two cases have been seen clinically with a partial lesion involving only the lateral two rays. When the cadaveric foot was twisted into plantarflexion and eversion, the first bone to be displaced was the first metatarsal, which rotated on its plantar aspect so that the dorsum of the bone swung medially away from the medial cuneiform (Fig. 11.130). Further strain caused dorsilateral displacement of the four lesser metatarsals, beginning laterally and progressing medially (Fig. 11.131). This parallels clinical experience.

In experiments involving plantarflexion only, two alternative lesions could be produced. Either the second metatarsal base became subluxated dorsally out of its little mortise between the cuneiforms (Fig. 11.136) or the first metatarsal fractured

Table 11.22   Incidence of the types of tarsometatarsal injuries. (Figures are numbers of cases.)

	Number of cases analysed	P1	P2	S1	S2	PF
del Sel (1953)	7		2	3	2	
Aitken & Poulson (1963)	9		1	1	6	1
Cassebaum (1963)	14		2	2	9	1
Wiley (1971)	10	2		5	2	1
D. Wilson (1972)	22	4	2	5	7	4
D. Wilson (additional cases)*	6			2	3	1
Fourteen other authors	32	4	6	9	13	
Totals	100	10	13	27	42	8

Note   The other authors included in the above are: Easton (1938); Jazikoff (1939); Huet & Lecoeur (1946); Imaz & D'Ovidio (1946); Botreau-Roussel (1947); Oliver (1947); Geckeler (1949); Holstein & Joldersma (1950); Rudge (1951); Montis (1956); Collett & Andrews (1958); Granberry & Lipscomb (1962); Jeffreys (1963); English (1964).
* Including cases of Mr H.D.W. Powell FRCS, High Wycombe General Hospital.

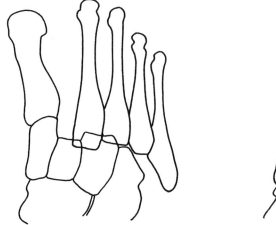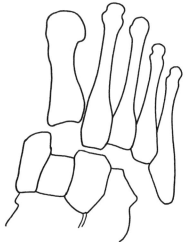

Fig. 11.132 (*Left*) S1 type tarsometatarsal dislocation.

Fig. 11.133 (*Right*) S2 type tarsometatarsal dislocation.

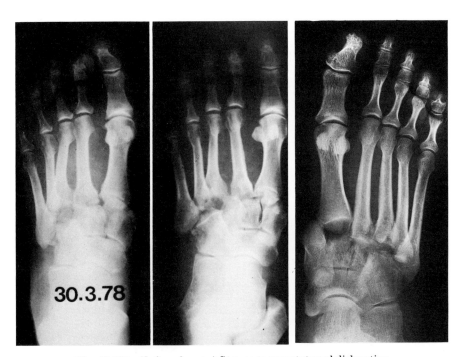

Fig. 11.134 (*Left and centre*) S1 type tarsometatarsal dislocation.

Fig. 11.135 (*Right*) S2 type tarsometatarsal dislocation.

through its base into the first cuneiform-metatarsal joint. This latter, coronal fracture–dislocation left a triangular fragment of the metatarsal attached inferiorly, while the remainder of the base of the bone displaced on to the dorsum of the tarsal (Figs. 11.137, 11.138). These types are seen clinically, but are less common than the other types.

Two-thirds of tarsometatarsal injuries are caused in road traffic accidents, commonly to front-seat passengers in cars, whose feet lie in plantarflexion on the sloping floor under the dash. Forefoot rotation is then added when the trunk is

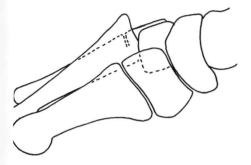

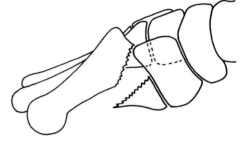

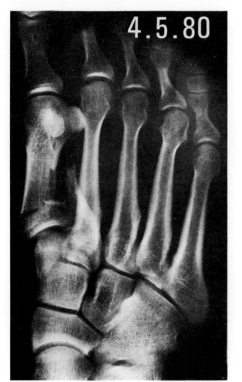

Fig. 11.136 (*Above left*) PF type dorsal subluxation of the base of the second metatarsal.

Fig. 11.137 (*Above right*) **and Fig. 11.138** PF type coronal fracture–dislocation of the base of the first metatarsal.

thrown to one side. Classically these injuries were common during cavalry accidents, in which the rider's foot was moulded into plantarflexion around the flank of the fallen horse. Other accidents which have been incriminated include falls downstairs or from capsizing stools (when the foot meets the ground in the toe-pointing position) or backward falls with the foot entrapped (in a hole or under a vehicle wheel).

The clinical picture of these injuries is of a grossly swollen and bruised foot on which the patient cannot bear weight. The deformity due to the displacements of the metatarsal bases may be seen and felt early after the injury, but is soon concealed by soft-tissue oedema. Radiographs must be taken in the dorsiplantar, oblique and true lateral planes to demonstrate all possible combinations of displacement. A true lateral view of the opposite, normal foot is essential in the child suspected of the plantar–flexion type of injury.

Treatment should aim at accurate, stable reduction. The dislocations are not intrinsically stable and reduction, even if good initially, may be difficult to maintain, especially when swelling subsides and the plaster cast loosens. Because of the importance of gaining and maintaining impeccable reduction, open operation and internal fixation of the joints with Kirschner wires is recommended (del Sel 1955; Granberry & Lipscomb 1962; Cassebaum 1963; English 1964; Wilson

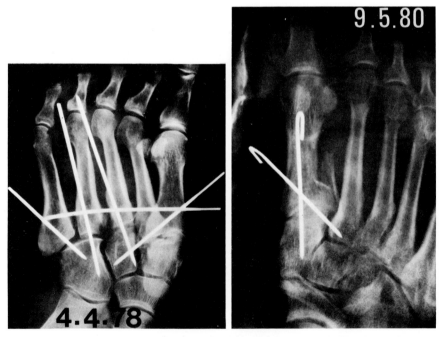

Fig. 11.139   (*Left*) Same as Fig. 11.134 after internal fixation with Kirschner wires.

Fig. 11.140   (*Right*) Same as Fig. 11.138 after internal fixation with Kirschner wires.

1972). The operation is not difficult to perform through one or two short longitudinal incisions on the top of the foot (Figs. 11.139, 11.140). A non-weight-bearing cast is applied for six weeks and the Kirschner wires are removed when the cast is taken off and before the patient walks without protection. A valgus arch support is a help in the rehabilitation period.

The results of treatment depend on the quality of the reduction and the degree of residual deformity. Pain, although seldom severe or incapacitating, can be a problem and is more common in cases with poor reduction and misshapen feet. Poor reduction is common after conservative management (Table 11.23; Figs. 11.141,

Table 11.23 Results of treatment of tarsometatarsal injuries.

	Cassebaum (1963)	D.Wilson (1972) and additional cases
*Radiological quality of reduction**		
Conservative managment		
Number analysed		15
Number satisfactory		7
% satisfactory		47%
Planned open reduction		
Number analysed		2
Number satisfactory		2
% satisfactory		100%
Clinical—deformity		
Conservative management		
Number analysed	7	13
Number satisfactory†	3	4
% satisfactory	43%	31%
Planned open reduction		
Number analysed	4	6
Number satisfactory	3	4
% satisfactory	75%	67%
Clinical—pain		
Conservative management		
Number analysed	7	16
Slight or no pain	5	11
% satisfactory	71%	69%
Planned open reduction		
Number analysed	4	5
Slight or no pain	4	4
% satisfactory	100%	80%

* Satisfactory = under 4 mm residual displacement on radiograph
† No deformity

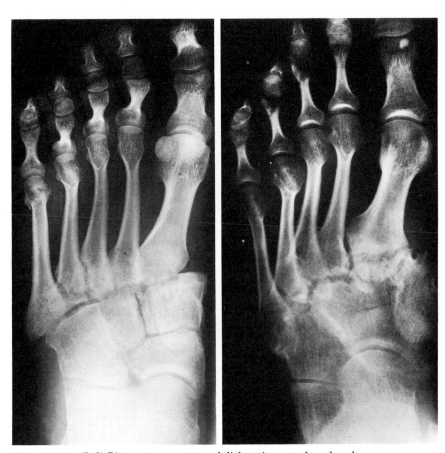

Fig. 11.141 *(Left)* S2 type tarsometatarsal dislocation, poorly reduced.

Fig. 11.142 *(Right)* Same as Fig. 11.141. Late result of a poorly reduced S2 dislocation.

11.142) and may be associated with marked deformity. In 4 cases from 16 (25%) treated conservatively, there was notable deformity (Wilson 1972) and 3 of these 4 patients had had to change their occupation and to give up active hobbies because of their feet. The majority of cases (e.g. 13 of 15 reviewed (87%) Wilson 1972) are likely to develop bony bosses around the tarsometatarsal joints, respresenting either residual bony displacements or osteophytes. Some stiffness is to be expected in almost all feet. Approximately half of all injured feet will have half or less of the normal range of tarsal motion. Also, a similar degree of stiffness is common in the metatarsophalangeal joint of the great toe on the affected side. The method of treatment adopted has little influence on this stiffness. Some residual limp is common. Radiological evidence of osteoarthritis in the damaged joints is universal, even in cases with anatomical reduction, but it is not necessarily related to symptoms.

Two other syndromes associated with the tarsometatarsal region deserve mention: English (1964) described the association of irreducible dislocation of a lesser metatarsophalangeal joint with dislocation of the base of an adjacent

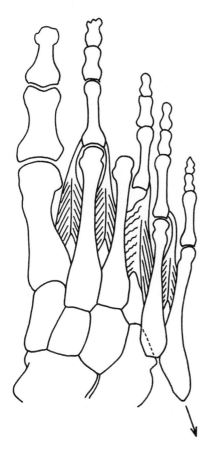

Fig. 11.143 The 'linked toe' syndrome of English (1964). The dislocation at the metatarsophalangeal joint of the middle toe cannot be reduced until the pull of the dorsal, bipennate interosseous muscle of the third interspace is relieved by reduction and stabilization of the proximally displaced tarsometatarsal joints of the fourth and fifth rays.

metatarsal. He found that it proved impossible to maintain reduction of the distal joint until the proximal lesion was properly reduced and stabilized (by Kirschner wire fixation). He ascribed this 'linked toe' phenomenon to the tether between the phalanx and the adjacent metatarsal provided by the dorsal, bipennate interosseous muscle (Fig. 11.143). The arrangement maintains a proximal pull of the toe while the metatarsal remains displaced and prohibits the necessary elongation for reduction of the toe joint.

Cassebaum (1963) drew attention to sprains of the tarsometatarsal region, in which the clinical disturbance was in excess of the normal or near normal radiological appearance. These sprains are notable insults to the foot and need proper treatment if prolonged, low-grade disability is to be avoided. A plaster cast for 4 weeks, followed by graduated rehabilitation is worthwhile. Early, unprotected use of the foot is not advisable. Clinical judgement of the severity of the injury to the foot should override the radiological assessment.

METATARSUS AND TOES

Certain injuries of the metatarsals and of the toes deserve special attention, but in general these common injuries cause little difficulty in either diagnosis or treatment. The common injuries are illustrated in Fig. 11.144 and the particular ones in Fig. 11.145.

Metatarsal fractures

Fractures of the metatarsals arise from direct violence, commonly after the fall of weights on to the forefoot or crushing under vehicle wheels, or from indirect trauma during twisting injuries. The former produces transverse or comminuted fractures of the distal shafts or necks of the bones, while twists cause spiral fracture of the shaft of the fifth metatarsal or avulsion of its styloid (probably the commonest fracture in the foot). In the majority of cases, simple immobilization in either a below-knee walking cast or in adhesive strapping for 3–4 weeks is sufficient treatment. 'Mal-union rarely results in disability. . . .' and '. . . non-union does not occur' (Apley 1968).

Fracture of the metatarsal neck with gross displacement

Occasionally the metatarsal head is markedly displaced from the shaft fragment and becomes excessively prominent in the sole, leading to secondary metatarsalgia (Milch 1942; Watson-Jones 1956). If closed manipulation fails, open reduction through one or two short longitudinal incisions and fixation with Kirschner wires is indicated. The wires may be inserted through the metatarsal head with the toes in extreme dorsiflexion (Smith 1963) or better along the axis of the toe, traversing all the phalanges (London 1979). Alternatively, if the fracture is in the distal shaft

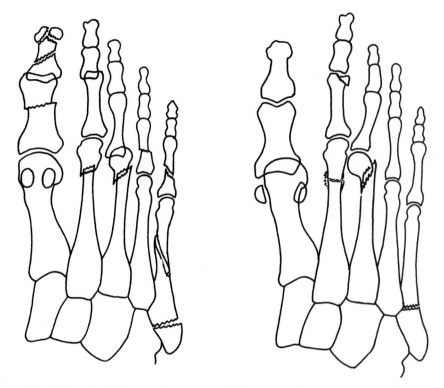

Fig. 11.144 (*Left*) Common fractures and dislocations of the metatarsus and toes.

Fig. 11.145 (*Right*) Particular injuries of the metatarsus and toes.

rather than in the neck, two wires may be inserted in a curved path through the side of the metatarsal head (Campbell Reid 1979). The wires should remain *in situ* for six weeks and weight-bearing should be delayed until after their removal lest slight joint movements fracture the wires.

Fractures of the proximal end of the fifth metatarsal

Stewart (1960) divided fractures of the proximal part of the fifth metatarsal into five types (Table 11.24) and Fig 11.146(A)–(D). There is a difference in prognosis among among these types (Dameron 1975).

Fractures of the proximal tubercule (styloid) of the fifth metatarsal Styloid fractures were described by Jones (1902). They are due usually to forced plantarflexion and inversion and the styloid is avulsed by peroneus brevis. The fracture line enters the cubometatarsal joint. Displacement is variable, but usually not marked.

Occasionally fracture of the styloid of the fifth metatarsal is associated with transverse fracture of the lateral malleolus of the ankle. In these cases the inversion injury has taken place with the ankle in dorsiflexion or neutral position. The malleolus is avulsed by the calcaneofibular ligament and the styloid by the peroneus brevis (Pearson 1961). In cases of avulsion of the styloid of the fifth metatarsal, the prognosis is excellent. Union takes place within two months in 99% of cases with simple treatment (Dameron 1975) and clinical symptoms and disability settle in 3–6 weeks. It is not difficult to distinguish the oblique or transverse, jagged fracture, entering the adjacent joint (Fig. 11.146B), from the longitudinal, smoothly outlined, scale-like epiphysis of the adolescent (Fig. 11.147). This secondary centre lies on the plantar and lateral aspect of the flare of the base of the fifth metatarsal. The epiphysis is never seen under the age of 8 years, normally appearing in girls of 9–11 years and in boys of 11–14 years of age. The cycle between the appearance of the epiphysis and its union to the main bone is usually complete in two years (83%) and always within three years. Union is complete by the age of 12–13 years in girls and 15–16 years in boys (Dameron 1975). Many persons never develop the epiphysis. Similarly confusion should not arise between fractures and accessory bones, such as the os peronaeum (in peroneus longus in 8–15% of feet) or the os vesalianum pedis (at the insertion of peroneus brevis in 0·1% of feet; O'Rahilly 1953).

Fractures of the extreme proximal shaft of the fifth metatarsal Dameron (1975) drew attention to the troublesome transverse fracture in the fifth metatarsal at the distal limit of the intermetatarsal joint 4–5, about 1.5–2.0 cm distal to the tuberosity (Fig. 11.146). It occurs in a younger age group than the styloid avulsion fracture (Table

Table 11.24   Fractures of the proximal part of the fifth metatarsal. (From Stewart 1960)

Fracture	No. of cases	%
Indirect trauma		
Fracture at the junction of the shaft and the base, at the distal limit of the intermetatarsal joint 4/5	8	$16\frac{1}{2}$
Comminuted fracture	6	12
Oblique fracture entering the cubometatarsal joint	21	43
Transverse fracture proximal to the cubometatarsal joint	11	$22\frac{1}{2}$
Direct trauma		
Fracture due to direct trauma	3	6
Total	49	

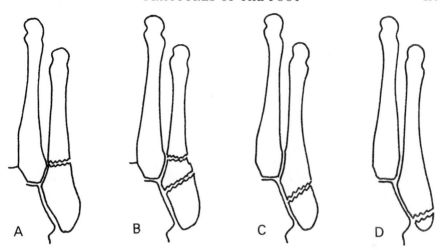

Fig. 11.146   (A)–(D) The four types of fracture at the base of the fifth metatarsal caused by indirect violence (Stewart 1960).

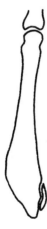

Fig. 11.147   Normal epiphysis at the base of the fifth metatarsal.

11.25), commonly in the athletic and it carries a surprisingly high risk of non-union. Of Dameron's 20 cases, 12 (60%) united in 2–12 months and 3 (15%) within 21 months with conservative treatment. Five (25%) required bone grafts to secure union (complete within 8–10 weeks of operation). Not all non-unions were symptomatic. On the basis of his experience, he recommended early operation for this injury in the athlete and symptomatic treatment in those of sedentary habit.

Dameron (1975) drew attention to the rare occurrence of an epiphysis-like, transverse lucency in the position of these fractures in the fifth metatarsal, found coincidentally in patients with history neither of injury nor of symptoms from the foot (Fig. 11.148). It is uncertain if this lucency represents an anomalous epiphysis

Table 11.25 Age groups associated with fractures of the proximal part of the fifth metatarsal. (From Dameron 1975)

Fracture	% of cases in the age range 15–21 years
Avulsion of the styloid of the fifth metatarsal	17
Transverse fracture of the extreme proximal shaft of the fifth metatarsal	70

or an un-united, forgotten stress fracture. We have chanced to see one such case, present on both sides.

Stress fractures of the metatarsals

Stress fracture of the second or third metatarsal shafts in Army recruits ('march fracture') is too well known to merit elaboration.

Stress fractures can occur in the proximal shaft of the fifth metatarsal and also in circumstances unrelated to military training. The lesions occur in patients with rheumatoid arthritis (Miller *et al* 1967), after Keller's excision arthroplasty of the great toe (Ford & Gilula 1977) and during rehabilitation in patients recently released from lower limb plaster casts (e.g. following tibial fracture or first metatarsal osteotomy).

Phalanges and toe joints

Metatarsophalangeal joints

Dislocation of the metatarsophalangeal joints of the lesser toes is a common manifestation of degenerative disease of the forefoot and may be associated with hammer toe or claw toe. Traumatic dislocation is uncommon. The 'linked toe' syndrome is discussed on p. 291 and, except for that and dislocation of the metatarsophalangeal joint of the great toe (see below), reduction is not usually difficult.

Dislocation of the metatarsophalangeal joint of the great toe This dislocation is an uncommon injury, but is important as it is frequently irreducible by closed manipulation. The proximal phalanx of the hallux is displaced on to the dorsum of the metatarsal head. The metatarsophalangeal joint lies in hyperextension and the interphalangeal joint in flexion. The injury has been ascribed to hyperextension of the joint when the plantar surface of the toe impacts against an obstruction (Salamon *et al* 1974; Giannikas *et al* 1975). The plantar capsule (volar plate) is

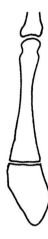

Fig. 11.148 Transverse, epiphysis-like lucency described by Dameron (1975).

avulsed from the underside of the metatarsal neck and follows the base of the phalanx dorsally. The lateral capsule (collateral ligaments) remain intact and hold the volar capsule tightly across the dorsum of the metatarsal head, blocking reduction. Usually the sesamoids are displaced and lie dorsal or lateral to the metatarsal head (Figs. 11.145, 11.149). Flexor hallucis longus is displaced lateral to the metatarsal head.

Open reduction through a transverse, plantar incision is necessary, but the joint remains stable once it is reduced.

Interphalangeal joints Dislocation of the interphalangeal joint of the great toe or of a lesser toe is more common than the corresponding injury at metatarsophalangeal level. (Fig. 11.144). Reduction is easy and stable. Occasionally fracture-dislocation occurs, an oblique fracture separating one condyle of the head of the proximal phalanx (Fig. 11.145).

In the lesser toes exact reduction is unnecessary and support of the injured toe by simple strapping to its neighbour to control marked deformity is sufficient. In the great toe, notable deformity should be prevented and it may be necessary to secure the displaced condyle by operation and fixation with a short Kirschner wire or a mini-screw.

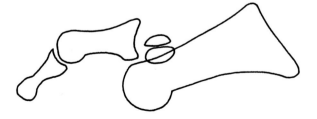

Fig. 11.149 Dorsal dislocation of the metatarsophalangeal joint of the great toe. Lateral view. See also Fig. 11.145.

Phalangeal fractures   Fracture of the phalanges, especially the terminal phalanx of the great toe, is common after the dropping of heavy objects on to the toes. Commonly there is no significant bony displacement and the main feature is of soft-tissue swelling and bruising and subungual haematoma. A period of rest in a below-knee walking plaster cast with a protective toe platform may be needed to relieve symptoms.

Fracture of the proximal phalanx of the little toe is a common result of stubbing the bare foot against furniture. Both this and similar injuries in the other lesser toes may be managed with simple strapping.

Sesamoids

The hallux invariably has two sesamoids (absence of the tibial sesamoid in 0·3% of persons is described). Similarities to the patella have been noted by various authors. Fractures of the sesamoids have been ascribed both to crushing injuries (the bone being split between the metatarsal head and the ground) and to hyperextension injuries (the bone being pulled asunder). Confusion with multipartite sesamoid is common. The radiological features said to be characteristic of fracture (Figs. 11.150, 11.151 Hubay 1949; Golding 1960) are: separation of the pieces; jagged edges to the pieces; evidence of attempts at healing (callus formation).

The relative size of the fragments and the appearance of the sesamoids in the opposite foot are little help, as multipartite sesamoids are very variable in their appearance. The tibial sesamoid of the hallux is the more commonly fractured. Clinical features are of swelling, bruising and local tenderness. Conservative management with relief of pressure with pads or in a walking cast usually allows pain to settle. If the bone remains painful, it may be excised. Multipartite sesamoids are common on the tibial side (one person in ten), but are rare on the fibular side (Table 11.26). Ossification in the sesamoids may occur from one, two or

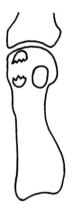

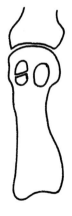

Fig. 11.150   (*Left*) Fracture of the tibial sesamoid.

Fig. 11.151   (*Right*) Bipartite tibial sesamoid.

Table 11.26 Percentage occurrence of multipartite sesamoids of the hallux. (From Hubay 1949.)

	%	
	Tibial	Fibular
286 males	13.6	2.8
224 females	17.9	1.8
Totals	15.5	2.4

multiple centres, but the radiological incidence of the consequent multipartite appearance falls with age as the centres tend to coalesce.

Gottlieb (1943), Golding (1960) and Devas (1963) also ascribe fractures of the sesamoids to 'microtrauma' or the stress mechanism.

ACKNOWLEDGEMENTS

The author is grateful to Mr C. Gilson MSc and the staff of the Department of Medical Illustration of the Royal Free Hospital for the photographs.

REFERENCES

AARON D.A.R. (1974) Intra-articular fractures of the os calcis. *Journal of Bone and Joint Surgery* **56B**, 567.

AITKEN A.P. (1963) Fractures of the os calcis—treatment by closed reduction. *Clinical Orthopaedics* **30**, 67–75.

AITKEN A.P. & POULSON D. (1963) Dislocations of the tarsometatarsal joint. *Journal of Bone and Joint Surgery* **45A**, 246–60.

ALLEN J.H. (1955) The open reduction of fractures of the os calcis. *Annals of Surgery* **141**, 890–900.

ANTHONSEN W. (1943) An oblique projection of roentgen examination of the talo-calcaneal joint, particularly regarding intra-articular fracture of the calcaneus. *Acta Radiologica* **24**, 306–10.

APLEY A.G. (1968) *A System of Orthopaedics and Fractures*, 3rd edn. Butterworth, London.

ASHHURST A.P.C. (1926) Divergent dislocation of the metatarsus. *Annals of Surgery* **83**, 132–4.

BERNARD L. & ODEGARD J.K. (1970) Conservative approach in the treatment of fractures of the calcaneus. *Journal of Bone and Joint Surgery* **52A**, 1689.

BERMAN S. (1924) Complete dislocation of the tarsal scaphoid. *Journal of the American Medical Association* **83**, 181–2.

BERNDT A.L. & HARTY M. (1959) Transchondral fractures (osteochondritis dissicans) of the talus. *Journal of Bone and Joint Surgery* **41A**, 988–1020.

BIGELOW D.R. (1974) Fractures of the processus lateralis tali. *Journal of Bone and Joint Surgery* **56B**, 587.

BIRT D. & TOWNSEND R. (1976) Major talar fractures. *Journal of Bone and Joint Surgery* **58B,** 138.

BLAIR H.C. (1943) Comminuted fractures and fracture dislocations of the body of the astralagus. *American Journal of Surgery (NS)* **59,** 37–43.

BOHLER L. (1931) Diagnosis, pathology and treatment of fractures of the os calcis. *Journal of Bone and Joint Surgery* **13,** 75–89.

BOHLER L. (1958) *The Treatment of Fractures* Vol. 3, 5th edn. Grune & Stratton, New York.

BOTREAU-ROUSSEL P-J. (1947) Luxation de metatarse traitee par manoeuvres orthopaediques. *Memoires de l'Academie Chirurgie* **73,** 115–17.

BURWELL H.N. & CHARNLEY A.D. (1965) The treatment of displaced fractures at the ankle by rigid internal fixation and early joint movement. *Journal of Bone and Joint Surgery* **47B,** 634–60.

CAMPBELL-REID D.A. (1979) Operative treatment of fractures of the hand. In Robb & Smith, *Operative Surgery—Orthopaedics,* 3rd edn. Butterworth, London.

CANALE S.T. & KELLY F.B. (1978) Fractures of the neck of the talus. *Journal of Bone and Joint Surgery* **60A,** 143–56.

CASSEBAUM W.H. (1963) Lisfranc fracture-dislocations. *Clinical Orthopaedics* **30,** 116–28.

CLARK K.C. (1973) *Positioning in Radiography* Vol. 1, 9th edn. William Heinemann Medical Books, London.

COLTART W.D. (1952) Aviator's astragalus. *Journal of Bone and Joint Surgery* **34B,** 545–66.

DACHTLER H.W. (1931) Fractures of the anterior superior portion of the os calcis due to indirect violence. *American Journal of Roentgenology* **25,** 629–31.

DAMERON T.B. (1975) Fractures and anatomical variations of the proximal portion of the fifth metatarsal. *Journal of Bone and Joint Surgery* **57A,** 788–792.

DAY A.J. (1947) The treatment of injuries to the tarsal navicular. *Journal of Bone and Joint Surgery* **29,** 359–66.

DETENBECK L.C. & KELLY P.J. (1969) Total dislocation of the talus. *Journal of Bone and Joint Surgery* **51A,** 283–8.

DEVAS M.B. (1961) Compression stress fractures in man and the greyhound. *Journal of Bone and Joint Surgery* **43B,** 540–51.

DEVAS M.B. (1963) Stress fractures in children. *Journal of Bone and Joint Surgery* **45B,** 528–541.

DEWAR F.P. & EVANS D.C. (1968) Occult fracture-subluxation of the mid-tarsal joint. *Journal of Bone and Joint Surgery* **50B,** 386–388.

DICK I.L. (1953) Primary fusion of the posterior subtalar joint in the treatment of fractures of the calcaneum. *Journal of Bone and Joint Surgery* **35B,** 375–80.

DIMON J.H. (1961) Isolated displaced fractures of the posterior facet of the talus. *Journal of Bone and Joint Surgery* **43A,** 275–81.

DRUMMOND D.S. & HASTINGS D.E. (1969) Total dislocation of the cuboid bone. *Journal of Bone and Joint Surgery* **51B,** 716–18.

DUNN A.R., JACOBS B. & CAMPBELL R.D. (1966) Fractures of the talus. *Journal of Trauma* **6,** 443–68.

EFTEKHAR N.M., LYDDON D.W. & STEVENS J. (1969) An unusual fracture-dislocation of the tarsal navicular. *Journal of Bone and Joint Surgery* **51A,** 577–81.

EICHENHOLTZ S.N. & LEVINE D.B. (1964) Fractures of the tarsal navicular bone. *Clinical Orthopaedics* **34,** 142–57.

ENGLISH T.A. (1964) Dislocations of the metatarsal bone and adjacent toe. *Journal of Bone and Joint Surgery* **46B,** 700–4.

EVANS M. (1968) Fractures of the calcaneus. *Journal of Bone and Joint Surgery* **50B,** 884.

ESSEX-LOPRESTI P. (1952) The mechanism, reduction technique and results in fractures of the os calcis. *British Journal of Surgery* **39,** 395–419.

FORD L.T. & GILULA L.A. (1977) Stress fractures of the middle metatarsals following the Keller operation. *Journal of Bone and Joint Surgery* **59A,** 117–18.

GALLIE W.E. (1943) Subastragalar arthrodesis in fractures of the os calcis. *Journal of Bone and Joint Surgery* **25**, 731–6.

GECKELER E.O. (1949) Dislocations and fracture dislocations of the foot: transfixation with Kirschner wires. *Surgery* **25**, 730–3.

GER R. (1971) The technique of muscle transposition in the operative treatment of traumatic and ulcerative lesions of the leg. *Journal of Trauma* **11**, 502–10.

GIANNIKAS A.C., PAPACHRISTOU G., PAPAVASILIOU N., NIKIFORIDIS P. & HARTOFILAKIDIS-GAROFALIDIS G. (1975) Dorsal dislocation of the first metatarsophalangeal joint. *Journal of Bone and Joint Surgery* **57B**, 384–6.

GOLDING C. (1960) The sesamoids of the hallux. Museum pages V. *Journal of Bone and Joint Surgery* **42B**, 840–3.

GOTTLIEB A. (1943) Diseased tibial sesamoid of the big toe joint. *Western Journal of Surgery* **51**, 193–5.

GRANBERRY W.M. & LIPSCOMB P.R. (1962) Dislocation of the tarsometatarsal joints. *Surgery, Gynaecology and Obstetrics* **114**, 467–9.

HALIBURTON R.A., SULLIVAN C.R., KELLY P.J. & PETERSON L.F.A. (1958) The extra-osseous and intra-osseous blood supply of the talus. *Journal of Bone and Joint Surgery* **40A**, 1115–20.

HARRIS R.I. (1963) Fractures of the os calcis: treatment by early subtalar arthrodesis. *Clinical Orthopaedics* **30**, 100–10.

HAWKINS L.G. (1965) Fracture of the lateral process of the talus. *Journal of Bone and Joint Surgery* **47A**, 1170–5.

HAWKINS L.G. (1970) Fractures of the neck of the talus. *Journal of Bone and Joint Surgery* **52A**, 991–1002.

HERMAN O.J. (1937) Conservative therapy for fractures of the os calcis. *Journal of Bone and Joint Surgery* **19**, 709–18.

HERMEL M.B. & GERSHON-COHEN J. (1953) The nutcracker fracture of the cuboid by indirect violence. *Radiology* **60**, 850–4.

HOLSTEIN A. & JOLDERSMA R.D. (1950) Dislocation of the first cuneiform in tarsometatarsal fracture-dislocation. *Journal of Bone and Joint Surgery* **32A**, 419–21.

HUBAY C. (1949) Sesamoid bones of the hands and feet. *American Journal of Roentgenology* **61**, 493–505.

HUET P. & LECOEUR P. (1946) Sur 4 cas de luxation tarso-metatarsienne. *Memoires de l'Academie Chirurgie* **72**, 124–9.

HULLINGER C.W. (1944) Insufficiency fracture of the calcaneus. *Journal of Bone and Joint Surgery* **26**, 751–7.

IMAZ J.I. & D'OVIDIO E.C. (1946) Luxacion bipolar del primer metatarsiano. *Revista de la Sanidad Militar* **XLV(3)**, 337–47.

ISBISTER J.F.St.C. (1974) Calcaneo-fibular abutment following crush fracture of the calcaneus. *Journal of Bone and Joint Surgery* **56B**, 274–8, 567–8.

JASIKOFF D. (1939) Luxations de l'articulation de Lisfranc. *Revue d'orthopedie* **26**, 126–34.

JEFFREYS T.E. (1963) Lisfranc's fracture-dislocation. *Journal of Bone and Joint Surgery* **45B**, 546–51.

JONES R. (1902) Fracture of the base of the fifth metatarsal by indirect violence. *Annals of Surgery* **35**, 697–700.

KALAMCHI A. & EVANS J.G. (1977) Posterior sub-talar fusion (Modified Gallie's procedure). *Journal of Bone and Joint Surgery* **59B**, 287–9.

KENWRIGHT J. & TAYLOR R.G. (1970) Major injuries of the talus. *Journal of Bone and Joint Surgery* **52B**, 36–48.

LANCE E.M., CAREY K.J., JR. & WADE P.A. (1963) Fractures of the os calcis: treatment by early mobilisation. *Clinical Orthopaedics* **30**, 76–90.

LARSON R.L., SULLIVAN C.R. & JANES J.M. (1961) Trauma, surgery and circulation of the talus—what are the risks of avascular necrosis? *Journal of Trauma* **1**, 13–21.

LEABHART J.W. (1959) Stress fractures of the calcaneus. *Journal of Bone and Joint Surgery* **41A**, 1285–90.

LEITNER B. (1955) The mechanism of total dislocation of the talus. *Journal of Bone and Joint Surgery* **37A**, 89–95.

LONDON P.S. (1979) Principles of fracture treatment. In Robb & Smith: *Operative Surgery— Orthopaedics 1*, 3rd edn. Butterworth, London.

LOWY M. (1969) Avulsion fractures of the calcaneus. *Journal of Bone and Joint Surgery* **51B**, 494–7.

MAIN B.J. & JOWETT R.L. (1975) Injuries of the mid-tarsal joint. *Journal of Bone and Joint Surgery* **57B**, 89–97.

MARKS K.L. (1952) Flake fractures of the talus progressing to osteochondritis dissicans. *Journal of Bone and Joint Surgery* **34B**, 90–2.

MATTERI R.E. & FRYMOYER J.W. (1973) Fractures of the calcaneus in young children. *Journal of Bone and Joint Surgery* **55A**, 1091–4.

MAXFIELD J.E. & McDERMOTT F.J. (1955) Experiences with the Palmer open reduction of fractures of the calcaneus. *Journal of Bone and Joint Surgery* **37A**, 99–106.

McKEEVER F.M. (1963) Treatment of complications of fractures and dislocations of the talus. *Clinical Orthopaedics* **30**, 45–52.

McLAUGHLIN H.L. (1963) Treatment of late complications after os calcis fractures. *Clinical Orthopaedics* **30**, 111–15.

McREYNOLDS I.S. (1972) Open reduction and internal fixation of calcaneal fractures. *Journal of Bone and Joint Surgery* **54B**, 176–7.

MILCH H. (1942) Operative reduction of metatarsal fractures. *Medical Record* **155**, 85–6.

MILLER O.L. & BAKER L.D. (1939) Fracture and fracture-dislocation of the astragalus. *Southern Medical Journal* **32**, 125–36.

MILLER B., MARKHEIM H.R. & TOWBIN M.N. (1967) Multiple stress fractures in rheumatoid arthritis. *Journal of Bone and Joint Surgery* **49A**, 1408–14.

MINDELL E.R., CISEK E.E., KARTALIAN G. & DZIOB J.M. (1963) Late results of injuries to the talus. *Journal of Bone and Joint Surgery* **45A**, 221–45.

MITCHELL J.I. (1936) Total dislocation of the astragalus. *Journal of Bone and Joint Surgery* **18**, 212–14.

MONTIS G.F. (1956) Su di un caso di lussazione della Lisfranc. *Ateneo Parmense* **27**, 272–6.

MORESTIN H. (1902) Traitment operatoire de l'ecrasement du calcaneum. *Bulletins et Memoires de la Societe Anatomique de Paris* 6° Serie, **IV**, 225–9.

MORRIS H.D., HAND W.L. & DUNN A.W. (1971) The modified Blair fusion for fractures of the talus. *Journal of Bone and Joint Surgery* **53A**, 1289–97.

MORRISON G.M. (1937) Fractures of the bones of the feet. *American Journal of Surgery* (NS) **38**, 721–6.

MUKHERJEE S.K. & YOUNG A.B. (1973) Dome fractures of the talus. *Journal of Bone and Joint Surgery* **55B**, 319–26.

MUKHERJEE S.K., PRINGLE R.M. & BAXTER A.D. (1974) Fracture of the lateral process of the talus. *Journal of Bone and Joint Surgery* **56B**, 263–73.

MULFINGER G.L. & TRUETA J. (1970) The blood supply of the talus. *Journal of Bone and Joint Surgery* **52B**, 160–7.

NADE S. & MONAHAN P.R.W. (1972) Fracture of the calcaneus—a study of the long term prognosis. *Journal of Bone and Joint Surgery* **54B**, 177.

NEWCOMB W.J. & BRAV E.A. (1948) Complete dislocation of the talus. *Journal of Bone and Joint Surgery* **30A**, 872–4.

NISBET, N.W. (1954) Dome fracture of the talus. *Journal of Bone and Joint Surgery* **36B**, 244–6.

NOBLE J. & McQUILLAN W.M. (1979) Early posterior subtalar fusion in the treatment of fractures of the os calcis. *Journal of Bone and Joint Surgery* **61B**, 90.

NOVOTNY H. (1953) Subluxatio tarso-metatarsea. *Acta Chirurgica Scandinavica* **105**, 467–73.

OLIVER E. (1947) Traumatisme du pied ou malformation congenital? (Luxation homolaterale dorsale externe totale du metatarse). *Memoires de l'Academie Chirurgie* **73**, 117–20.

OMBREDANNE L. (1902) Contribution a l'etude des fractures d'astragale. *Revue de Chirurgie* **26**, 177–95.

O'RAHILLY R. (1953) A survey of carpal and tarsal anomalies. *Journal of Bone and Joint Surgery* **35A**, 626–42.

ORTICOCHEA M. (1972) The musculo-cutaneous flap method—an immediate and heroic substitute for the method of delay. *British Journal of Plastic Surgery* **25**, 106–10.

PALMER I. (1948) The mechanism and treatment of fractures of the calcaneus. *Journal of Bone and Joint Surgery* **30A**, 2–8.

PEARSON J.R. (1961) Combined fracture of the base of the fifth metatarsal and the lateral malleolus. *Journal of Bone and Joint Surgery* **43A**, 513–16.

PENHALLOW D.P. (1937) A complete compound subastragalar dislocation of the tarsal bones. *Journal of Bone and Joint Surgery* **19**, 514–17.

PENHALLOW D.P. (1937) An unusual fracture-dislocation of the tarsal scaphoid. *Journal of Bone and Joint Surgery* **19**, 517–19.

PENNEL G.F. (1963) Fractures of the talus. *Clinical Orthopaedics* **30**, 53–63.

PETERSON L. & GOLDIE I.F. (1975) The arterial supply of the talus. A study on the relationship to experimental ta. :r fractures. *Acta Orthopaedica Scandinavica* **46**, 1026–34.

PETERSON L. & ROMANUS B. (1976) Fracture of the collum tali—an experimental study. *Journal of Biomechanics* **9**, 277–9.

PETERSON, L., GOLDIE I. & LINDELL D. (1974) The arterial supply of the talus. *Acta Orthopaedica Scandinavica* **45**, 260–70.

PETERSON L., GOLDIE I.F. & IRSTAM L. (1977) Fracture of the neck of the talus. *Acta Orthopaedica Scandinavica* **48**, 696–706.

QUENU E. & KUSS G. (1909) Etude sur les luxations du metetarse (Luxations metatarso-tarsiennes). *Revue de Chirurgie* **39**, 1–72, 281–336, 720–91, 1093–1134; **40**, 104–41.

ROBERTS N. (1968) Fractures of the calcaneus. *Journal of Bone and Joint Surgery* **50B**, 884.

ROSENBERG N.J. (1965) Fractures of the talar dome. *Journal of Bone and Joint Surgery* **47A**, 1279.

RUDGE O. (1951) Luxacao totale tarso-metatarsiana. *Revista Brasileira de Cirurgia* **22**, 277–86.

SALAMON P.B., GELBERMAN R.H. & HUFFER J.M. (1974) Dorsal dislocation of the metatarso-phalangeal joint of the great toe. *Journal of Bone and Joint Surgery* **56A**, 1073–5.

SCHROCK R.D. (1952) Fractures of the foot: Fractures and dislocations of the astragalus. *American Academy of Orthopaedic Surgeons. Inst. Course Lect. Ann Arbor* **9**, 361–8.

SEL J.M. DEL (1953) El tratamiento quirurgico de la fractura-luxacion de Lisfranc. *Revista de la Asociacion Medica Argentina* **67**, 276–9.

SEL J.M. DEL (1955) The surgical treatment of tarsometatarsal fracture-dislocations. *Journal of Bone and Joint Surgery* **37B**, 203–7.

SMITH H. (1963) *Campbell's Operative Orthopaedics*, 4th edn. C.V. Mosby, St Louis.

SOEUR R. & REMY R. (1975) Fractures of the calcaneum with displacement of the thalamic portion. *Journal of Bone and Joint Surgery* **57B**, 413–21.

STEWART I.M. (1960) Jones's fracture: Fracture of the base of the fifth metatarsal. *Clinical Orthopaedics* **16**, 190–8.

THOMAS H.McK. (1969) Calcaneal fracture in childhood. *British Journal of Surgery* **56**, 664–6.

TOWNE L.C., BLAZINA M.E. & COZEN L.N. (1970) Fatigue fracture of the tarsal navicular. *Journal of Bone and Joint Surgery* **52A**, 376–8.

WARRICK C.K. & BREMNER A.E. (1953) Fractures of the calcaneum. *Journal of Bone and Joint Surgery* **35B**, 33–45.

WATSON-JONES Sir R. (1956) *Fractures and Joint Injuries*, 4th edn. E. & S. Livingstone, Edinburgh.

WESTHUES H. (1934) Zur Behandlung der Calcaneusfraktur. *Zentralblatt fur chirurgie.* **61**, iii, 2231.

WILSON D.W. (1972) Injuries of the tarso-metatarsal joints. *Journal of Bone and Joint Surgery* **54B,** 677–86.

WILSON J.N. (1976) In Watson-Jones *Fractures and Joint Injuries.* 5th edn. Churchill Livingstone, Edinburgh.

WILSON P.D. (1933) Fractures and dislocations of the tarsal bones. *Southern Medical Journal* **XXVI,** 833–45.

12

The Radiology and Radiography
of the Foot

P. RENTON & W.J. STRIPP

1 RADIOLOGY OF THE NORMAL FOOT

The radiologist has a mental image of what constitutes a normal foot. Such a normal foot is, however, more difficult to define in words. According to Gamble and Yale (1975), a normal foot is 'a mobile framework of individual bones of correct conformation that are aligned for maximal structural stability and functional efficiency'. This definition is both radiological and clinical. Steel *et al* (1980) prefer the term 'painless foot'. Such a foot, besides being painless, has no history of significant pain or disability, has not been operated upon, and is without skin or soft tissue lesions. This definition is looser and clinical, and need not be associated with 'normal' anatomy.

The structure or form of the foot is determined by the shape of its individual bones and adjacent articular surfaces. Movements of the foot are pre-determined by the shape of the bones and joints. Variations of form, whether inherent or acquired, alter and deform structural relationships and thereby alter function.

The foot, a dynamic chain or linkage of interdependent bones, is designed for both stance and locomotion. Radiographs in the non-weight-bearing situation do demonstrate bone and joint relationships. Radiographs taken while weight-bearing, however, demonstrate the foot in a locked and static, yet simultaneously kinetic and functional, situation, giving a truer impression of the bony and soft tissue complex under stress. Such a film must be more informative as to the normality of the foot since the movement or deformity created in weight-bearing reflects normal or abnormal structure of bone and mobility at joints.

Other advantages also accrue from examination while weight-bearing. Better comparison can be made, both between patients and, on successive examinations, of the same patient. The erect or weight-bearing posture allows greater standardization of radiographs. Small variations in position of both x-ray tube and patient can cause distortion of the image. Ideally, all examinations should be reproducible. Unless contraindicated by painful pathology, the patient finds the erect posture naturally easier to adopt than some of the contortions necessary for recumbent views. It is also usually quicker for the radiographer, especially if some form of simple footstand-film holder is available. Such a stand also facilitates immobilization during exposure (Gamble & Yale 1975).

The need for standard and easily reproducible views has already been stressed. A standard tube–film distance and centring technique are essential, and the foot–film distance must be minimized. The erect or weight-bearing posture places the foot at about 90° to the leg on all occasions, aiding reproducibility. Radiographic distortion of normal relationships can also be minimized by examining and centring on each foot individually. Centring between two feet on an anteroposterior projection causes poor visualization of the lateral parts of the foot because of obliquity of both beam and foot laterally (Fig. 12.1).

Integrity of the hindfoot can be said to be present when certain features are seen radiologically on the lateral view (Fig. 12.2).

The joint between the plafond of the distal tibia and the trochlear surface of the talus is clearly visualized. Anteriorly the head of the talus is smooth and round as it extends to the talonavicular joint. The superior surfaces of the talus, navicular and medial cuneiform lie in a straight line (the inferior surfaces of these three bones also lie in a straight line, parallel to the upper line).

The midtarsal joint line separates talus and calcaneum from navicular and cuboid. Gamble and Yale (1975) emphasize that this line is a continuous 'cyma'. This word, derived from the Greek for a wave, is used in architectural practice for a moulding which is concave in its upper part, convex below. An intact cyma indicates integrity of the talonavicular and calcaneocuboid joints.

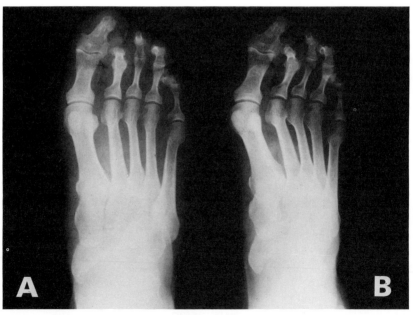

Fig. 12.1   (A) With the beam centred directly over the foot the metatarsal bases and adjacent tarsal bones are much more clearly shown than in (B). This is half of the examination of both feet with the tube centred between the feet. Marked overlap of metatarsal bases and adjacent tarsal bones is seen. The midtarsal joint can be seen as a continuous line or cyma.

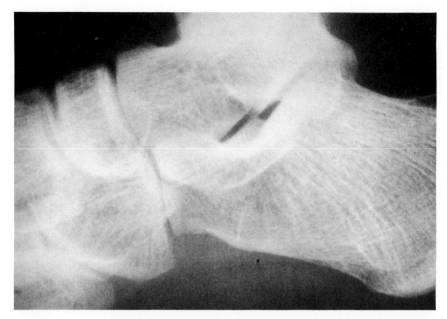

Fig. 12.2   Normal lateral hindfoot showing a cyma between calcaneum, talus, navicular and cuboid.

The talus and calcaneum overlap where the anterior process of the calcaneum projects superiorly. Elsewhere spaces are seen between the two bones:

1   Posteriorly, between the posterior calcaneal facet on the talus and the posterior facet on the calcaneum.

2   At the sinus tarsi. This lucency lies above the sustentaculum tali. A groove in the inferior talus, the sulcus tali, between its posterior and middle facets, lies above a groove on the superior surface of the calcaneum, the sulcus calcanei, between its posterior and middle facets. The two grooves together form a tunnel, the canalis tarsi, containing the interosseous ligament. As the canal is oblique, only the anterior portion, the sinus tarsi, is seen on a lateral view.

3   Anterior to the sinus tarsi, the joint space formed by the two opposing middle facets may be seen.

The line of the body of the talus is normally parallel with the weight-supporting plane, and is drawn through the posterior subtalar joint to just above the sinus tarsi (Gamble & Yale 1975).

The calcaneum bears weight on its posterior tuberosity and provides attachment for both plantar fascia and Achilles tendon. Distally it articulates with the cuboid and, though radiographically an anterior process overlaps the talus, this portion of the calcaneum lies laterally and is not actually in contact with the talus.

The sustentaculum tali is represented on the lateral view by an area of increased density antero-inferior to the sinus tarsi, beneath the middle facet of the subtalar joint and the superimposed shadow of the lateral process of the talus. It varies in shape, but is generally rectangular.

The calcaneal pitch, or angle of inclination (Fig. 12.3; Table 12.1) is the angle between the weight-bearing plane and the inferior surface of the calcaneum. The greater the pitch, the greater the height of the foot framework. The pitch is similar for both feet.

The angle of Böhler lies between the plane of the posterosuperior surface of the calcaneum and the backward projection of the plane of the anterosuperior surface of the calcaneum. The angle may thus be decreased following fractures of the body of the bone (Fig. 12.4).

On routine anteroposterior views of the foot, the midtarsal joint is again seen as a cyma (Fig. 12.1). A film exposed for the fore- and midfoot shows little detail posterior to the cyma, though views of greater radiographic exposure display the hindfoot at the expense of the distal parts. Gamble and Yale (1965) use a 'composite' view in which a double exposure technique displays the entire foot on one film. This is said to be of particular value in displaying the linear relationship of hind-, mid- and forefoot in the sagittal plane. Using a composite radiograph, Gamble and Yale (1965) have shown that in foot-charting not one, but many lines have been used by different investigators to define the midline of the foot. Most of these lines seem to vary little and, in view of both radiographic and anatomical variation between different patients, the differences between lines may be of little importance. Certainly a line drawn from the middle of the posterior aspect of the calcaneum to a point between the second and third metatarsal heads provides an adequate base for

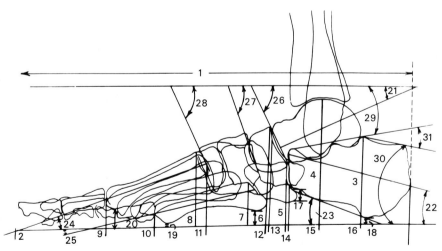

Fig. 12.3 Lateral view of the foot showing normal measurements as defined by Steel *et al* (1980) (see Table 12.1). The calcaneal angle of inclination is No. 23 on the illustration. (Reproduced with kind permission of the authors and publishers. Copyright 1980, the American Orthopaedic Foot Society.)

Table 12.1 Measurements from lateral radiograph and absolute left-right values. (From Steel *et al* (1980) with permission. Copyright 1980, the American Orthopaedic Foot Society.)

	Range	Distribution					Absolute value of left-right difference	Standard deviation of difference
		10%	25%	50%	75%	90%		
1 Metatarsal 2 length	6.7–9.3 cm	6.9 cm	7.3 cm	7.6 cm	8 cm	8.3 cm	0.10	0.09
2 Total length of foot	23–27.8 cm	23.5 cm	24.5 cm	25.2 cm	26 cm	26.7 cm	0.27	0.25
3 Calcaneus height	5.8–7.5 cm	5.9 cm	6.1 cm	6.3 cm	6.8 cm	6.9 cm	0.10	0.11
4 Talar dome height	7.3–9.5 cm	7.8 cm	8.1 cm	8.3 cm	8.9 cm	9.1 cm	0.16	0.15
5 Cuboid height	4–6 cm	4.6 cm	4.9 cm	5.1 cm	5.3 cm	5.6 cm	0.18	0.21
6 Navicular height	5.9–8.2 cm	6.2 cm	6.6 cm	6.9 cm	7.3 cm	7.6 cm	0.19	0.14
7 Metatarsal 5 base height	2.3–3.8 cm	2.9 cm	3.1 cm	3.3 cm	3.4 cm	3.6 cm	0.16	0.16
8 Metatarsal 1 base height	4.3–6.6 cm	4.8 cm	5.2 cm	5.4 cm	6 cm	6.2 cm	0.22	0.20
9 Calcaneus-distal metatarsal 1 length	16.4–20 cm	17.1 cm	17.6 cm	18.3 cm	18.9 cm	19.6 cm	0.30	0.29
10 Calcaneus-distal metatarsal 5 length	12.5–18.1 cm	14.3 cm	14.9 cm	15.6 cm	15.9 cm	16.9 cm	0.43	0.38
11 Calcaneus-proximal metatarsal 1 length	11.6–14.5 cm	12.1 cm	12.6 cm	13 cm	13.3 cm	13.8 cm	0.29	0.43
12 Calcaneus-proximal metatarsal 5 length	8.1–10.7 cm	8.8 cm	9.1 cm	9.6 cm	10 cm	10.3 cm	0.26	0.19
13 Calcaneus-proximal navicular length	7.7–10.3 cm	8.2 cm	8.6 cm	8.8 cm	9.2 cm	9.6 cm	0.20	0.18
14 Calcaneus-proximal cuboid length	6.5–9.6 cm	7.1 cm	7.4 cm	7.7 cm	8.1 cm	8.4 cm	0.26	0.41
15 Calcaneus-talar dome apex length	3.6–6.7 cm	4.8 cm	5.2 cm	5.5 cm	5.8 cm	5.9 cm	0.29	0.35
16 Calcaneus-calcaneus maximum height length	2.7–5.6 cm	3 cm	3.1 cm	3.3 cm	3.6 cm	3.8 cm	0.23	0.29

17 Calcaneus-cuboid articular surface difference	0.1–1.4 cm	0.4 cm	0.6 cm	0.7 cm	0.9 cm	1 cm	0.11	0.11
18 Calcaneus-soft tissue pad height	0.4–1.7 cm	0.7 cm	0.9 cm	1 cm	1.2 cm	1.3 cm	0.07	0.10
19 Metatarsal head 5 soft tissue pad height	0.1–1.6 cm	0.3 cm	0.6 cm	0.6 cm	0.8 cm	0.9 cm	0.08	0.08
20 Metatarsal head 1 soft tissue pad height	0.7–2.5 cm	1.1 cm	1.5 cm	1.7 cm	2.1 cm	2.2 cm	0.14	0.13
21 Talus-base reference angle	14–36°	18°	22°	24.5°	27°	30°	2.90	2.38
22 Calcaneus-base reference angle	15–39°	18°	24°	28°	31°	33°	2.80	2.07
23 Calcaneus angle of inclination	11–38°	16°	20°	22°	26°	28°	2.55	2.46
24 Metatarsal 1 shaft-base reference angle	16–30°	17°	20°	22°	23°	26°	1.70	1.45
25 Metatarsal 5 shaft-base reference angle	7–25°	8°	10°	12.5°	15°	17°	1.53	1.24
26 Proximal navicular articular surface angle	54–74°	59°	62°	63°	66°	68°	2.95	2.41
27 Proximal cuneiform 1 articular surface angle	51–78°	58°	62°	65.5°	69°	73°	2.68	2.09
28 Proximal metatarsal 1 articular surface angle	55–72°	59°	62°	63°	65°	67°	2.35	1.79
29 Calcaneus anterosuperior surface angle	2–30°	7°	10°	12.5°	16°	17°	2.28	2.71
30 Calcaneus posterosuperior surface angle	10–35°	15°	18°	22°	27°	30°	2.93	2.35
31 Böhler's angle	22–48°	27°	32°	35°	40°	44°	3.58	2.41

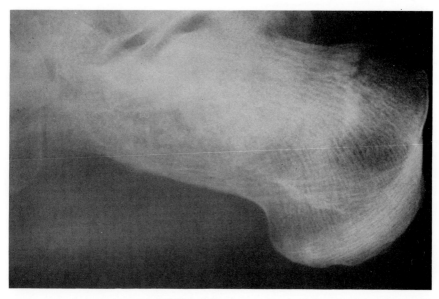

Fig. 12.4   Decrease in the angle of Böhler following a calcaneal fracture, so that the superior plane of the calcaneum is now nearly straight.

references purposes. A line through the midpoint of the talar head makes an angle with this midline and defines the relationship between talus and midline.

The talocalcaneal angle, on the other hand, in adults lies between the bisector of the talar head and the bisector of the distal calcaneum between the calcaneocuboid joint margins (Gamble & Yale 1975). In children, a line through the long axis of the talus points to the head of the first metatarsal, and a line through the long axis of the calcaneum points to the head of the fourth metatarsal. The talocalcaneal angle between these two lines varies in the normal, gradually decreasing from infancy to five or more years. The lines of the metatarsal shafts are roughly parallel in infants (Davis & Hatt 1955). The long axes of talus and first metatarsal also form an angle, as do those between the first metatarsal and proximal phalanx of the hallux.

Though many measurements and angles have been described in the literature, their usage must be critically assessed. Radiographic techniques vary, not only between departments, but often between different patients or even the same patient on different occasions. Different lines are used to define angles which clearly then cannot mean the same thing. Hlavac (1967) has shown that varying the position of the foot alters angular measurements. Thus, if the foot is pronated, the talocalcaneal angle (as he defines it!) increases, the angle between a metatarsal and adjacent phalangeal shaft increases, the cyma line breaks anteriorly and the entire foot apparently increases in length and breadth. On the lateral view the calcaneal pitch decreases in pronation, the sustentaculum tali becomes lower, broader and less well-defined, and the lateral tuberosity of the calcaneum no longer visible.

A very complete analysis of radiographic measurements of the normal adult foot has recently been performed. Using 41 pairs of adult female feet, Steel *et al* (1980) were apparently able to demonstrate that, while Böhler's angle has been described as normal between 28° and 40°, in 21% of their 'normal' feet the angle was over 40°, and in 9% less than 28° (Fig. 12.3; Table 12.1). The angle between the first metatarsal and proximal phalanx should normally be 0–10° (Gamble & Yale 1975). A much wider variation (0–32°) in 'normals' was seen by Steel *et al*, however (Fig. 12.5; Table 12.2). Measurements can be used as part of a general radiographic and clinical assessment of the foot but should not be used, therefore, to impose a rigid standard of normality by which all else must be judged.

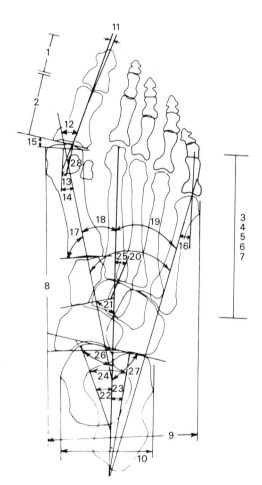

Fig. 12.5 Normal measurements of the AP foot, as defined by Steel *et al* (1980) (see Table 12.2). The metatarsal 1–phalangeal 1 angle is No. 12 on the illustration. (Reproduced with kind permission of the authors and publishers. Copyright 1980, the American Orthopaedic Foot Society).

FOOT DEVELOPMENT

Development of the foot *in utero* has been described (Gardner *et al* 1959). Ossification of the calcaneum is seen, though not of course radiologically, as early as thirteen weeks. Certainly at five months gestation, an ossific nucleus for the calcaneum is radiologically visible. Two centres of ossification apparently arise which have usually fused by birth, though bifid centres occasionally persist (Meschan 1970). The talus may be visualized from six months on, though its appearance is more variable and it may even appear after birth. Antenatal radiography of the fetus to determine maturity using heel and knee ossification is no longer practised since the advent of ultrasound. The cuboid and lateral cuneiform are also occasionally ossified before birth. Late on in gestation, the female foot matures more rapidly than the male and so is more advanced at birth (Hoerr *et al* 1962). These authors in their *Atlas of Skeletal Development of the Foot* show a male foot at 40 weeks gestation with well-developed talus and calcaneum, and an irregular cluster of bony nodules forming the cuboid, aligned with the long axis of the calcaneum. The shafts or diaphyses of the metatarsals are present, having begun ossification in the third fetal month, and modelled, as are the proximal phalanges. The distal phalanges are small but visible. Middle phalangeal ossification is still spreading laterally, but that of the little toe does not appear till seven months of age on the standard male. As the authors state, unless children are examined frequently, the time at which ossification is noted is later than its actual occurrence. Often, but not invariably, when bigger samples are used in studies to determine onset of ossification, onset is noted earlier. The standard deviation must also be taken into account. Children who have been seriously ill also distort any sample, growth being retarded, while apparently in those children who naturally mature more slowly, the short bones of the foot develop more slowly than the tarsal bones. Hoerr *et al* list the order of onset of ossification of foot bones seen in boys, and give the mean age (in months) for the onset of ossification (Fig. 12.6).

Biphalangism

Variations in the digital skeleton of the foot were analysed in 1800 school children and 500 adults by Venning (1960).

The incidence of biphalangism of the post-axial toes is the same in both the twelve week fetus and the adult, indicating that there are no grounds for describing such terminal interphalangeal joints as 'having fused'. The fifth toe is far more frequently biphalangeal (35–45% in Europeans; Fig. 12.7) than the fourth toe (< 5%), third toe (< 2%) or second toe (< 1.5%, if ever). Biphalangism also shows racial variation. Japanese show biphalangism of the fifth toe in 70–80% of cases. Toes with two phalanges are more common in females and are usually symmetrical. Where asymmetry is present, the left foot is more often affected.

Venning notes that the number of phalanges is determined by the presence or absence of the middle phalanx which, in turn, may or may not have an epiphysis.

Table 12.2 Measurements from anteroposterior radiograph and absolute left-right values. (From Steel *et al* (1980) with permission. Copyright 1980, the American Orthopaedic Foot Society.)

	Range	Distribution						Absolute value of left-right difference	Standard deviation of difference
		10%	25%	50%	75%	90%			
1 Distal phalanx 1 length	1.9–2.8 cm	2 cm	2.2 cm	2.3 cm	2.4 cm	2.5 cm		0.14	0.12
2 Proximal phalanx 1 length	2.1–3.5 cm	2.5 cm	2.7 cm	2.9 cm	3.2 cm	3.2 cm		0.10	0.17
3 Metatarsal 1 length	5.6–7.9 cm	5.8 cm	6.2 cm	6.4 cm	6.7 cm	7 cm		0.09	0.07
4 Metatarsal 2 length	6.7–9.3 cm	6.9 cm	7.3 cm	7.7 cm	8 cm	8.4 cm		0.10	0.09
5 Metatatsal 3 length	6.2–8.8 cm	6.7 cm	7 cm	7.3 cm	7.5 cm	7.9 cm		0.23	0.78
6 Metatarsal 4 length	6.3–8.4 cm	6.6 cm	6.9 cm	7 cm	7.4 cm	7.6 cm		0.12	0.12
7 Metatarsal 5 length	6.5–8.4 cm	6.7 cm	6.9 cm	7.2 cm	7.5 cm	7.8 cm		0.11	0.09
8 Metatarsal 1 phalangeal 1 length ratio	1–1.4 cm	1.1 cm	1.2 cm	1.2 cm	1.3 cm	1.3 cm		0.03	0.06
9 Metatarsal head 1–5 length (forefoot width)	7.1–9 cm	7.5 cm	7.9 cm	8.1 cm	8.5 cm	8.6 cm		0.17	0.14
10 Talocalcaneal length (hindfoot width)	4–5.5 cm	4.3 cm	4.6 cm	4.8 cm	4.9 cm	5.1 cm		0.18	0.17
11 Interphalangeal 1 angle	6–24°	9°	11°	14.5°	18°	20°		3.10	2.83
12 Metatarsal 1-phalangeal 1 angle	0–32°	6°	9°	12°	16°	18°		2.68	2.35
13 Proximal phalanx 1-proximal articular surface angle	0–10°	1°	3°	3.5°	6°	7°		2.35	1.86
14 Metatarsal 1 distal-articular surface angle	0–15°	0°	2°	3°	7°	8°		2.85	2.44
15 Angle on incongruity	−4–24°	0°	1°	3°	5°	11°		3.43	3.37
16 Metatarsal 5-phalangeal 5 angle	1–21°	2°	3°	7.5°	12°	14°		2.60	2.56

17 Metatarsal-proximal articular surface angle	0–15°	0°	1°	3°	5°	12°	3.20	2.96
18 Intermetatarsal 1-2 angle	4–23°	5°	7°	7°	8°	10°	1.53	2.44
19 Intermetatarsal 2-5 angle	8–21°	9°	12°	14°	17°	18°	2.15	1.93
20 Intermetatarsal 1-5 angle	14–35°	17°	20°	22°	25°	27°	2.20	2.33
21 Cuneiform 1 proximal articular surface-metatarsal 2 shaft angle	84–122°	89°	95°	98°	105°	108°	5.30	4.94
22 Talometatarsal 2 shaft angle	6–42°	11°	15°	22°	27°	32°	4.30	3.68
23 Calcaneus-metatarsal 2 shaft angle	3–35°	6°	12°	14°	18°	26°	5.25	4.43
24 Hindfoot angle	15–63°	20°	26°	37°	47°	54°	5.98	4.88
25 Forefoot adductus angle	−13–13°	−4°	−2°	2°	4°	8°	4.03	2.69
26 Navicular proximal articular surface-metatarsal 2 shaft angle	76–107°	82°	88°	90.5°	93°	100°	5.08	3.63
27 Distal hindfoot articular surface-metatarsal 2 shaft angle	44–122°	99°	104°	108°	111°	117°	5.75	11.80
28 Tibialward sesamoid position	1–7	1	2	2	3	5	0.68	0.76

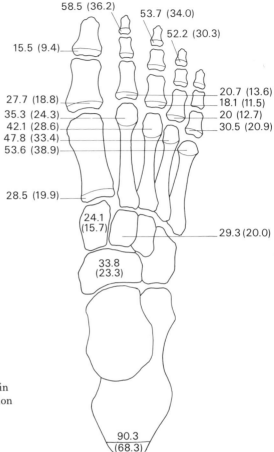

Fig. 12.6   AP diagram of the foot
showing the times of appearance (in
months) of the centres of ossification
for boys (girls in brackets). (From
Hoerr *et al* (1962), with kind
permission of Charles C. Thomas,
Springfield, Illinois.)

Just as in biphalangism, middle phalangeal epiphyses are more often missing in
females, and on the left, and the abnormality is lateral, and not medial, to a more
normal form. While middle phalanges generally become shorter toward the lateral
aspect of the foot, they are also shorter in those feet in which biphalangeal fifth
toes are seen (Fig. 12.7). There is thus a progression of anomalies, ending in
biphalangism, maximal laterally, resulting from the size of the middle phalanx.
The author quotes work to show that before segmentation at a joint can take place,
adequate amounts of skeletal tissue must be present at both sides of the
presumptive joint.

RHEUMATOID ARTHRITIS AND ITS VARIANTS

The radiological changes at joints in adult rheumatoid arthritis have been
summarized by Jacobs (1975). They are:

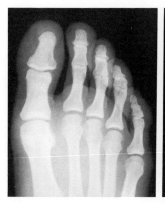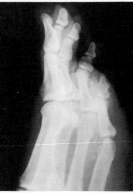

Fig. 12.7 Biphalangism of the little toe with failure of segmentation of the distal interphalangeal joint and a progressive increase in length of the middle phalanges, proceeding medially.

1 Soft tissue changes.
2 Osteoporosis.
3 Joint space changes and alignment deformities.
4 Periostitis.
5 Erosions.
6 Secondary osteoarthritis.

Analysis of the radiograph in rheumatoid disease must be systematic. A magnifying glass should be used to assess early cortical changes.

Soft tissue swelling in the forefoot is obvious clinically but is also seen radiologically, especially by comparison with the contralateral (normal) foot. Swelling may be seen over the outer surfaces of the first and fifth metatarsophalangeal joints when inflammation is present in the bursae adjacent to those joints (Fig. 12.8). Swelling over the remaining metatarsophalangeal joints may be seen as a soft tissue projection into adjacent web spaces. Soft tissue swelling also shows as a local increase in density around the joint, again visible by comparison with a normal joint. Diffuse soft tissue swelling over all the metatarsal heads may be seen on lateral views.

Osteoporosis may be generalized, or local and subarticular. With local inflammation of a joint, demineralization is localized to the bone around the joint (Fig. 12.8). This is seen in rheumatoid arthritis and especially in tuberculous arthritis. Generalized demineralization involving the entire foot is seen less often in early rheumatoid disease, though disuse atrophy may cause this change, as may steroid therapy.

The radiological visualization of osteoporosis depends in part on film quality. There is inevitably some variation between examinations so that assessment of minor changes of bone density may be difficult. Comparison between normal and abnormal joints in the same patient is helpful. The use on a film of a 'normal' phalanx embedded in wax, or an aluminium wedge for direct densitometry has never been widespread. The interpretation of osteoporosis is subjective and osteoporosis may only be identifiable after 25–50% loss of mineral. In osteoporosis

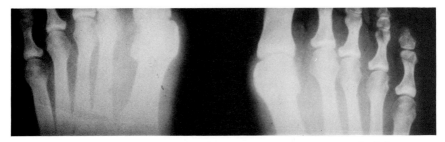

Fig. 12.8 A soft tissue x-ray shows marked soft tissue swelling over the left great toe metatarsal head and fifth toe metatarsal head. By comparison with the right foot the great toe metatarsophalangeal joint is narrowed. Marked subcortical osteoporosis is seen at the remaining metatarsal heads, especially the fifth on both sides.

due to hyperparathyroidism, for instance, correlation between two radiologists in grading osteoporosis in the peripheral skeleton was 53% when clearly normal films were excluded from the study, rising to 71% if normals were included (Genant *et al* 1973). Kellgren and Lawrence (1957) found 'substantial' agreement between observers in the assessment of osteoporosis in rheumatoid disease. Using a grading of 0 (none) to 4 (severe) in 19 sample films extracted from a population survey, seen by 60 observers, 50% of films were identically graded. On no film was there a difference between observers of two grades. Fletcher and Rowley (1952), using three observers, found a difference of opinion not only between the three, but also with the same observer on different occasions. They found osteoporosis in 65% of patients with rheumatoid disease, the incidence varying with the length of history of the disease. In those with three months duration of disease only 40% were affected, while in those with ten years of disease 78% were affected. Brook and Corbett (1977) found osteoporosis on presentation in 27% of rheumatoid patients, but in 76% of patients at two years.

Fletcher and Rowley also demonstrated an increasing incidence of osteoporosis with age, in 48% of 25 cases below thirty, and in 88% of 24 cases at 60. This is presumably related to duration of disease, bone loss in the post-menopausal female (the usual sex incidence for rheumatoid disease is around $M:F = 1:3$) and, presumably, steroid therapy.

Total foot osteoporosis is less common (35%) than juxta-articular porosis (65%), which is especially seen in cases of more recent onset. The figure given seems high for total osteoporosis. In the hand, a figure of 5% has been quoted (Thould & Simon 1966).

Young *et al* (1980) correlated clinical activity of disease with radiological progression. No statistical correlation was found between clinical activity over a three year period and juxta-articular porosis, though they do note that patients on long term steroids developed severe osteoporosis. Active disease apparently flourished in the absence of osteoporosis, while of those with osteoporosis, 25% were inactive.

Brook and Corbett, however, showed elsewhere (1977) that of 52 osteoporotic patients, 50 developed erosions. Clearly, therefore, osteoporosis is a precursor of erosive disease. Indeed, I believe that marked subarticular osteoporosis actually *hides* early erosions. Erosive bone loss is hidden in the generalized subarticular demineralization. Initial films showing local osteoporosis turn out later to have an erosion which more or less matches the earlier osteoporotic area in size.

Martel *et al* (1980) have described the earliest sites of cortical erosions. They occur on the 'bare areas' between the attachment of the joint capsule and the edge of the articular cartilage (Fig. 12.9). In the hand, the bare areas are larger on the proximal than on the distal joint surface at all the joints of a ray. Cartilage is not distributed evenly along joint surfaces, being thicker at the centre of a metacarpal head than at the periphery and, reciprocally, thicker at the periphery of the base of a proximal phalanx. At proximal interphalangeal and distal interphalangeal joints, however, cartilage is thicker on the periphery at the proximal side of the joint and centrally on the distal surface. The anatomy of the joint bare areas and distribution of cartilage are felt by Martel *et al* to be of great importance in the development of joint erosions.

It has long been recognized that the feet are involved earlier and more frequently than the hands in rheumatoid arthritis. Fletcher and Rowley found that at six months 19% of metatarsophalangeal joints were abnormal, but only 9% of metacarpophalangeal joints—the fifth metatarsophalangeal joint being most often affected. Calabro (1962) quotes similar figures at onset. Overall in the disease, the

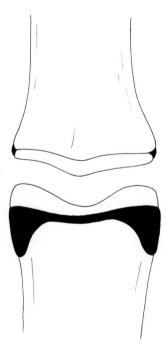

Fig. 12.9 'Bare areas' between the attachment of the joint capsule and the edge of the articular cartilage are shown shaded black. Note the absence of symmetry of cartilage distribution over joint surfaces. (After Martel *et al* 1980.)

feet may be eroded in some 90% of adult cases. Thould and Simon assessed the hands and feet of 105 patients with rheumatoid arthritis, unselected for duration of disease. 91% had bone changes in the feet, but only 75% had changes in the hands, i.e. 16% had abnormal feet with normal hands. Interestingly, 35% of this latter group had a negative latex fixation, as opposed to 9% of those with both hands and feet involved; no cases had normal feet with abnormal hands. Brook and Corbett describe a similar tendency. They show erosions appearing first of all in the feet (35.8%), then in the hands (16.4%) and simultaneously in both in 47.8%, but this must be related to their radiological examination which was at yearly intervals. 38% of their patients had erosions only at the metatarsophalangeal joints. As in the hands, the distal interphalangeal joints are only infrequently affected in rheumatoid arthritis though, in the feet, changes at these joints cannot easily be seen due to flexion deformities.

Using magnification techniques it is probable that smaller erosions can be seen earlier. Early cortical loss, which may be continuous or interrupted (giving a 'dot-dash' pattern), has been described. Linear subcortical porosis has also been shown to progress to erosion at metatarsal heads (Fletcher & Rowley 1952).

It has been pointed out that the feet, and especially the metatarsal heads, are the most common site of erosive change. There is agreement as to which heads are most commonly involved (Thould & Simon 1966; Fletcher & Rowley 1952), the order of involvement being 5, 3, 2, 4, 1. Some 60–70% of fifth metatarsal heads erode, while only 25–30% of first metatarsal heads are thus changed. The higher the latex test titre, the more erosions develop. With progression of the disease, the tendency is to symmetry between feet. Early disease shows a degree of asymmetry with a right-sided predominance.

The metatarsal head erodes before the base of the distal phalanx. This may relate to a larger bare area on the metatarsal head. The predilection is apparently for the anteromedial border of the head to be initially eroded in the foot.

Abnormalities of alignment

In patients with rheumatoid disease, abnormalities of alignment are seen in the fore-, mid- and hindfeet. Just as ulnar deviation is recognized in the hand, so fibular fibular deviation occurs at the metatarsophalangeal joints in the feet. In particular, hallux valgus was found in 59% of feet at risk (Kirkup *et al* 1977). Using an angle of over 11° for the great toe proximal phalanx on metatarsal shaft to diagnose hallux valgus, Vidigal *et al* (1975) made the diagnosis in 70% of cases.

Of feet with hallux valgus, 86% had erosions at the metatarsophalangeal joint, but there is, in any case, an increase in the valgus angle, especially in the female, with increase in age (Fig. 12.10).

Dislocation of hallux sesamoids between first and second metatarsal heads occurs, which may be seen on the anteroposterior (Fig. 12.10) and on the tangential radiograph of the forefoot (Gheith & Dixon 1973). By this method, partial or complete dislocation was shown in 71% of consecutive patients with rheumatoid

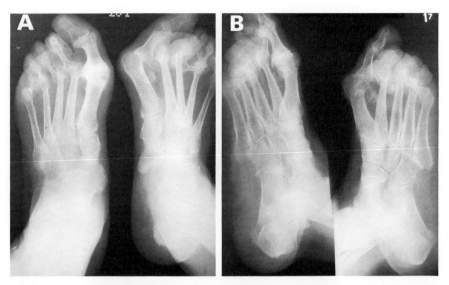

Fig. 12.10 (A) and (B) Rheumatoid arthritis showing bilateral hallux valgus with lateral drift of the phalanges and dislocation of the hallux sesamoids. There is marked osteoporosis overall. Joint narrowing is pronounced at the left tarsus together with secondary degenerative change, while the right tarsus shows more normal joints. Tarsal erosions are not common despite the severity of the disease. The metatarsal heads, however, are showing signs of absorption, especially where they are bearing a disproportionate amount of weight, as at the right second and third metatarsal heads.

arthritis. The sesamoids act as markers for the flexor hallucis tendon. Weakening of the fibrous structures around joints allows tendons to shift laterally. Together with lateral sesamoid dislocation, the space between first and second, and fourth and fifth, metatarsal heads increases as the intermetatarsal ligaments are weakened by inflammation, possibly because of local bursitis. The foot spreads and the metatarsal heads prolapse, as seen on the tangential view in 66%. The metatarsal heads, especially the second and third, become subcutaneous and the sesamoids and metatarsal heads, already eroded, undergo further osteolysis. The soft tissue fibro-fatty cushion, clearly seen on the tangential view, is almost invariably thinned or displaced.

While hallux valgus is the commonest acquired deformity of the great toe in rheumatoid arthritis, hallux rigidus was found in 28%, chisel toes in 22% and hallux elevatus in 11% (Kirkup *et al* 1977).

Radiological changes in the mid- and hindfoot

Changes behind the forefoot receive less attention, yet rigid flat foot is common in rheumatoid arthritis and increases with duration of disease (Calabro 1962) so that it is eventually present in up to 50% of females (Fig. 12.11).

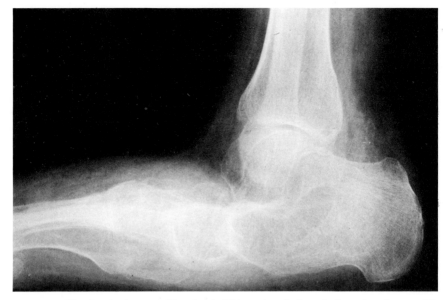

Fig. 12.11   Flat foot in rheumatoid arthritis. This patient had marked erosive change of the metatarsophalangeal joints.

Excluding the calcaneum, Resnick (1976) found radiographic abnormality in the talocalcaneonavicular joint in 39% of the feet of 50 rheumatoid patients (he defines this joint as formed by the anterior facets on the talus and calcaneum, proximal surface of the navicular and the plantar calcaneonavicular ligament; Fig. 12.12). Joint narrowing occurred in all cases, but fusion in only two. The predilection was for the talonavicular portion of the joint, and osteophytosis at the dorsum of that joint was also commonly seen. Most patients with change at the calcaneocuboid joint (26% of total) also had changes at the talocalcaneonavicular joint. Erosive change was more common at the calcaneocuboid joint, but the usual tarsal changes of joint narrowing and osteophytosis were also present.

The tarsometatarsal joints were abnormal in 36% of feet. Usually both medial and lateral compartments of the joint were involved. Narrowing was again common, but fusion uncommon, and erosions were seen only in 4 of 27 affected feet.

The subtalar joint was abnormal in 29% (13 of 45) feet. 50% of these also had ankle joint abnormality. The small joints of the midfoot (intercuneiform, cuboidonavicular, etc.) showed change in 28%.

It seems then that change at the mid- and hindfoot consists firstly of joint narrowing, reactive sclerosis and osteophytosis (Fig. 12.10), rather than erosions (Fig. 12.12). Fusion, as in the forefoot in rheumatoid arthritis, remains uncommon. Vidigal *et al* (1975) found subtalar involvement in 32% of feet in patients with rheumatoid arthritis, almost inevitably in the presence of midtarsal and metatarsophalangeal joint involvement. Similarly, the involvement of the midtarsal joints

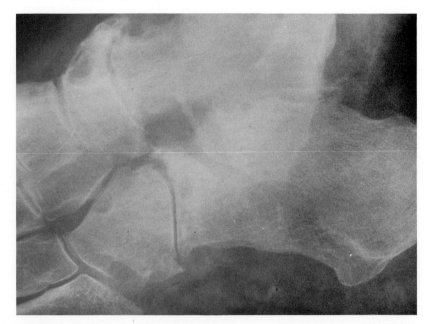

Fig. 12.12   Erosive change is seen at the talocalcaneonavicular joints, as well as around the cuboid, associated with joint narrowing and secondary osteophytosis.

(in 62% of feet—not further subdivided as in Resnick's paper) occurred ten times more often with metatarsophalangeal joint disease than without. The ankle joint proper was involved in 26% of feet, again much more often with metatarsophalan-geal and midtarsal disease than not (Fig. 12.13). The concomitant of subtalar disease, a valgus hindfoot, was seen clinically in 55 of 204 feet, but varus deformity in only two feet. Kirkup (1974) examined 50 adults with hindfoot symptoms in rheumatoid arthritis. 53 of 100 feet had valgus deformity and only four varus. Valgus deformity is explained as a combination of horizontal deviation following subluxation of talo-navicular and calcaneo-cuboid joints, and vertical deviation following subluxation at the subtalar and ankle joints. Fibular stress changes and fractures may then result. Hindfoot disease was present in those with chronic rheumatoid disease (duration 4–43 years). 25 tarsi were found to be fused, on average after 19 years of disease, but the ankle was fused in only three cases. It was again found that when ankle disease is present, tarsal change is nearly always present, but the tarsus is involved alone in 35% of cases.

The calcaneum in erosive disease

Bywaters (1954) and Resnick *et al* (1977) have demonstrated the anatomy of the calcaneal region. The Achilles tendon inserts 2 cm below the upper surface of the calcaneum. The retrocalcaneal bursa is situated between the two, enveloped in a

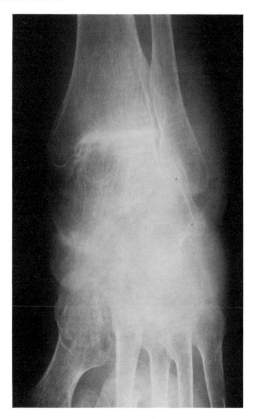

Fig. 12.13 Marked soft tissue
swelling is seen over the malleoli
together with narrowing of the ankle
joint proper, but no obvious erosion.
There is narrowing of the midtarsal
and tarsometatarsal joints in this
patient with longstanding
rheumatoid disease.

thin layer of synovium which extends upwards to cover the inferior projection of
the pre-Achilles fat pad (Fig. 12.14). The back of the calcaneum is covered by
fibrocartilage which degenerates with age, though the underlying bone usually
retains its cortex.

The Achilles tendon is easily visualized and on average is some 6 mm thick at
the level of the calcaneum. The retrocalcaneal recess shows as a lucency between
the back of the calcaneum and Achilles tendon, for some 2–10 mm below the top of
the calcaneum (Fig. 12.15). It rarely extends above the calcaneum, but is
obliterated in dorsiflexion and exaggerated in plantar flexion. The plantar surface
of the calcaneum is covered by periosteum into which the Achilles tendon and
plantar fascia insert.

Bywaters found 2.4% of patients with rheumatoid arthritis to have heel pain
and radiological abnormality (presumably spurs and erosions) on the calcaneum.
Heel abnormalities, especially spurs, had apparently earlier been noted in systemic
diseases—syphilis, gonorrhoea, gout and 'rheumatism'—but the author demonstrated these changes in rheumatoid arthritis using clinical and radiologic–pathologic correlation. Clinically, the Achilles tendon was thicker, the underlying bursa

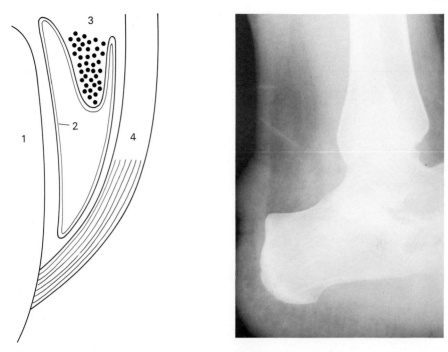

Fig. 12.14 (*Left*) Normal anatomy of the retrocalcaneal region. (1) calcaneum, (2) synovium lining the bursa, (3) inferior tip of the pre-Achilles fat pad, (4) Achilles tendon.

Fig. 12.15 (*Right*) Radiological demonstration of the Achilles tendon insertion into the back of calcaneum and the pre-Achilles fat pad, which lies above the calcaneum posteriorly. The insertion of the plantar fascia into the inferior aspect of the calcaneum is also seen.

large and tender, and the plantar surface of the bone tender. Pathologically, the lesions resembled rheumatoid tissue. Bywaters also pointed out that the earliest radiological changes were in the soft tissues, the tendon becoming thicker on the lateral radiograph and the lucent region anterior to it obliterated by inflammation. The underlying bone loses density, becomes fuzzy and eventually erodes above the upper end of the Achilles insertion (Fig. 12.16). Plantar lesions show erosion of bone, often behind the spur, which usually is involved and eventually lengthens (Fig. 12.17).

Resnick *et al* (1977) analysed the calcaneal lesions in rheumatoid arthritis, ankylosing spondylitis, psoriatic arthritis and Reiter's syndrome, and also examined 'normal' controls. 22% of heels in his control group had spurs, which increased in frequency with increasing age. They were plantar in 16%, posterior in 11% and on both sites in 4%. Generally smooth and well-defined in outline, they were usually less than 4 mm in size and generally smaller on the plantar surface.

1   64 rheumatoid patients then had their 128 heels radiographed.
2   47 heels (37% overall) were abnormal.

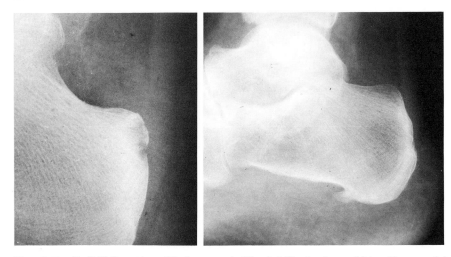

Fig. 12.16 (*Left*) Obliteration of the lower part of the Achilles tendon and fat pad by synovial inflammation in rheumatoid arthritis, associated with erosion in the region of the tendinous insertion.

Fig. 12.17 (*Right*) Rheumatoid arthritis. The Achilles tendon is still well visualized and the pre-Achilles fat pad well seen. There is a plantar spur which looks 'benign' but the bone behind it is eroding and the plantar fascia is not well seen. There is also a talar beak.

3   17 of the 47 heels (13% overall) had well-defined plantar-posterior spurs similar to those in the control population with *no other* abnormality.

4   26 of the 47 heels (20% overall) had abnormality of the retrocalcaneal recess and 7 of the 47 heels (5% overall) had tendon thickening.

5   24 of the 47 heels (18% overall) had erosions.

6   44 further spurs were shown as *additional* findings (in those patients other than with the well-defined spurs (3) above), together with retrocalcaneal recess abnormality, tendon thickening and erosion. Plantar spurs were then more common (2:1). These spurs were irregular in margin, but not particularly larger than the 'benign' spurs mentioned above.

Half of the abnormal heels ((4) above) had an abnormal retrocalcaneal recess. It now extended, on average, 2 mm above the level of the calcaneum, while the Achilles tendon was 7.5 mm thick on average at that level (normal = 6.0 mm).

Other papers (see below) have also assessed calcaneal abnormalities in rheumatoid (and other) disease. Information is presented so differently in the various studies that it is often difficult to make valid comparisons between them, even if the populations assessed would have been similar. Thus, the average duration of disease in Resnick's series was 16 years, and that of Gerster *et al* (1977) nine years.

In 100 patients with rheumatoid arthritis (presumably with 200 heels), 4% showed clinical evidence of 'achillobursitis' (Gerster *et al* 1977). Using xeroradiography, he was then able to demonstrate the enlarged bursa actually indenting the anterior surface of the Achilles tendon. Erosions are then shown developing anterior to the bursa above the tendon insertion. Thickening of the plantar fascia at the sites of erosion is also demonstrated, so that the heel pad thickness (*vide infra*) is increased. This author found well-defined spurs in 20% of patients, posterior erosions in 6%, plantar erosions in 1% and irregular spurs in 4%, equally divided between sites. It is important to note that this paper emphasizes the absence of clinical correlation between simple spurs and heel pain.

Mason *et al* (1959) observed simple plantar spurs in 39% of 81 rheumatoid *patients* and erosions in 21%, mainly posterior. This author and his colleagues also distinguish between the benign spur and the irregular form, due in part to a diffuse periostitis. They believe these changes to be common posteriorly (21% of patients) but not on the plantar surface (4%). They also describe how a 'benign' spur becomes irregular on follow-up (Fig. 12.18), while Resnick *et al* (1977) observed how irregular plantar spurs become better defined on subsequent examination (Fig. 12.19). Spur formation and morphology is clearly therefore subject to dynamic change, which would account for the increased number of rheumatoid arthritis patients with spurs, compared with a control population, possibly depending on duration and activity of disease, and also compatible with Gerster's observation of

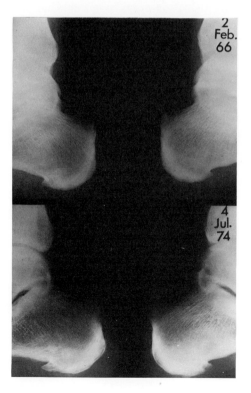

2
Feb.
66

4
Jul.
74

Fig. 12.18 Reiter's syndrome. The initial films showed plantar spurs which looked benign and which may be seen in normal patients. Eight years later the spurs have become larger, eroded and very fluffy. There were posterior erosions in the region of the Achilles tendon insertion on the initial film and there is now posterior spur formation. (By courtesy of Dr H.I. Jory, Queen Elizabeth II Hospital, Welwyn Garden City.)

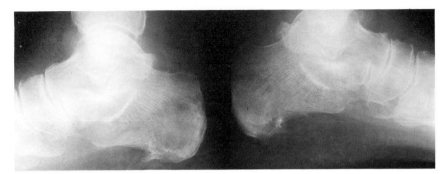

Fig. 12.19 This patient with chronic rheumatoid arthritis shows spurs which are larger than normal and misshapen, but nonetheless well-corticated. The demineralization posterior to both plantar spurs may have been the seat of previous erosive change, while the posterior aspect of the calcaneum may also have been eroded in the past. The fat anterior to the Achilles tendon is obliterated because of chronic synovitis.

lack of correlation between pain and simple spurs in patients with rheumatoid arthritis.

Resnick *et al* believe that the erosions on the heel may be situated in different sites in different diseases (Fig. 12.20; Table 12.3), and Mason *et al* also show cases which demonstrate this. That the design of most surveys is so variable has been mentioned. Unfortunately, even the terminology used to describe the spurs, for instance, varies.

According to Mason *et al* (1959) a very fluffy, dense, irregular and large spur is strongly suggestive of Reiter's syndrome. This periostitis occurred in 20% of their patients with Reiter's syndrome (Figs. 12.18, 12.21). Only a further three patients (4%) with rheumatoid arthritis and two (5%) with ankylosing spondylitis had this

Fig. 12.20 Target areas for spurs and erosions in rheumatoid disease and its variants (after Resnick *et al* 1977). (1) superior surface, (2) posterior surface above attachment of Achilles tendon, (3) posterior surface at attachment of Achilles tendon, (4) plantar surface at the attachment of plantar aponeurosis, (5) plantar surface anterior to attachment of aponeurosis. Rheumatoid arthritis mainly affects (1), (2), (3) and (4). Ankylosing spondylitis mainly affects (2), (3), (4) and (5). Psoriatic arthritis mainly affects (2), (3), (4) and (5). Reiter's syndrome mainly affects (1), (2) and (4). (With permission of the authors and the Editors of *Radiology*.)

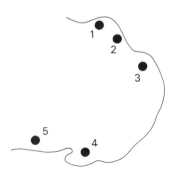

Table 12.3 Calcaneal target areas (after Resnick *et al* 1977; with kind permission of the authors and the publishers of *Radiology*).

	1	2	3	4	5
Rheumatoid arthritis	E	E	S(WD)	S(WD)	
Ankylosing spondylitis		E	S(WD)	E,S(WD/I)	P
Psoriasis		E	S(WD)	E,S(WD/I)	P
Reiter's syndrome	E	E		E,S(WD/I)	

E = erosions; S = spur; WD = well-defined; I = irregular;
P = periostitis.

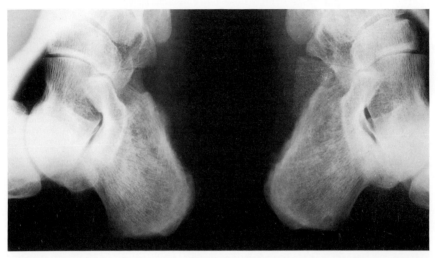

Fig. 12.21 Reiter's syndrome. A very fluffy dense irregular periostitis is demonstrated on the inferior surface of both calcaneal bones, together with erosive change on their posterior surface in the region of the Achilles tendon insertions.

gross 'plantar periostitis'. These five patients were then reviewed and, in most cases, the diagnosis changed. Gerster *et al* (1977) agree that irregular plantar spurs have their greatest incidence in Reiter's syndrome—plantar in 18% of patients but posterior in 0%—but also finds them in ankylosing spondylitis—plantar in 11.4% of patients and posterior in 2.8% (it will be noted that his equivalent figure for rheumatoid arthritis was 2% for each). Resnick *et al* (1977) also comment that bony proliferation is frequent in Reiter's syndrome, ankylosing spondylitis and psoriasis.

Psoriasis and arthritis

Martel *et al* (1980) studied the relative onset of arthritis and psoriasis in 44 patients. Five patients (11%) developed an initial arthritis with skin lesions appearing 2–15 years later. In 11 cases (25%) the two developed simultaneously and, in 28 cases (64%), psoriasis preceded arthritis by up to 36 years (mean 12 years). Wright (1961) notes that an association between psoriasis and arthritis was described as long ago as 1822. A number of different definitions of psoriatic arthropathy have been given, but the incidence of psoriatic arthritis in psoriasis varies from 1–5% (Wright 1978). In his study 121 patients with psoriasis had an erosive arthritis. Of these, 18 (15%) had a positive Rose–Waaler test. Their clinical and radiological features did not different from uncomplicated rheumatoid arthritis. In Peterson and Silbiger's radiological survey (1967), 28% of patients with arthritis and psoriasis had classical changes of rheumatoid arthritis.

Lack of osteoporosis has long been regarded as a feature of psoriatic arthropathy (Wright 1978) even where bone destruction is present and, indeed, one's own experience bears this out. Both the papers mentioned above, however, (Wright 1961; Martel *et al* 1980) found this to be uncommon. Lack of porosis was found in only three of Wright's patients. In only five of Martel's patients with severe destruction was regional osteoporosis not present. Presumably treatment, age, sex and immobilization are also involved.

Clearly, it is not possible to assess a specific disease without considering the whole skeleton. Sacro-iliitis, for instance, distinguishes ankylosing spondylitis from rheumatoid arthritis. A characteristic feature of psoriatic arthropathy, however, is its predilection for the distal interphalangeal joints of the toes, even more than those of the hands, while changes at the metatarsophalangeal joints are much more common in rheumatoid arthritis. Erosions at distal interphalangeal joints occurred in 17% of psoriatics and in 2% of control rheumatoid feet (Wright 1961) and in 55% of 'interphalangeal joints' excluding the great toe (Martel *et al* 1980). Psoriatic arthropathy shows a predilection for the great toe interphalangeal joint, which may be especially severely affected, in 70% (Martel *et al* 1980), in 17% (Wright 1961) or 35% (Peterson & Silbiger 1967) (Fig. 12.22). Erosions in psoriatic arthropathy may resemble rheumatoid erosions early on in the disease, but bone proliferation and even subsequent ankylosis eventually alter their appearance. The 'bare area' erosions at the base of the distal interphalangeal joint give an appearance likened to 'mouse ears' (Fig. 12.22), when articular cartilage is relatively spared (Martel *et al* 1980). Periosteal new bone apposition may be smooth or irregular (Martel *et al* 1980; Peterson & Silbiger 1967) and is commonly seen in up to 70% of patients (Martel *et al* 1980). Interphalangeal joint ankylosis, uncommon in rheumatoid arthritis, is seen in 12–15%, while the interphalangeal joints may be widened (35%), especially at the great toe, at the site of marked subjacent bone loss. Peterson and Silbiger found no definite correlation between psoriatic nail changes and distal interphalangeal joint disease. Wright, however, showed that erosion of the tips of the terminal phalanges, especially in the feet, was only seen with nail changes, though conversely, as expected, nail changes without arthritis were more common.

Lack of symmetry is a feature of psoriatic arthropathy which may also be seen early on in rheumatoid arthritis. Psoriatic arthropathy may not only be asymmetri-

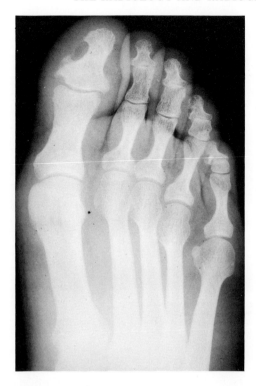

Fig. 12.22 Psoriatic arthropathy.
The distal interphalangeal joint of
the great toe is affected while the
metatarsophalangeal joint is spared.
There is little osteoporosis. New
bone formation is probably present,
as well as a large marginal erosion.

cal, but unilateral, or even may affect only one ray (Martel *et al* 1980) so that a
swollen, sausage-like finger or toe can be seen both clinically and radiologically
due to affliction of both the tendon sheaths and joints. Where asymmetry is present
it may be most marked at the metatarsophalangeal joints (42% of patients with
these joints involved (Wright 1961)).

Reiter's syndrome

Reiter's syndrome has many radiological and clinical features in common with
psoriatic arthropathy, but the latter is not associated with urethritis, nor
apparently usually with arthritis mutilans. Reiter's syndrome affects the feet
rather than the hands, while the converse is generally true in psoriatic arthropathy. Mason *et al* (1959) found a peripheral arthropathy in the feet of 48% and
hands of 28% of cases of Reiter's syndrome. The disease is also much more severe in
the feet. Sholkoff *et al* (1970) found soft tissue swelling and interphalangeal joint
erosion in 24 great toes of 45 patients with Reiter's syndrome, and 48 metatarsophalangeal joints, but in no distal interphalangeal joints. Again, asymmetry occurs in
Reiter's syndrome (Fig. 12.23).

Mason *et al* (1959) had formed a clinical impression that periosteal new bone
formation was common in Reiter's syndrome, but their survey did not bear out this

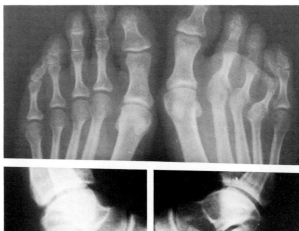
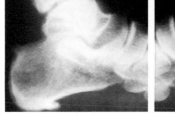
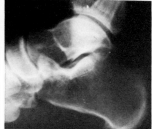

Fig. 12.23 Reiter's syndrome. The metatarsophalangeal joints are affected by an erosive arthropathy and the distal interphalangeal joints are spared, in contradistinction to psoriasis. There is asymmetry, and osteoporosis is not prominent. Irregular plantar spurs are present together with posterior erosions and spur formation.

impression, apart from at the calcaneum. Periostitis was present in half their patients at the malleoli, but they found it in only 8% of patients at the metatarsals, and never on the phalanges. Sholkoff *et al* (1970) concur that periostitis is found at the distal tibia and fibula, but also found it frequently along metatarsal shafts. The periostitis may be rather more linear in acute cases or fluffy and irregular in chronic cases (Peterson & Silbiger 1967; Fig. 12.24).

Again, asymmetry occurs, and osteoporosis is not inevitable.

The sacro-iliac joints and thoracolumbar regions are affected in psoriatic arthropathy, Reiter's syndrome and ankylosing spondylitis, though Patton (1976) has demonstrated some differences in the pattern of new bone formation around disc spaces in ankylosing spondylitis on the one hand, and Reiter's syndrome and psoriatic arthropathy on the other. Comparison between rheumatoid arthritis and ankylosing spondylitis (Dilsen 1962) and Reiter's syndrome, rheumatoid arthritis and ankylosing spondylitis (Mason *et al* 1959) confirm the paucity of metatarsophalangeal joint involvement in ankylosing spondylitis. Hand lesions in ankylosing spondylitis are also uncommon. Though 24% of cases of ankylosing spondylitis showed a peripheral arthropathy in the feet (Mason *et al* 1959), 'minimal' radiographic involvement in ankylosing spondylitis was seen in another series at metatarsophalangeal joints (10%; Dilsen 1962). 'In most patients with ankylosing spondylitis the great predominance and early appearance of sacro-iliac changes and mild involvement of feet is in contrast to the severe affection of feet and late development of sacro-iliitis in Reiter's syndrome' (Mason *et al* 1959).

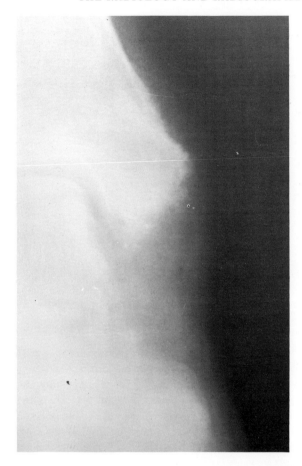

Fig. 12.24 Psoriatic arthropathy. Irregular fluffy periostitis is present at the medial malleolus of the distal tibia. Similar appearances are found in Reiter's syndrome.

THE FOOT IN JOINT DISEASE OF CHILDREN

Ansell and Kent (1977) and Ansell (1980) have written comprehensive accounts of the clinical, immunological and radiological features of rheumatic disorders in children. The radiological changes seen in juvenile chronic polyarthritis vary with age of onset and type of disease, for this group of diseases is heterogenous. 10% of these children are IgM rheumatoid factor positive. The disease in these children is similar to adult-type rheumatoid arthritis. Osteoporosis around metatarsophalangeal and interphalangeal joints and periostitis along the shafts of the short tubular bones are seen early on, and rheumatoid-type erosions are seen after one year in all these patients (Fig. 12.25). Of those who are IgM negative, the mode of onset may be systemic (20%), mono or pauci-articular (64%) or polyarticular (18%) in type. These children, who are by far the largest group, are seronegative, and their disease was previously known as Still's disease.

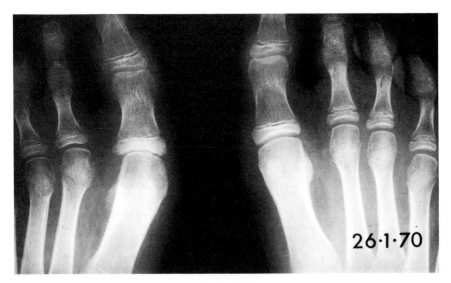

Fig. 12.25 Seropositive rheumatoid arthritis in a 14-year-old boy. Marked soft tissue swelling and osteoporosis is demonstrated with cartilage loss at the left metatarsophalangeal joint of the great toe and erosive change at the metatarsal head and adjacent second metatarsal head. The right fourth metatarsal neck shows faint periostitis.

Systemic disease has little bone change. In those children with polyarthritis, however, 45% have involvement of the tarsus and ankle. Soft tissue swelling and osteoporosis are seen around joints together with phalangeal shaft periostitis and overgrowth of the tarsal bones. Should disease persist the tarsal bones take on a curious angular shape, so that the normally curved contours are lost. Joint spaces are narrowed, so that the now angular bones are crowded together. In severe cases, the developing ossification centres, especially that for the navicular, may be so irregular that avascular necrosis might be suggested (Fig. 12.26). The tarsal centres may even vanish altogether, only to reappear later. Ankylosis may also develop. Erosive change, if it appears at all, is late and minor—rather the epiphyses become squared, large and prematurely fused, so that rays end up shortened.

Pauci-articular disease is probably due to a number of different disease entities (Ansell 1980). 17% turn out to have juvenile ankylosing spondylitis and 4% psoriatic arthropathy. 14% are seropositive for rheumatoid factor and the remainder (65%) end up as a truly seronegative juvenile chronic arthritis.

The age of onset of juvenile ankylosing spondylitis is around ten years. The tarsus, ankle or toe interphalangeal joints are involved first. Plantar fasciitis leads to calcaneal spur formation, while bursal inflammation at the Achilles tendon insertion may lead to erosions on, or premature fusion of, the calcaneal apophysis. Sacro-iliitis follows later, after 5–15 years. Most of these patients have HLA-B27 specificity.

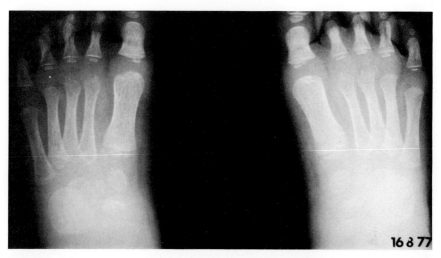

16 8 77

Fig. 12.26 The bones of the foot are demineralized and hypoplastic but show accelerated skeletal development in terms of ossification. The tarsal bones are angular, crowded together and irregular. There is no erosive change.

Psoriasis and arthritis have been seen in children from one year of age on, mainly in females. Some patients have the typical patterns of adult disease, and others resemble juvenile chronic arthritis.

TARSAL COALITION

Cowell (1972) gives a history of the literature of tarsal coalition. It is found in two major forms. Calcaneonavicular coalition was first described anatomically by Cruveiller in 1829, and Zuckerkandl described talocalcaneal coalition in 1877. In a remarkable pathological and radiological *Atlas of Variations of the Bones of the Hand and Foot*, published just twelve years after the discovery of the Roentgen ray, Dwight (1907) demonstrated two examples of calcaneonavicular synostosis, which he noted to be 1 cm broad. In one example, the foot is obliquely projected on a radiograph and the synostosis is especially well shown. Slomann (1926) demonstrated calcaneonavicular coalition radiologically by an oblique view with the foot at 45° to the 'plate'. He also recognized that bony coalition could be complete—a synostosis—or incomplete, so that an amphiarthrosis existed between the prologations from the two bones, while a fibrous union between the two bones which might contain a 'secondary os calcis' was also described (Fig. 12.27). Slomann associated the bony change with a painful flat foot turned out in abduction. Seddon (1932) described eight possible variants of coalition.

Harris and Beath (1948) showed that most cases of peroneal spastic flat foot are due to tarsal coalition (Fig. 12.28). They found that the medial talocalcaneal bridge

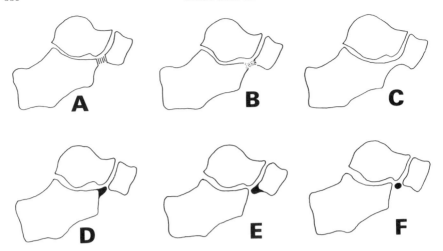

Fig. 12.27 Diagramatic representation of the types of union: (A) fibrous, (B) cartilaginous, (C) osseous, (D) prominent process on the calcaneum, (E) prominent process on the navicular and (F) separate calcaneonavicular ossicle (calcaneum secondarium).

was the most common anomaly. Other less common sites of fusion are posterior talocalcaneal bridge, cubonavicular fusion (Del Sel & Grand 1958), talonavicular fusion and calcaneocuboid fusion (Harris 1965). A 'block' tarsus may also exist, as does naviculocuneiform synostosis (Lusby 1959) and anterior talocalcaneal facet fusion (Cowell 1972).

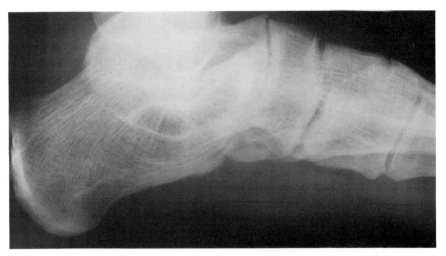

Fig. 12.28 Peroneal spastic flat foot due to tarsal coalition. Calcaneonavicular synostosis can be partially visualized on the lateral view, which also shows flattening of the longitudinal arch and the beginnings of a small talar beak. None of the normal joint spaces between the calcaneum and the talus are demonstrated and the sinus tarsi is not seen. The lateral process of the talus is broadened.

Table 12.4   Causes of spastic flat foot (after Outland & Murphy 1960, with permission).

Congenital

TARSAL ANOMALIES

Intertarsal bridges, possibly mediated by an accessory tarsal bone
    Calcaneonavicular bar
    Anterior talocalcaneal bar (talosustentacular)
    Calcaneocuboid bar
    Posterior talocalcaneal bar
    Malformation of the sustentaculum or of the talus that acts as a
    block to motion
Tarsal synostoses due to incomplete segmentation
    Combined anterior and posterior talocalcaneal synostosis
    Combined tarsal and phalangeal (hand) synostosis
    Calcaneocuboid, talosustentacular and posterior talocalcaneal
    synostosis and scoliosis
Anomaly of the navicular

OSTEOCHONDRODYSTROPHY (MORQUIO'S DISEASE)

Acquired

Gallie subtalar arthrodesis
Tuberculosis of the tarsus
Rheumatoid arthritis involving the tarsus
Osteoarthritis superimposed on a burned-out rheumatoid arthritis
Non-specific tarsal synovitis
Trauma
Occupational strain

In their paper, Harris and Beath found that 2% of Canadian Army recruits had a 'peroneal spastic flat foot'. They also described how the coalition could be complete and bony, or partial with a fibrous, cartilaginous or arthrodial bond.

The following lesions have been implicated in the production of spastic flat foot (Outland & Murphy 1960; Table 12.4). In the papers of Jack (1954) and Chambers (1950), calcaneonavicular fusion was more common than talocalcaneal (Table 12.5). Slomann believed that calcaneonavicular coalition was due to the

Table 12.5   Incidence of causes of peroneal spastic flat foot in the literature.

Authors	Cases	TCF	CNF	Both	Other	No bony lesion
Harris & Beath (1948)	17	12	3	0		2
Webster & Roberts (1951)	21	4	8	2		7
Jack (1954)	30	11	12	0		7
Chambers (1950)	17	12	3		2 (RA)	
Harris (1965)	102	66	29		7	

presence of an os calcaneum secondarium, said to be present in 1% of the population (Fig. 12.27f). The medial talocalcaneal bridge has also been said to occur when the os sustentaculare fails to separate and eventually forms a bridge between the two bones (Harris 1965). There are, however, many reports of talocalcaneal and calcaneonavicular fusions in embryos and fetuses (O'Rahilly 1953, 1960; Harris 1965) so that it seems that fusions are more likely to be due to failure of separation of mesenchyme. O'Rahilly (1953) states that ossification of individual elements in a single cartilaginous primordium, instead of in the normal two, may well predispose to subsequent fusion of the two osseous elements. Moreover, since the initial element of fusion—failure of segmentation—takes place in cartilage *in utero*, demonstration of accessory bones in children is irrelevant to the problem. In cats and dogs, indeed, the scapholunate develops in a single cartilaginous element from ossific centres which later fuse.

Clearly, some cases of fusion are acquired (see Table 12.4). The clinical features which follow tarsal coalition are deformity, rigidity, pain and spasm in the peroneal muscles. The lesions are apparently autosomal dominant in inheritance (Jayakumar & Cowell 1977).

Since the cartilaginous or fibrous bonds are not ossified at birth, no plain film changes can then be seen. Talonavicular coalitions ossify at 3–5 years, calcaneonavicular coalitions at 8–12 years, and talocalcaneal coalitions at 12–16 years (Jayakumar & Cowell). Adequate movement between tarsal bones is apparently possible with a fibrous link, while a cartilaginous link gives greater restriction of movement and an osseous band gives complete loss of joint motion. Symptoms therefore are gradual in onset in the second decade.

There are two compartments of the talocalcaneal joint, the anterior and the posterior. The anterior compartment has a middle and anterior facet, which may be fused into one. As previously noted, most tarsal coalitions are at the middle facet. The posterior compartment has its (posterior) facet. The axial or ski-jump view (Korvin–Harris view) usually demonstrates the middle facet well. It also demonstrates the posterior facet in most cases, as both lie in the same plane on this view (Fig. 12.29). Harris originally utilized a 45° tilt for the axial view. If this does not satisfactorily demonstrate the middle and posterior facets, then the appropriate angle of inclination of the middle facet to the weight-bearing plane can be drawn on a lateral view of the foot. This angle is then utilized for the axial projection. An alternative is to take views decreasing by 5°, 40°, 35° and 30°. In the presence of disease, such as fusion, the two facets (middle and posterior) are no longer necessarily parallel on the axial view. With the usual middle facet coalition, the middle facet may become oblique, while the posterior remain transverse (Jayakumar and Cowell). Should the parallelism of the two facets be lost, multiple axial views at different angles will, in any case, be necessary. The two joints normally show similar alignment but are centrally discontinuous since they lie in different compartments (Cowell 1972). The axial view does not show the anterior facet because of the overlap of the distal leg, nor is it seen on a lateral view, as it is inclined downward and medially (Beckly *et al* 1975) and so is oblique to the lateral

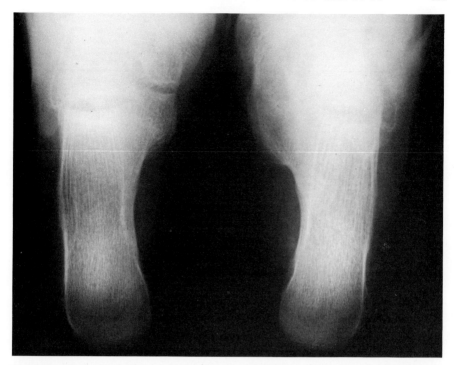

Fig. 12.29   The axial, or Korvin–Harris, view. On the left, the middle and posterior facets are well demonstrated, while on the right there is congenital total fusion of the middle facet.

beam. In order to demonstrate the anterior facet, Conway and Cowell (1969) utilized lateral tomography of the foot. This demonstrates the anterior facet and, as a bonus, confirms abnormality of the middle facet and also demonstrates the posterior facet. Their method requires four exposures, but only one if a multiplane box cassette is available. It was not recommended if coalition was visible on conventional views but if the clinical signs are positive and the plain radiographs negative, occult coalition may be demonstrated. Caution is recommended in the interpretation of lateral tomograms, as the obliquity of the joint means that it does not lie in the same plane as the lateral tomographic cut. This malalignment is accentuated with valgus flat foot and calcaneal rotation and a false impression of coalition may be formed and mistakenly operated on (Beckly et al 1975).

Other approaches to the subtalar joint include that described by Anthonsen (1943). This requires a double tube tilt which cannot always be performed with standard equipment. This view demonstrates the posterior and medial facets and sinus tarsi very well. Isherwood (1961) recommends the oblique lateral view for the anterior joint, the medial oblique axial view to show the middle joint and give a tangential view of the convexity of the posterior joint, and a lateral oblique axial view to show the posterior joint.

The radiological signs of coalition may be divided into the primary and the secondary.

Primary signs

A normal joint presents two normal, thinly corticated parallel joint surfaces to the beam and a joint space of uniform width. Total bony coalition can clearly be seen as bony union, or a solid bar of bone.

Calcaneonavicular coalition is often seen as a bar of bone over 1 cm in width (Fig. 12.30). When the union is fibrous or cartilaginous, the two bones are in closer apposition, arthritic changes will be seen between them, and the talar head may be hypoplastic (Conway & Cowell 1969). The navicular on the side of the coalition may be larger (Chambers 1950; Fig. 12.31).

The pathomechanics of the hindfoot with these fusions have been well-documented.

In dorsiflexion, for the navicular to glide upwards over the talar head the calcaneum must first move forwards on the talus. If this movement is restricted by coalition, the navicular moves with a hinge-like motion, impacts on the head of the talus and remoulds it. Restriction of subtalar movement is clearly greater with subtalar fusion than with calcaneonavicular fusion, but if fusion is only partial the changes of remodelling are lessened (Outland & Murphy 1960). Jayakumar and Cowell (1977) believe that restriction of the subtalar joint forces the navicular over the talar head, elevating the talonavicular ligament and periosteum, beneath which new bone is laid down. A large spur then forms, seen on the lateral view at

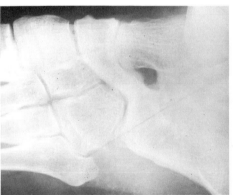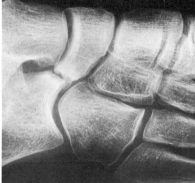

Fig. 12.30 (*Left*) Calcaneonavicular coalition. Total bony union is demonstrated, as well as bony beaks on the upper surfaces of navicular and talus. The head of the talus may well be small.

Fig. 12.31 (*Right*) Calcaneonavicular coalition. Fibrous or cartilaginous, rather than osseous, union between the bones is seen with osteoarthritic changes of the opposing bone surfaces and an enlarged navicular.

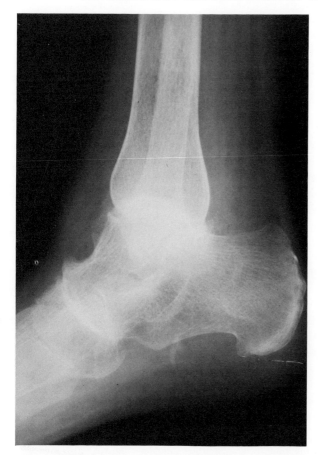

Fig. 12.32 Flat foot in
rheumatoid arthritis
with the formation of a
large talar beak.

the distal talus and, to a lesser extent, on the upper proximal navicular (Fig. 12.32).
This spur cannot be held to be a form of osteoarthritis as it is not around the entire
joint (Outland & Murphy 1960). In addition, the normal gliding movement of the
talus on the calcaneum is restricted on the medial aspect of the joint at the site of
coalition. The medial restriction puts the heel into valgus and the foot flattens
(Conway & Cowell 1969). It is interesting to note that Dwight (1907) demonstrates a
large 'trochlear process near (the) head of astragulus'—which is clearly our
spur—and says 'except for a tendency to flatness, the foot is otherwise healthy'.

Secondary signs

Further secondary signs of talocalcaneal coalition include (Fig. 12.28):
1   Broadening of the lateral process of the talus which impinges on the sulcus
calcanei on a lateral view, and also narrowing of the posterior facet (Conway &
Cowell 1969).

2 Obliteration of the space between sustentaculum tali and neck of the talus
(Harris 1965).

3 Failure to visualize the mid-subtalar joint on a lateral view, and gross
asymmetry of the anterior subtalar joint on the oblique lateral view of Isherwood.
This may be associated with concavity of the under surface of the neck of the talus
on the affected side (Beckly *et al* 1975).

THE POINTED TUBULAR BONE

In an article under this title, Gondos (1972) points out that a pointed tubular bone
in the foot is observed in those diseases which cause a sensory neuropathic
osteopathy or arthropathy. Because of the radiological change, the appearances
have also been likened to 'pencilling', 'a licked candy stick', an 'icicle' or 'sucked
barley sugar'. In fact, only some 50% of patients with such appearances in Gondos'
series had a sensory neuropathic arthropathy. Felson (1970) indicates a difference
between 'neuropathic arthropathy'—related to loss of deep pain sense secondary
to a central or peripheral nervous disorder—and 'neurotrophic bone change' in
which a neurovascular abnormality may be the causative factor. He lists some
causes of both (Table 12.6). Some diseases cause both types of lesion, though
possibly the joining together of the terms 'neuropathic' and 'arthropathy' rather
than 'osteopathy' creates a rather artificial distinction. In any case, the pointed
tubular bone is seen in both types of disease.

Table 12.6 Conditions causing neuropathic joints and neuropathic joint changes. (From
Felson (1970), with permission.)

Neuropathic joint	Neurotrophic bone changes
Tabes dorsalis	Scleroderma, dermatomyositis
Diabetic myelopathy or neuropathy	Diabetes
	Peripheral nerve injury
Spinal cord or peripheral nerve injury	Leprosy
	Frostbite, burn
Leprosy	Syringomyelia
Multiple sclerosis	Other spinal cord diseases
Syringomyelia	Arterial disease: Raynaud's,
Other spinal cord diseases (inflammatory, pernicious anaemia, meningocele)	Buerger's, arteriosclerosis obliterans
	Congenital indifference to pain
Cushing's disease, steroid therapy	Rheumatoid arthritis
	Psoriasis
Congenital indifference to pain	Congenital acro-osteolysis, pyknodysostosis
	Tropical ulcer

There may or may not be a justification for saying that as the end results in so many different conditions are so similar, a basic process must be at least common to some, if not all, of them. The literature generally is not helpful as to the basis of this appearance, but leprosy and diabetes in particular may provide reasonable models for any discussion. Certainly, osseous change in leprosy has been investigated and, because of the frequent amputations, radiologic–pathologic correlations have been performed.

The incidence of bony change in leprosy varies from 3–5% (Enna *et al* 1971) through 15% (Reeder 1970) to anything from 50–90% (Lechat 1962). There is general agreement on the division of radiological lesions (Paterson 1961; Lechat 1962) into:

1   Specific changes of osteitis leprosa (14%). *M. leprae* is often found (85%) in the bone of lepers with lepromatous leprosy, but not necessarily related to visible change. Granulomas, however, cause areas of focal cortical or medullary lysis, or subarticular cysts which cause articular collapse and joint deformity.

2   Non-specific leprous osteitis (45%). These patients rarely, if ever, have Hansen bacilli in their marrow (Faget & Mayoral 1944). According to Lechat, this form is always associated with evidence of damage to nerves. Resorption of bone may be at the distal phalanges, or more proximally at the metatarsophalangeal joints (curiously termed 'metatarsophalangeal osteoarthritis' by Lechat) and both may be complicated by ulceration and secondary infection.

3   Osteoporosis.

Distal atrophy of the phalanges was seen in 27% of amputation specimens (Skinsnes *et al* 1972). These lesions on histology showed focal thinning of the cortex, with fibrous tissue extending from the periosteal region into the marrow together with increased osteoclastic activity. Barnetson (1951), in a similar earlier study, while also describing invasion of the distal phalangeal cortex and marrow by connective tissue, was unable, however, to show increased osteoclastic activity.

Abnormalities of the nerves and blood vessels were found in nearly every amputated foot examined by Skinsnes *et al* (1972). Nerves showed chronic inflammatory infiltrates or fibrosis, while arteries showed varying degrees of medial and intimal thickening and luminal narrowing which, when of marked severity, was always associated with resorptive changes at the metatarsophalangeal joints or with 'chronic osteitis or periostitis' (defined as a non-infectious inflammatory cell infiltration and fibrosis in periosteum, cortex or spongiosa, associated with increased bone turnover).

Faget and Mayoral (1944) and Enna *et al* (1971) believe that, at least in part, absorption of bone occurs because of alteration in the extrinsic factors acting upon it. Thus, absorption of the proximal phalanx occurs with the rigid clawed toes of the denervated weight-bearing foot. Enna observes that distal absorption does not occur in the denervated clawed hand, when it is useless, but occurs in the foot when the toes are deformed and rigid. Similarly, at the metatarsophalangeal joints, claw toes and drop foot resulting in abnormal forces on the bone are, in part, responsible for resorption at the site of greatest pressure, often the first metatarsal head.

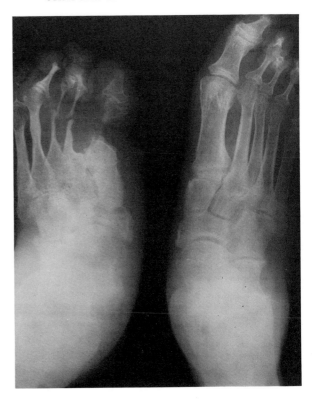

Fig. 12.33 Leprosy. Pointed tubular bones are demonstrated. Abnormalities are seen at the metatarsals, proximal and distal phalanges in this patient with longstanding non-specific leprous osteitis. Overall, there is sclerosis of bone in the affected regions.

Longitudinal bone resorption then leaves small phalangeal remnants with flail toes (Fig. 12.33). An imbalance between tensile and compressive force, possibly by varying the electric potentials on the bone surface, may lead to an abnormal balance between osteoblasts and osteoclasts, so that the form and function of the bone is altered. Examination of Skinsnes' speciments does indeed show that the edges of the whittled bone are often thickened and sclerotic, possibly the result of adaptions to new stresses, with resultant new bone formation.

Plantar ulceration and infection of the soft tissues and bone is also important. Hallux valgus, an abnormal situation of the tibial sesamoid, and abnormal weight-bearing on denervated and devitalized soft tissue all cause ulceration and secondary osteomyelitis. Changes of pyogenic osteomyelitis were found in 35% of Skinsnes' amputation specimens. Sequestra and involucra were rare, but a 'cloudy' disintegration was seen together with osteoporosis. 43% of specimens had soft tissue ulceration and infection, usually plantar. Gondos, indeed, does not believe that a pointed bone is the result of absorption or atrophy, but is part of a reparative process, the result of new bone formation and healing following destruction, fragmentation, periostitis, etc. (Fig. 12.34). He provides examples to show this and also points to the example of the stumps following below-knee amputation, where a

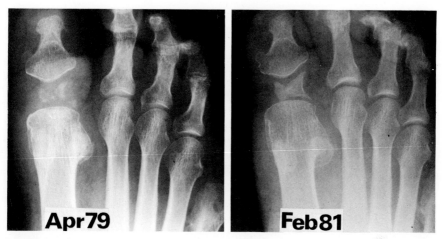

Fig. 12.34 Leprosy. Disintegration of the proximal phalanx of the great toe is shown in April 1979. By 1981 healing had taken place, giving the bony remnants a sclerotic and rather pointed appearance.

pointed end may develop on the fibula rather than, or earlier than, on the remaining tibia. This is, he says, because the smaller the tubular bone initially, the more likely it is to be pointed. Thus, he points out, in syringomyelia the phalanges end up pointed, while the humeral head does not. This is perhaps not the best example to give, as the size of the arteries and thickness of local soft tissues are vastly different in the two areas. Radiologically, the 'point' is shown on the lateral views often to be wedge-shaped, that is, the bone is not pointed in all planes.

That blood vessels and nerves are abnormal has already been mentioned. Barnetson (1951) has shown that while dilatation of peripheral vessels in the neuropathies is not diminished in response to *local* stimulation, there is failure of *reflex* (contralateral) vasodilatation, as measured by absence of a rise in skin temperature, corresponding in degree to the extent of bone change and neuritis. This he presumed to be due to destruction of vasomotor nerve fibres. There is also marked variation in extremity temperature in a patient with leprosy, and anaesthetic feet are warmer, on average, than normal feet. Skinsnes believes that hypervascularity with stasis and oedema (passive hyperaemia) is associated with osteoblastic activity while hyperaemia with rapid blood flow (active hyperaemia) is associated with osteoclastic activity. High oxygen concentrations (60–95%) stimulate osteoclasis, and a low oxygen concentration (35%) stimulates bone formation. In leprosy he believes the two are not in balance, though clearly the balance is on the side of bone resorption overall.

Barnetson quotes varying findings at angiography in leprosy in the literature, including (1) a rich and patent arterial network, even at an ulcer. Faget and Mayoral describe (2) little change in the arterial supply in neural leprosy with 'no causal relationship between the arterial supply of the hands and feet and the degree of neurotrophic bone absorption'. With mixed and lepromatous leprosy cases, however, their lipiodol post-mortem angiograms beautifully demonstrate irregular and interrupted digital arteries.

Paterson (1961) demonstrated (3) diminution of vascular end loops in the presence of pulp resorption, (4) hyperaemia in areas of local inflammation and (5) a considerable increase in the circulation time in the fingers (to 30–120 seconds), or arteriovenous shunts at the levels of proximal phalanges.

Pointed tubular bones also occur in rheumatoid arthritis (Fig. 12.35) and it is of interest to note that Laws *et al* (1963), in an angiographic study of 67 patients with connective tissue disorders, mainly rheumatoid arthritis, found digital artery occlusion, narrowing and tortuosity in 68% of patients with rheumatoid arthritis, pulp filling being especially defective. Hyperaemia at sites of synovial inflammation was seen in 60%. Occlusive lesions were always present in those patients who had a peripheral neuropathy, suggesting possible ischaemia of peripheral nerves, and in 60% of those digits with erosive change. Histologically, gross intimal thickening and sclerosis were found.

Patients with primary Raynaud's phenomenon also showed occlusive lesions, indistinguishable from rheumatoid arthritis on angiography, as did those with scleroderma, calcinosis circumscripta and ankylosing spondylitis with peripheral arthropathy (all also with raynaudism), and those with psoriatic arthropathy and disseminated lupus erythematosus (without raynaudism). Similarly, in frostbite, another cause of a pointed tubular bone, vasoconstriction and thrombosis are seen early on, giving segmental obstructions which may persist, as well as local vasodilatation with increased permeability of blood vessels and local oedema (Gralino *et al* 1976).

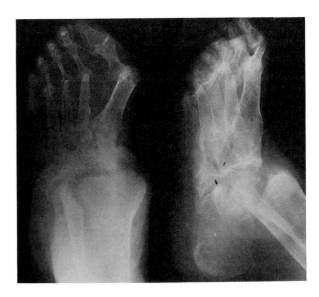

Fig. 12.35 Rheumatoid arthritis. Gross osteoporosis and hallux valgus with pointed tubular bones, giving a cup and pencil deformity at the metatarsophalangeal joints. Marked destruction of the tarsus is seen with partial fusion distally and, proximally, an appearance resembling neuropathic destruction of the tarsus. The patient had also been on steroids. The talus has almost totally been resorbed.

THE DIABETIC FOOT

In a review of the films of the feet of 1501 diabetic patients, Geoffroy *et al* (1979) found a 'destructive osteolytic pattern' in just under 5%. The appearances were those of 'pencilling' at distal phalanges or around metatarsophalangeal joints (Fig. 12.36). A few patients (< 1 per cent) showed reconstitution and hardening of the articular surfaces after a period of 'invisibility', giving a more sclerotic form of a pointed bone.

Gondos (1968) investigated 38 cases of diabetic osteopathy. 97% had involvement of metatarsals and/or phalanges, but the tarsal bones were involved in only 1% (Fig. 12.36). This author also again states his belief that the pointed bone is the end result of a healing process, depending partly on the shape of the bone following destruction. Should there be direct contact with an opposing neighbouring bone, a pointed bone-end does not develop.

In another series of 90 patients with diabetic osteoarthropathy, 56% were male (Clouse *et al* 1974)—a greater male bias than in Geoffroy's series. As in most series, the right foot was more commonly affected. Duration of diabetic disease varied from 8 months to 43 years. *All the patients had a peripheral neuropathy.* The metatarsals were affected in 84%, the phalanges in 42% and the tarsus was heavily affected in 63%.

Avascular bone retains a normal radiographic density. This is seen, for instance, after scaphoid fractures when the proximal pole, devoid of its blood supply, remains normal in density while the remainder of the carpus becomes demineralized. From this it can be inferred that in diabetes soft tissue necrosis accompanied by radiologically normal bone indicates the presence of ischaemia, even though necrosis of bone may be histologically visible, while soft tissue necrosis and diabetic osteopathy indicate the presence of a neuropathy. In one series of patients with ischaemia and soft tissue necrosis, but normal bones radiologically, only some 15% had palpable foot pulses. 70% had intermittent claudication and only 11% (two patients) had a neuropathy. According to Catterall (1972), the solitary black toe of the infected ischaemic diabetic foot usually progresses to a below-knee amputation within the year. Even the patient with an uninfected ischaemic foot usually submits to amputation, the only decision being as to the level. A neuropathic sore or ulcer, however, often heals without surgery.

Bone destruction therefore usually takes place in feet which have an adequate blood supply. Since, according to Staple (1973), 72% of feet of patients with diabetic osteoarthropathy show bone sclerosis, 38% bone resorption and 15% subchondral osteoporosis, a reasonable circulation must be present in many cases of osteoarthropathy. The radiographic appearance of the diabetic neuropathic foot cannot then be easily differentiated from that of any other form of neuropathic foot, though the presence of arterial calcification may be helpful. Osteomyelitis may mimic diabetic osteopathy and, should secondary infection supervene, perhaps via an ulcer on the plantar surface of the great toe metatarsal head, the processes of osteoporosis and destruction are accelerated (Fig. 12.37). Where skin ulceration is

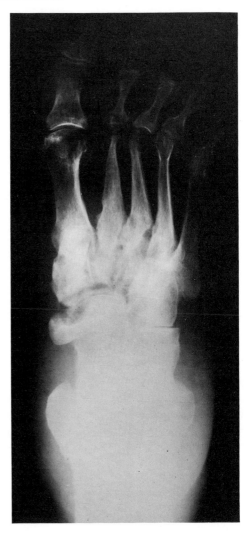

Fig. 12.36 Diabetes. Pointed tubular bones are seen at the second and third metatarsals. Bony density there is diminished as well as at the bases of the adjacent phalanges. The tarsal bones show a mixture of sclerosis and lysis and there is bone destruction, especially around the navicular. This foot was not painful. (By courtesy of Dr R.O. Murray, Royal National Orthopaedic Hospital, London.)

absent, however, osteomyelitis is unlikely. In diabetic osteopathy, pathological speciments show no gross signs of osteomyelitis.

Infection in soft tissues may be seen with swelling, loss of fat planes due to oedema and, if gas-producing organisms are present, vaguely spherical collections of gas are seen extending proximally (Fig. 12.38). Trophic ulcers show as gas-containing defects within localized soft tissue swellings, usually on pressure points, as in leprosy.

Two forms of vascular calcification may be seen in the thigh and calf. Mönkeberg's medial sclerosis is seen in young diabetics and elderly non-diabetics.

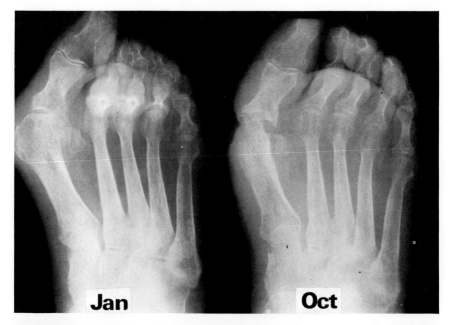

Fig. 12.37 Diabetic osteopathy. A large soft tissue defect is present over the head of the great toe metatarsal and, on the second film, the metatarsophalangeal joint of the great toe is being destroyed. There is marked osteoporosis throughout the foot. The changes are those of osteomyelitis rather than neuropathy.

It appears as a smooth continuous pipe-like calcification, but is usually not associated with loss of foot pulses.

Atheromatous calcification is rather more patchy and less evenly distributed. As it is intimal, the lumina are more likely to be occluded. The dorsalis pedis artery is often calcified—in 25% in the series of Geoffroy *et al*, but vascular calcification was seen in 78% in the series of Clouse *et al*, and in 50% in that of Kraft *et al* (1975). According to Staple, angiography in the young atheromatous diabetic reveals vasculo-occlusive disease maximal in popliteal artery branches, and only with increasing age are the more proximal major vessels thus affected.

A neuropathic arthropathy has also been seen in alcoholics with a polyarthropathy. Ulcers over the first and fifth metatarsal heads led to infection, but peripheral pulses were preserved. Phalangeal narrowing was seen leading to resorption of distal and middle phalanges and pointing of the distal metatarsals (Thornhill *et al* 1973).

The aetiology of the pointed bone is not clear, but a neural abnormality alone, or in combination with organic blood vessel changes, is commonly present. The distal arteries may be totally or partially occluded or there may be some abnormality of local blood flow due to disruption of the vascular reflex arc in the peripheral nerves (at least in diabetes and leprosy). Abnormalities of blood flow

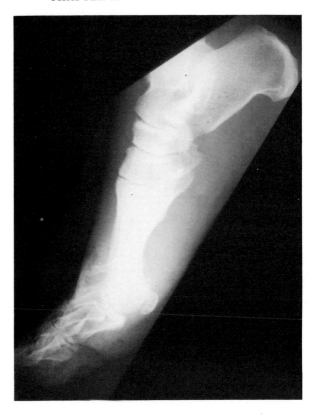

Fig. 12.38 Gas is demonstrated in the soft tissues around the metatarsal heads in a diabetic patient.

and local changes in oxygen tension may stimulate osteoclastic or blastic activity. Local pressure changes may resorb bone, possibly through changes of electric potential at bone surfaces altering osteoclastic/blastic balance. Infection destroys bone in insensitive areas and then local release of lactic and other acids may cause further resorption of bone, so that the tubular bone may be the result of healing and osteoblastic activity. The end stages of histology with fibrous tissue, little vascular reaction and variable amounts of osteoclastic acitivity are a reflection of healing rather than of that which caused the bone change in the first place. This change will have taken place slowly over a long time, and is certainly multifactorial.

NEUROPATHIC DESTRUCTION OF THE TARSUS

It has been shown above that the forefoot is more frequently involved than the tarsus in patients with diabetic neuropathy. Neuropathic destruction of the hindfoot requires loss of pain sensation together with an episode of trauma or infection for its initiation. If the foot is anaesthetic but the muscles acting on it spared (unlike the situation in polio or paraplegia), tarsal disintegration can occur

(Harris & Brand 1966). Ligamentous laxity may also follow sepsis. Laxity of joint capsules may lead to instability of tarsal joints, or a fracture may occur in bone weakened by past or current infection. Lack of pain or position sense permits a wide range of abnormal movement on already abnormal bones and joints, so that fractures and fragmentation result. Harris and Brand noted five specific patterns of tarsal destruction in leprosy (Fig. 12.39).

Pattern one: posterior pillar

Following a fall on the heel, the calcaneum fractures and collapses. The posterior pillar of the heel fails and stress on the anterior pillar is now vertical, through the talus and flattened calcaneum, which is deformed into recurvatum by body weight and the pull of the Achilles tendon.

Pattern two: disintegration of the talus

The talus may fracture *ab initio*, or calcaneal deformity may lead to subtalar joint degenerative change and eventual instability, so that the talus is destroyed from below (Fig. 12.35).

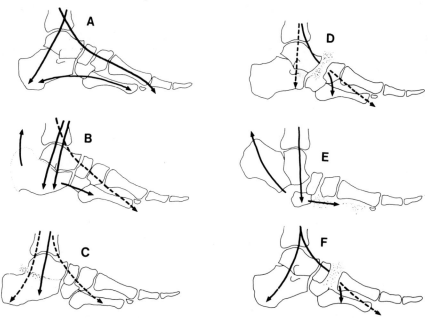

Fig. 12.39 Patterns of neuropathic destruction of the tarsus. (From Harris and Brand (1966), with kind permission of the Editor of the *Journal of Bone and Joint Surgery*.) (A) Normal distribution of stresses. (B) Pattern 1—collapse of the posterior pillar. (C) Pattern 2—disintegration of the talus. (D) Pattern 3—navicular disintegration. (E) Pattern 4—destruction of the lateral ray. (F) Pattern 5—fracture and disintegration of the cuneiform bones.

Pattern three: navicular disintegration

Increased osteophytosis and sclerosis on the dorsum of the midfoot are, according to Harris and Brand (1966), signs of strain on the upper surface of the tarsus. These changes follow weakening of plantar tension following, for instance, paralysis of the intrinsic muscles. Eventual disintegration of the navicular and the head of the talus occurs. The talus articulates with the cuneiform bones, the medial arch flattens and the talus anteriorly becomes the site of plantar pressure ulceration (Fig. 12.40).

Pattern four: destruction of the lateral ray

This apparently mainly follows infection at the base of the fifth metatarsal in leprosy, with varus deviation. A perforating ulcer is followed by septic destruction of the lateral ray (Fig. 12.41).

Pattern five: cuneiform fracture

This lesion is apparently uncommon. Disintegration follows direct trauma to these bones. In diabetes and syphilis, in addition, pes valgus rather than varus results as the peronei are intact. The tarsal bones may then be displaced medially and the base of the fifth metatarsal no longer articulates with the cuboid, which is shifted medially.

BONE TUMOURS IN THE FOOT

Tumours, benign or malignant, primary or secondary, are rare in the foot. In Dahlin's series of 4277 primary benign and malignant bone tumours, there were 35 benign and 38 malignant tumours in the foot (Dahlin 1978). In the smaller study of 1402 primary tumours and tumour-like lesions of the Netherlands Committee on

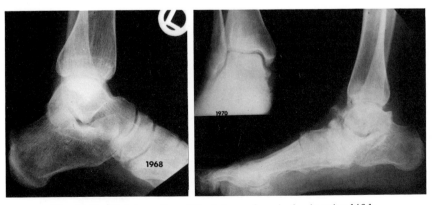

Fig. 12.40 Disintegration of the talus and navicular in spina bifida.

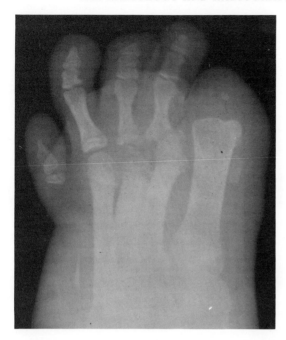

Fig. 12.41 Destruction of the lateral ray in leprosy.

Bone Tumours (1966), there were eight malignant, 25 benign and 8 'benign tumour-like' in the foot. The breakdown by tumour types is given in Table 12.7.

Osteoid osteoma

This occurs mainly in males, usually in the second and third decades. Classical symptoms are of pain, especially at night, relieved by aspirin, often of 1–2 years duration. The usual size is less than 1.5 cm diameter. A fairly typical appearance is of a radiolucent nidus with a sclerotic margin which increases in density the nearer the tumour lies to the cortex and periosteum. The radiolucent nidus itself undergoes sclerosis and the lesion may radiologically mimic a Brodie's abscess. The osteoid osteoma usually shows marked increase in uptake of isotope on a bone scan. The lucent nidus is hypervascular on an angiogram. In the tarsus their radiological diagnosis is difficult. In a site of little periosteum, such as the talus, which has many articular facets and so is largely covered by cartilage, little reactive sclerosis is to be seen and the relatively lucent tumour is often missed. A long history of a painful foot with no obvious plain film lesion, especially in a young adult, deserves a bone scan (Fig. 12.42).

In a metatarsal, an osteoid osteoma may simulate a stress fracture or Looser's zone.

Table 12.7 Types of tumours seen in the foot in two separate surveys.

	D	N
Benign		
BONE		
Osteoid osteoma	8	6
Osteoblastoma	1	7
CARTILAGE		
Exostosis	5 ⎫	
Enchondroma	9 ⎭	1
Chondroblastoma	1	2
Chondromyxoid fibroma	7	1
FIBROUS TISSUE		
Fibrous dysplasia	NQ	1
CYSTS		
Simple bone cyst	NQ	2
Aneurysmal bone cyst	5	3
Giant-cell tumour	3	1
Malignant		
Osteosarcoma	9	1
Chondrosarcoma	6	4
Fibrosarcoma	2	1
Ewing's tumour	16	1
Malignant lymphoma	3	NQ

N = 1402 patients (Netherland Committee on Bone Tumours)
NQ = not quoted
D = 4227 patients (Dahlin)

Benign osteoblastoma

Arbitrarily, this tumour is separated from osteoid osteoma by its size. It is by definition over 1.5 cm in diameter and, because radiologically it can appear similar to an osteoid osteoma, it has been called a giant osteoid osteoma. Pain is not quite as well localized, nor mainly at night. The lesions are up to 10 cm in diameter, but are often surrounded by less sclerosis unless of really long standing. Once again, the central nidus ossifies so that an infective lesion or cartilaginous tumour may be simulated.

Osteocartilaginous exostosis (Fig. 12.43)

In Dahlin's series these comprised 40% of all benign bone tumours. They are usually solitary and less often multiple, in the latter case there is a 10% incidence

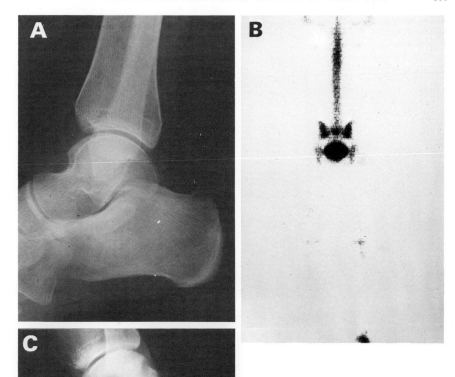

Fig. 12.42 Osteoid osteoma of the calcaneum. The lateral view of the foot (A) shows no abnormality in a 14-year-old girl who had night pain, relieved by aspirin, for the previous 18 months. The bone scan (B) demonstrates marked increase in uptake in the left heel. Lateral tomography of the calcaneum (C) demonstrates the osteoid osteoma as an area of sclerosis with a central lucency beneath the sulcus calcanei.

of chondrosarcoma. They may also be associated with polyposis coli. At their attachment the bone shaft is poorly modelled and broad. The cortex of the exostosis is continuous with that of the underlying bone. Their growth ceases at skeletal maturity. The lesions present early in the foot because of limited room for their expansion, usually in the second decade of life.

Enchondroma
Single or multiple enchondromas are common in the hand, but less common in the

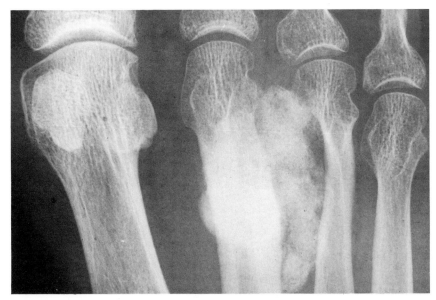

Fig. 12.43 Osteocartilaginous exostosis. A large osseous excrescence arises from the shaft of the second metatarsal which shows local abnormal modelling. The chronicity of the lesion is demonstrated by erosion of the shaft of the adjacent third metatarsal.

foot. They are usually seen in the metatarsals and phalanges. The tumour thins the cortex, so that the pain of a fracture may be the presenting feature. If pain occurs in the absence of a fracture, malignancy may have supervened. Of 26 patients with multiple chondromatosis in Dahlin's series, one developed chondrosarcoma in a metatarsal.

Osteogenic sarcoma

In the foot the more common site is in the tarsus, though metatarsals may also be affected. Though usually seen at 5–25 years of age, Norman (1970) reported two cases occurring in the foot in the fifth decade. The radiological features of these tumours are well described elsewhere, but they may vary greatly in the amount of destruction, expansion and tumour new bone they cause. In Dahlin's series, 3% of osteogenic sarcomas arose on pre-existing Paget's disease, which is itself a cause of a painful, dense, enlarged bone (Fig. 12.44). Acute change in size, pain or bone density must raise the possibility of malignant degeneration. In the same series, 3.6% of osteogenic sarcomas arose after irradiation.

Ewing's tumour

This tumour occurs more commonly in the hindfoot than the forefoot, at 5–25 years. Below this age group, neuroblastoma or leukaemia may give a similar radiological

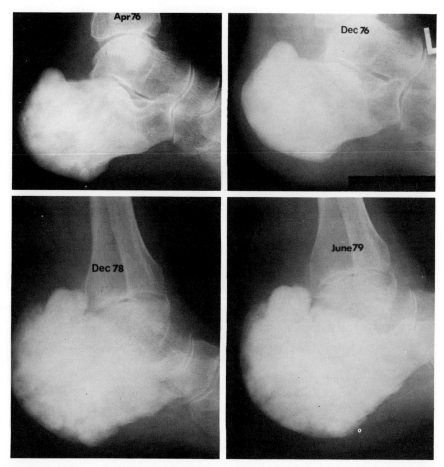

Fig. 12.44 Osteogenic sarcoma of the calcaneum arising on Paget's disease. The initial film (April 1976) shows characteristic features of Paget's disease. The posterior part of the calcaneum is enlarged and has a sclerotic coarse trabecular pattern which does not extend to the anterior portion of the bone. By December 1978 marked enlargement had taken place and in the film taken in 1979 almost the entire bone is affected. The marked enlargement and unremitting pain of the lesion should make one suspect the development of osteogenic sarcoma on pre-existing Paget's disease.

appearance. Osteolysis is patchy, often involving the greater part of the bone, and sclerosis is often less than is the case with osteogenic sarcoma. Periostitis is also much finer and lamellar, rather than coarse as in osteogenic sarcoma.

Giant-cell tumour (Fig. 12.45)

This characteristically arises in the articular region of a bone after epiphyseal (or

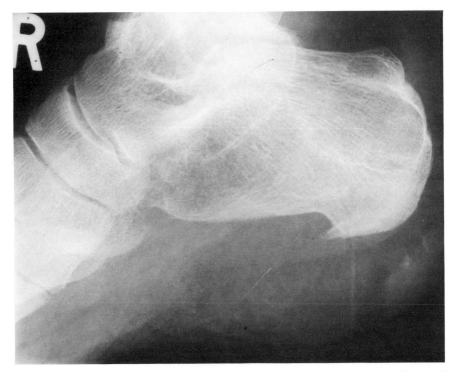

Fig. 12.45 Giant-cell tumour in hyperparathyroidism involving the calcaneum. Giant-cell tumours, whether occurring in hyperparathyroidism or not, are not common in this bone. Characteristically, a giant-cell tumour occurs in the adult skeleton and extends to an articular surface.

apophyseal) fusion. The lesions are mainly radiolucent with a fairly thin rim of quite poorly-defined reactive sclerosis. Few cases have been seen in the foot, mainly arising in the hindfoot. Multiple 'giant-cell tumours' may be seen in hyperparathyroidism, inevitably associated with subperiosteal bone resorption in untreated cases.

Aneurysmal bone cyst (Fig. 12.46)

This lesion tends to occur in the first and second decades, that is, earlier than the giant-cell tumour, but it is apparently slightly more common in the foot, even though a less common tumour overall. A well-circumscribed tumour, often grossly expansile, thins the cortex so that it often is barely visible, but residual trabeculation remains. There may be a periostitis at the bone-tumour interface. I believe that this lesion absolutely lives up to its name as far as diagnosis is concerned—it is an aneurysmally cystic bone tumour. While it is typically eccentric in a large bone, in a thin bone it rapidly reaches both adjacent cortices.

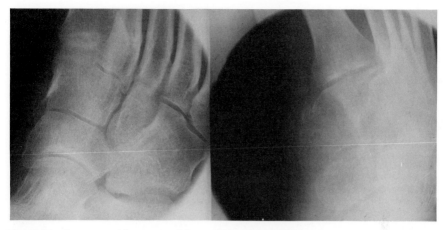

Fig. 12.46 Aneurysmal bone cyst of the medial cuneiform. There is little to distinguish this lesion from a giant-cell tumour, though the former usually occurs in a younger age group and often is larger. This cyst has undergone a pathological fracture.

Simple bone cyst

This is a distinctly unusual diagnosis to make in the foot or, for that matter, anywhere outside the upper humerus or femur. The lesion occasionally occurs in the calcaneum. The age of incidence is characteristic. It hardly ever appears after epiphyseal fusion and most cases are aged below 15 years, with a male predominance. They do not usually present unless a pathological fracture occurs, and do not expand the bone as does an aneurysmal bone cyst. This should not be confused with a normal variant, the 'simulated calcaneal cyst', which is situated between the major trabecular pillars anteriorly in the calcaneum.

The difficulties in the diagnosis of tumours of the foot are that they are uncommon and the bones are small. Tumours therefore rapidly 'fill' available space, soon reach, breach or expand the cortex, and those diagnostic features which are helpful elsewhere become lost. Many tumours thus end up looking similar, making biopsy crucial.

Metastatic tumours

Generally they are much more common than primary tumours and are often multiple. They tend to occur in an older age group (40+) and occur only rarely outside the red marrow areas in an adult, so are seldom seen in the feet, even less so than in the hand. Few case reports exist of metastases to feet, but in most cases the lesions originate in the lung (Mulvey 1964). As far as the hand in concerned, occasional deposits come from kidney, bladder, testis, parotid and colon (Kerin 1958). Peripheral metastases do not cross joint margins but usually leave a thinned expanded cortex or a fairly well-defined local soft tissue mass. Periostitis is uncommon (Fig. 12.47).

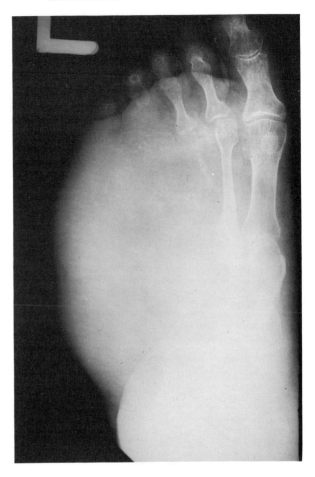

Fig. 12.47 Metastasis to foot from carcinoma of the uterus. A discrete soft tissue mass containing remnants of foot bones with some preservation of the articular margins. There is also, however, neo-ossification within this secondary deposit. This feature does occur with pelvic primary malignant tumours. primary malignant tumours.

ACCESSORY BONES OF THE FOOT

Supernumary centres of ossification occur in the foot more frequently than in any part of the body, far more often than in the hand.

Accessory bones have been defined as, 'inconstant, independent, well-defined bones—in an otherwise normally developed foot—the existence of which is not due to a recent minor fracture or other pathological condition no matter whether these bones bear no, or a less, or more intimate relationship to the constant bones, or entirely replace them because of a division of the latter into several segments' (Trolle 1948). In practical terms they should be identified to distinguish them from fractures. Occasionally the seat of disease, they may themselves be a cause of pain. Their identification in a 'normal' foot should also be a matter of pride and interest to those interested in osteology (Fig. 12.48).

Many large anatomical, radiological and embryological studies of the accessoria have been performed. Excellent summaries of all these surveys may be found in the works of Trolle (1948), O'Rahilly (1953) and Köhler and Zimmer (1968).

The accessoria are encountered as separate cartilages in the fetal foot. Their incidence varies from series to series since the number of feet examined is usually small when compared with the incidence of the rare varieties of accessoria. Since accessoria ossify with increasing age, their radiological incidence also increases with age.

Trolle lists 35 accessoria of the feet (his Nos. 13 and 19–21 are sesamoids at the metatarsophalangeal joints and phalanges). O'Rahilly says there are 'about thirty'. Köhler and Zimmer show 17 on the lateral view and 12 on the anteroposterior view of the hindfoot, but some are seen on both views. Hoerr *et al* (1962) state

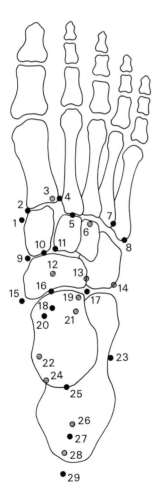

Fig. 12.48   Tarsal accessoria. After Trolle (1948) and O'Rahilly (1953). Trolle does not list Nos. 12, 27 and 28, but does show an os tuberis calcanei (which could be similar to No. 28). (Black = dorsal, hatched = more plantar). (1) Os sesamoideum tibialis anterior, (2) Os cuneo-metatarsale I tibiale, (3) Os cuneo-metatarsale I plantare, (4) Os intermetatarsale I, (5) Os cuneometatarsale II dorsale, (6) Os unci, (7) Os intermetatarsale IV, (8) Os Vesalianum, (9) Os paracuneiforme, (10) Os naviculocuneiforme I dorsale, (11) Os intercuneiforme, (12) Os sesamoideum tibialis posterior (according to Trolle, this may be the same as No. 15), (13) Os cuboideum secundarium, (14) Os peroneum, (15) Os tibiale (externum), (16) Os talonaviculare dorsale, (17) Os calcaneus secundarius, (18) Os supertalare, (19) Os trochleae, (20) Os talotibiale dorsale, (21) Os in sinu tarsi, (22) Os sustentaculi proprium, (23) Calcaneus accessorius, (24) Os talocalcaneare posterior, (25) Os trigonum, (26) Os aponeurosis plantaris, (27) Os supracalcaneum, (28) Os subcalcaneum, (29) Os tendinis Achillis.

that over 50 have been described, but only 20 of these occur as frequently as 1%. Their incidence varies from 18–30% in adults to 7% in children, exclusive of those seen at and distal to the metatarsophalangeal joints (Shands & Wertz 1953). In this last series the os tibiale externum was the most commonly seen accessory bone. This bone usually appears at about ten years and was seen in 37% of those with accessory bones. An os trigonum was seen in 32%, and a 'bony mass' at the base of the fifth metatarsal in 28% of those with accessory bones. Arho (quoted by Trolle 1948) found the os tibiale (externum) in 6.4% of 1074 feet, the os trigonum in 4.6% of feet, but the os peroneum in 8.3%, with no incidence at all for the 'os Vesalianum' (also the os subfibulare in 0.7%, os subtibiale in 0.7% and os intermetatarsale in 0.3%). Holle (again, in Trolle 1948) found the os trigonum (12.7%) more common than the os peroneum (9.5%), the os tibiale externum (7.9%) or the os subtibiale (1.5%).

There is some confusion in the early literature as to the nature of the 'bony mass' at the base of the fifth metatarsal. Holland (1928) gives an interesting history of this and other accessoria. The os Vesalianum was first described by Vesalius in 1568. In two drawings of an adult foot in the book of anatomical drawings of Vesalius, a small bone is shown at the tip of the tuberosity of the fifth metatarsal (Saunders & O'Malley 1950). Holland quoted more recent (!) investigators as describing this bone either as (i) a detached tuberosity of the fifth metatarsal or (ii) the proximal and external part of the tuberosity. The latter example, called the Vesalianum in Fig. 75 of Dwight's pioneering book, is clearly due, as shown by Holland, to the unfused apophysis for the base of the fifth metatarsal in the radiograph of a 13 year-old girl's foot. Dwight's Fig. 74 shows a prominent tuberosity which includes the 'Vesalianum' in an adult foot, that is, it no longer exists independently after fusion. At one time Holland was of the opinion that the os Vesalianum did not exist and that what Vesalius had described was the sesamoid of the peroneus longus. Later, however, he became of the opinion that either a small fragment of bone could exist just adjacent to the tip of the tuberosity, as described in 1568, but was rare, or that the whole tuberosity could be separately ossified, so that the bony shaft would be minus a tuberosity without it. In any case, the appearance should not be confused with that of an old, or recent, fracture of the tuberosity nor, since the original drawing of the foot by Vesalius is that of an adult, with the unfused apophysis. The separate apophysis may persist in an adult following trauma. Köhler and Zimmer show an os Vesalianum in a 17-year-old boy, but quote Neiss as doubting if it exists at all! (Fig. 12.49).

The incidence of sesamoids at metatarsal heads have been well documented. Accroding to Köhler and Zimmer, two are regularly seen at the head of the first metatarsal, with one at the head of the fifth, and one at the head of the second. Rarely, two at the head of the fifth metatarsal and one at the fourth may be seen and, quite rarely, a sesamoid at the medial side of the head of the third metatarsal is found (Fig. 12.50). The great toe medial sesamoid is bipartite in up to 33% and the lateral in up to 4%. Division is more common in females. A bipartite sesamoid is much larger than its normal counterpart, and its parts are well-corticated all

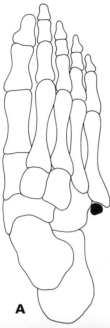

Fig. 12.49 (A) Os Vesalianum (after Vesalius 1586). Note that the epiphyses are all fused in this mature foot. (B) The apophysis at the base of the fifth metatarsal in the immature skeleton. According to Dwight (1907) this is the os Vesalianum. (C) Fracture of the base of the fifth metatarsal. The alignment of the fracture is usually transverse rather than oblique, as is the case with the apophysis, with which it is often confused. Non-union here, however, may lead to the appearance in (D). (D) Os Vesalianum according to Trolle (1948). A similar drawing is seen in Laquerriere and Drevon (1916) quoted by Holland (1928). It possibly consists of the whole tuberosity of the metatarsal developing separately.

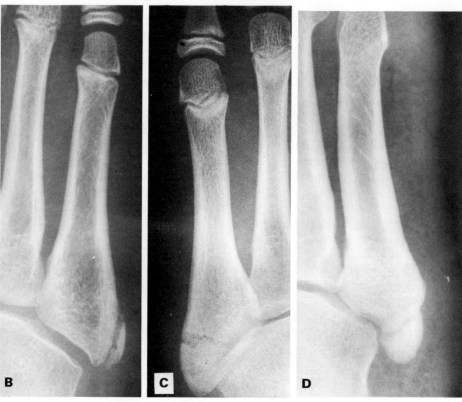

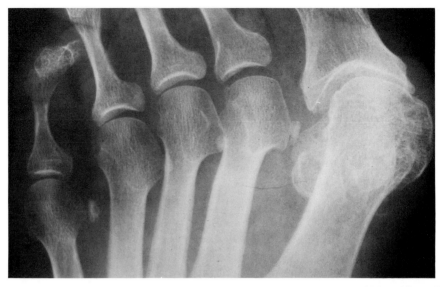

Fig. 12.50 Sesamoids at the metatarsal heads. Apart from the usual medial and lateral sesamoids at the great toe metatarsal head, sesamoids are also seen at the second, third, fourth and fifth metatarsal heads.

round. A fractured sesamoid is not corticated at its fracture line and is only slightly longer than its normal neighbours.

Resnick *et al* (1977) divide sesamoids into two types.

1   Adjacent to a joint, its tendon incorporated into the joint capsule and the sesamoid and opposing bone forming part of the articulation—such as the hallux sesamoid.

2   In a tendon, where it is angled about a bone and separated from the underlying bone by a synovial sac—such as the sesamoid of peroneus longus. Because of the intimate relationship of the sesamoid to the joint, it may become eroded in rheumatoid arthritis, gout and pyrophosphate disease, and may show whiskering or new bone formation in psoriasis and ankylosing spondylitis. Avascular necrosis may follow infection or trauma, or fusion to the underlying bone may result after septic arthritis. The sesamoids are enlarged in acromegaly and eroded in hyperparathyroidism. Osteoarthritic change is also often seen.

THICKNESS OF THE HEEL PAD IN HEALTH AND DISEASE

Steinbach and Russell (1964) measured the shortest distance between the calcaneum and the plantar surface of the skin, using a 40 inch focus–film distance. In 103 normal adult subjects, measurements ranged from 13–21 mm, with a mean of 17.9 mm in males and 17.8 mm in females. In 29 acromegalic patients, the heel pad thickness ranged from 17–34 mm, with a mean of 25.6 mm, and the thickness increased with age in acromegalics. Kho *et al* (1970), using a similar focus-film distance but emphasizing the necessity to avoid distortion of the heel, felt that the definition of thickness of the heel pad given above was too loose. They drew a line joining the anterior and posterior superior angles of the calcaneum, drew a further parallel line on the lowest point of the calcaneum and extended a perpendicular from that point to the skin (Fig. 12.51). They showed that, in controls, heel pad thickness increased with weight, but diminished with age. Their mean heel pad thickness was, in controls, 18.56 mm with a maximum of 25 mm in males and 23 mm in females, while no untreated acromegalic had a heel pad thickness of *less* than 18 mm (males) or 21 mm (females). Thickness in acromegalics is greater in those whose disease is long-standing (over 15 years) so that, in acromegalics, the measurements do not diminish with age. Jackson (1968) studied heel pad thickness in the obese. In those over 90 kg in weight, 65% had a thickness of more than 21 mm, while in those weighing from 125–185 kg, over 90% were over 21 mm in thickness. Puckette and Seymour (1967) had found that 40% of Negro patients had a thickness greater than 21 mm, but Raja *et al* (1980), in a study of 114 normal Kenyan Africans, found no significant difference between Negro and white normals. Their upper limit was 25 mm for males and 25 mm for females, with a mean of 20.65 mm. Their acromegalic

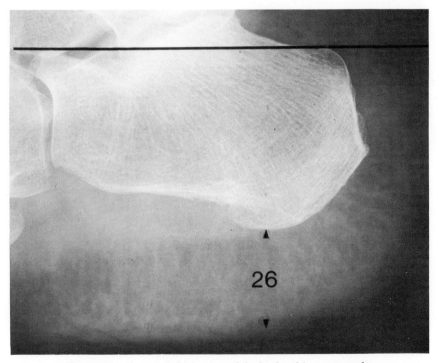

Fig. 12.51   Abnormal thickening of the heel pad in acromegaly.

patients were all grossly abnormal. Interestingly, 7 of 12 patients on long term (ten years) dilantin therapy, all white, had a heel pad thickness of over 20 mm (as against 1 of 43 controls; Kattan 1975). An increased thickness of the heel pad may also be seen in infection, myxoedema, after trauma, or any form of oedema, and in rheumatoid disease.

THREE CURIOUS CAUSES OF BIG FEET

Moore, in 1942, stated that macrodactyly is one of the rarer forms of congenital deformity seen in orthopaedic clinics. In a series of five cases of patients with overgrowth of bones, four showed definite or probable clinical stigmata of neurofibromatosis. His Case 2 was born with overgrowth of the lateral three left and two right toes, and also had cafe-au-lait spots and large lipomas on his trunk. Case 3 had overgrowth of the right leg with especially massive overgrowth of the first and second toes, cafe-au-lait spots and what seems to have been plexiform neurofibromas supplying the overgrown toes. This child also had marked naevus formation on the skin of the affected limb. The mother undoubtedly also had neurofibromatosis. Overgrowth of bone in neurofibromatosis is associated with enlargement of soft tissues which contain haemangiomatous and lymphangiomatous overgrowths in addition to plexiform neurofibromas (Fig. 12.52). McCarroll (1950), in a survey of 46 cases of neurofibromatosis, found bone enlargement in 14

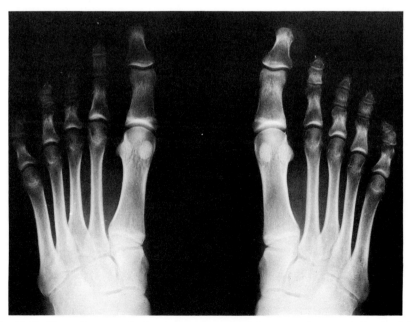

Fig. 12.52 Neurofibromatosis showing overgrowth of the great toes, especially the right.

(30%). In some cases, the soft tissues were enlarged, with plexiform neurofibromas supplying the overgrown part. Naevi were also present on the skin of the affected parts. Nineteen cases (41%) had blood vessel overgrowth and seven (15%) signs of lymphatic hyperplasia. Of even greater interest is the fact that two of his patients with undoubted neurofibromatosis—with overgrowth, cafe-au-lait spots and haemangiomas—*also* had melorheostosis. A theory was put forward that melorheostosis might have its origin in neurofibromatosis. Hall (1961) described a 15-year-old female with the undoubted bone and soft tissue changes of melorheostosis, but with port wine naevi and lymphoedema. There was no cutaneous evidence of neurofibromatosis, but undoubted overgrowth of the right lower limb was present on radiology, both in length and girth. No arteriovenous aneurysms were present, as were, however, in the case of melorheostosis of Murray (1951) which was otherwise typical.

Murray and McCredie (1979), thirty years later, have given an interesting theory as to the aetiology of melorheostosis. Radiologically, the disease is usually found in a single limb or side of the body, and constantly shows linear sclerotic densities affecting one segment of a bone, or bones, often in continuity. The flowing nature of the exostoses seen along the affected cortices is likened to melting candle wax. The disease crosses joints (Fig. 12.53) and para-articular ossification is then seen. This occurred in 25% of Murray and McCredie's series of 30 cases. The lesions are usually painful, and progress with age. The lower extremities are predominantly affected. According to Morris *et al* (1963), increased limb length occurs in 10% of cases and lymphoedema, haemangiomas and enlarged superficial blood vessels in 10%. It is the belief of Murray and McCredie that this curious disease of bone is related to the sclerotomes, that is, a zone of the skeleton supplied by individual spinal sensory nerves. It is thought that the approximation of the anatomical distribution of the bone lesions in melorheostosis to the sclerotomes suggests that the sensory nerve plays a vital role in the production of the bony lesions, just as in neurofibromatosis the nerves to an affected segment are often abnormal. As yet, the nature of the exciting factor is not clear, but it is of interest to note that the skin lesions of scleroderma, when seen in melorheostosis, are apparently to be found on the dermatome corresponding to the affected sclerotome.

Macrodystrophia lipomatosa is a rare condition which affects the foot mainly in a pre-axial distribution (Dennyson *et al* 1977). This also raises the possibility that the disease is due to a disorder of the nervous tissue, and some believe that the lesions are a feature of neurofibromatosis. Not only, however, is this disease not inherited (not in itself unusual, as many cases of neurofibromatosis are sporadic), but no histological evidence of neurofibromatosis seems to be found in cases affecting the foot, though nerves in affected feet are more 'prominent'. What is seen is enormous overgrowth, appearing soon after birth, both of bone and soft tissue. Most of the increased bulk is taken up by massive overgrowth of fibro-fatty tissue, clearly visible and diagnostic in a radiograph. This hypertrophy is mainly on the sole of the foot. Overgrowth of bones is seen radiologically to affect phalanges and, less often, the metatarsals. Marked exostosis-like growths give an almost

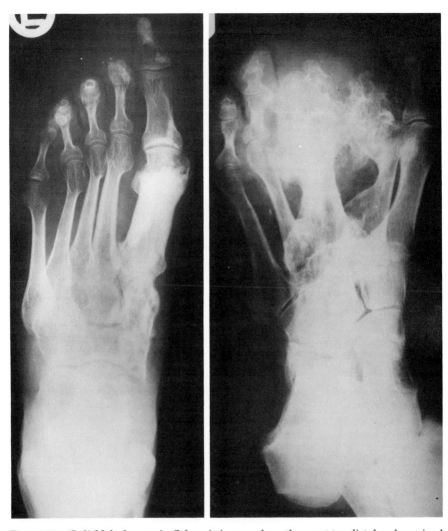

Fig. 12.53 (*Left*) Melorheostosis. Sclerosis is seen along the great toe distal and proximal phalanges, the metatarsal, medial cuneiform and medial portion of the navicular. Added bony density is seen, both on the outside of the cortex and within the medulla. The lesions have been said to resemble flowing candle-wax and, in this patient, are distributed along the L5 sclerotome.

Fig. 12.54 (*Right*) Macrodystrophia lipomatosa. The middle phalanx is enlarged and shows numerous osseous exostoses which deform the second ray. Fatty radiolucencies can be seen in the soft tissues distal to the second and third rays.

osteoarthritic appearance to the local joints due to the marked proliferation of new bone around them, and osteomata may be seen on long bone shafts (Fig. 12.54).

MORE TROPICAL FEET

The surgeon or radiologist who practises in any large town in England needs to have a good working knowledge of tropical diseases, not only because of local immigrant populations, but also because of the ease of intercontinental travel. Certainly thalassaemia and sickle-cell disease are now 'common' diseases of bone seen at University College Hospital, London, while leprosy is not uncommon at the Hospital for Tropical Diseases, London.

Ainhum (dactolysis spontanea) is seen, albeit uncommonly, in Southern USA (Fetterman *et al* 1967) and even in London. The incidence in Nigeria is just over 2% of the population, mainly apparently in Yorubas from the west (Cole 1965). According the Fetterman *et al*, the Yoruba word *ayun* (from which ainhum is derived) means to 'saw' or 'file', and the disease is a localized cause of pointing of a tubular bone. Most patients with it give a history of walking without shoes. Usually the fifth toe only is affected, but occasionally the fourth. Women are involved earlier than men, and the average age of patients is about 40 years.

A groove begins on the medial side of the base of the toe which spreads dorsally to surround the toe. The groove then deepens and fissures, and superadded infection may occur. Initially there is local thickening of the stratum corneum, but later gross hyperkeratosis and inflammation are seen. Blood vessels and nerves are said to be normal, though initially the lesions are painful and it is said that on plethysmography the involved toe has a greater blood flow than the normal (cf. diabetes, leprosy). As the band deepens, the distal toe becomes oedematous and ulcerated. The nail may point laterally and, though eversion of the fifth toe is often normal, it is apparently accentuated. Radiologically, bone is resorbed first at the medial aspect of the distal part of the proximal phalanx or base of the middle phalanx. Resorption is sharp and clean, and the underlying bone is sclerotic, so that the medulla becomes obliterated. The constriction and distal soft tissue swelling can be visualized. Eventually auto-amputation occurs, leaving a pointed proximal phalanx of the little toe (Fig. 12.55).

It is interesting to note that constriction bands (Streeter's bands) cause similar congenital lesions. These constriction bands, or rings, which are not apparently genetically determined, cause intra-uterine amputation of limbs or parts of limbs, often in association with clubfoot or cleft palate. In a fascinating study, Kino (1975) found the deformities to be twice as common in the upper limb but, in both hands and feet, the longest digits were involved—the first and second toes—rather than the shortest, as in ainhum. Radiologically, the lesions are identical. The author was able to induce similar lesions in fetal rats by performing amniocentesis and shows most elegant fetal foot films with constrictions narrowing bone shafts which even fuse together later on. Amniocentesis causes uterine

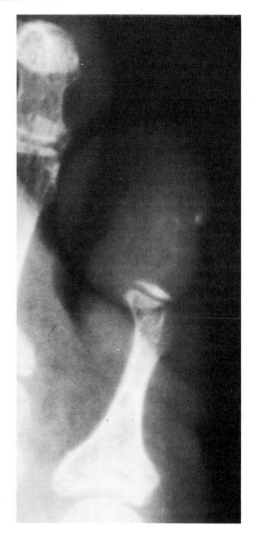

Fig. 12.55 Ainhum. Marked resorption of the distal and middle phalanges of the little toe is shown in this Nigerian patient together with the groove in the soft tissues.

defects into which limbs herniate. Haemorrhage then causes the amnion to adhere to ulcerated regions.

Madura foot

This lesion takes in name from the district of southern India in which it was first described in 1874 (Cockshott 1961). Mycetoma implantation occurs mainly in the feet in semi-desert regions with a definite dry season, throughout the tropical world. Thorns implant the causative organisms into the (bare) feet, though the knees and skull may also be affected. Different organisms are found in different parts of the world (Bohrer 1979)—*M. mycetomi* in the Middle East, Africa and India, *S. somaliensis* and *S. pelletieri* in Sudan and the Sahara. The radiological appearances may differ with the causative organism but very often secondary infection through a sinus track is superimposed on the initial mycetoma. Lesions due to *M. mycetomi* are localized, at least initially, while those due to *S. pelletieri* tend to disseminate rapidly to neighbouring bone and soft tissue.

Following implantation of the mycetoma into the foot, usually on the sole, soft tissue swelling may be seen radiologically, together with local loss or displacement of fat and soft tissue planes. The mycetomas may at first be limited by the plantar fascia, or the deep tissues may have been innoculated *ab initio*. In the bones, both destructive and productive changes occur. Extrinsic cortical erosions may be caused by large sacs of well-defined, black fungus balls containing *M. mycetomi* (Fig. 12.56). Indeed, according to Cockshott, the fungus balls can even be seen radiologically on occasion, especially if secondary infection has not taken place and fascial planes are merely displaced.

The cortex reacts to the extrinsic pressure with sclerosis and periostitis, but if the cortex is broken through the fungus spreads rapidly, causing small cystic lesions within the medulla with sinuses through the cortex. The medulla shows a marked amorphous reactive sclerosis with loss of the normal trabecular pattern (Davies 1958). A ragged periostitis occurs, of a rather coarse 'hair-on-end', rather than 'onion peel', type. Davies likens the changes of patchy peripheral bone destruction with sinuses and reactive sclerosis to a 'melting snow' appearance (Fig. 12.57). As the bones are resorbed, spaces between them increase in size, but ankylosis at joints can also result. Sequestra are not usually seen. Although the areas initially involved are usually the distal tarsus and adjacent bases of the metatarsals, spread of the disease may cause phalangeal bone loss, suggestive of neuropathic lesions (Bohrer), though neurological features are never present in this disease.

The duration of the disease and presence of secondary pyogenic osteomyelitis determine the final appearance. Irrespective of the initial causative organism the end results after many years may be identical.

Kaposi sarcoma

On occasion, the bone lesions of Kaposi sarcoma can resemble those seen in Madura foot, though in the latter the lesions are less well-defined (Davies 1958).

The lesion was first described by Moritz Kaposi in 1872. He was born in Kaposvar (from whence he took his name), but practised as a dermatologist in Vienna, succeeding his father-in-law in the Chair of Dermatology. Not surprisingly, considering Kaposi's Central European location, the disease was thought mainly to occur in Europeans of Russian or Polish Jewish background in 90% of cases, as well as in Italians (Gorham 1963). In such patients mainly males were affected, usually aged 40–70 years (Stout & Lattes 1967). The first reported case in a

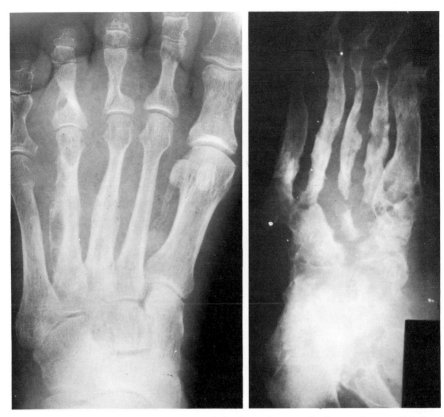

Fig. 12.56 (*Left*) Madura foot. In this relatively early case the bones show well-defined defects with periostitis corresponding to local soft tissue implantation by fungus spores.

Fig. 12.57 (*Right*) Madura foot. A 'melting snow' appearance due to patchy bone destruction, fusion and reactive sclerosis. Elsewhere joint spaces are increased. The appearances are remarkably similar to the pointed tubular bones seen earlier.

negro was in 1931 and it is now clear that the disease is fairly common in Uganda and Zaire in Africa, though it is uncommon in American negroes.

Certainly, in the African negro, the disease occurs in a younger age group (30–50 years).

Lesions are characteristically blue-red, on the legs especially, though they do occur elsewhere in the skin as well as in the gut, renal tract, lung, heart and liver. Over half the patients with skin change show osseous changes. Davies (1956) has classified the radiological changes.

1 Uniform osteoporosis (66%) in the feet.

2 Local osteoporosis with ill-defined margins, especially at phalanges of the feet (43%), but also in the tarsus (25%) so that parts of the bones look rubbed out and an appearance like a 'licked candy stick' is simulated.

3   Bone cysts, with clear-cut margins that lack reactive sclerosis, resembling lesions seen in sarcoid (25–33%).

4   Superficial cortical erosions which may be ill or well-defined, suggesting either malignant infiltration or pressure erosion (Fig. 12.58).

5   Complete loss of a bone.

Histological examination in cases of Kaposi sarcoma involving bone (Gorham) seem to show angiomatous change related to bone destruction in the absence of osteoclasts. The angiomatous tissue may look benign or sarcomatous, but Gorham feels that osteolysis may be brought about by arterial hyperaemia rather than malignant destruction, though presumably the localized extrinsic defects are the result of pressure atrophy.

Arteriography shows the nodules to be highly vascular with a malignant type

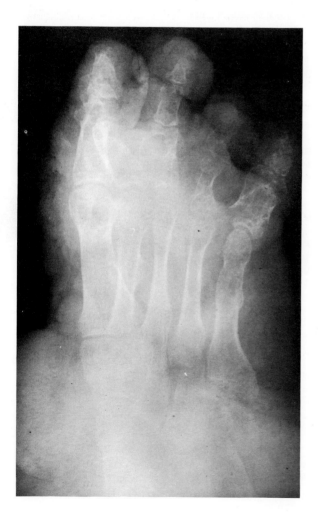

Fig. 12.58 Marked soft tissue swelling due to tumour masses and cystic erosion of bone are seen together with osteoporosis.

of tumour circulation, while lymphangiography shows the nodules to communi-
cate with the lymphatic system and the lymphatics to be obstructed. Nodules thus
demonstrated are shown adjacent to bony defects.

ACKNOWLEDGEMENT

The author acknowledges with gratitude the secretarial assistance of Miss
Veronika Aurens and the photographic assistance of Ms Uta Boundy, of the
Institute of Orthopaedics, London.

REFERENCES

ANSELL B.M. & KENT P.A. (1977) Radiological changes in juvenile chronic polyarthritis.
    Skeletal Radiology **1**, 129–44.
ANSELL B.M. (1980) *Rheumatoid Disorders in Childhood*. Butterworths, London.
ANTHONSEN W. (1943) An oblique projection for roentgen examination of the talo-calcaneal
    joint. *Acta Radiologica* **24**, 306–10.
BARNETSON J. (1951) Pathogenesis of bone changes in neural leprosy. *International Journal of
    Leprosy* **19**, 297–307.
BECKLY D.E., ANDERSON P.W. & PEDEGANA L.R. (1975) The radiology of the subtalar joint
    with special reference to talo-calcaneal coalition. *Clinical Radiology* **26**, 333–41.
BOHRER S.P. (1979) Bone Diseases. In Cockshott P. & Middlemiss H. (eds.), *Clinical Radiology
    in the Tropics*. Churchill Livingstone, Edinburgh.
BROOK A. & CORBETT M. (1977) Radiographic changes in early rheumatoid disease. *Annals of
    the Rheumatic Diseases* **36**, 71–3.
BYWATERS E.G.L. (1954) Heel lesions of rheumatoid arthritis. *Annals of the Rheumatic
    Diseases* **13**, 42–51.
CALABRO J.J. (1962) A critical evaluation of the diagnostic features of the feet in rheumatoid
    arthritis. *Arthritis and Rheumatism* **5**, 19–29.
CATTERALL R.C.F. (1972) The diabetic foot. *British Journal of hospital Medicine* **7**, 224–6.
CHAMBERS C.H. (1950) Congenital anomalies of the tarsal navicular with particular reference
    to calcaneo-navicular coalition. *British Journal of Radiology* **23**, 580–6.
CLOUSE N.E., GRAMM H.F., LEGG M. & FLOOD T. (1974) Diabetic osteoarthropathy. *American
    Journal of Roentgenology* **121**, 22–34.
COCKSHOTT P. (1961) In Middlemiss H. (ed.), *Tropical Medicine*. Heinemann, London.
COLE G.J. (1965) Ainhum. *Journal of Bone and Joint Surgery (Br)* **47B**, 43–51.
CONWAY J.J. & COWELL H.R. (1969) Tarsal coalition: clinical significance and roentgeno-
    graphic demonstration. *Radiology* **92**, 799–811.
COWELL H.R. (1972) Talo-calcaneal coalition and new causes of peroneal spastic flat foot.
    Clinical Orthopaedics and Related Research **85**, 16–22.
DAHLIN D.C. (1978) In *Bone Tumours*, 3rd edn. Charles Thomas, Springfield, Illinois.
DAVIES A.G.M. (1956) Bone changes in Kaposi's sarcoma. *Journal of the Faculty of
    Radiologists* **8**, 32–40.
DAVIES A.G.M. (1958) The bone changes of Madura foot. *Radiology* **70**, 841–7.
DAVIES L.A. & HATT W.S. (1955) Congenital abnormalities of the feet. *Radiology* **64**, 818–25.
DEL SEL J.M. & GRAND N.E. (1959) Cubonavicular synostosis. *Journal of Bone and Joint
    Surgery (Br)* **41B**, 149.

DENNYSON W.G., BEAR J.N. & BHOOLA K.D. (1977) Macrodactyly in the foot. *Journal of Bone and Joint Surgery (Br)* **59B**, 355–9.

DILSEN N., MCEWEN C., POPPEL M., GERSH W.J., DI TATA D. & CARMEL P. (1962) A comparative roentgenologic study of rheumatoid arthritis and rheumatoid (ankylosing) spondylosis. *Arthritis and Rheumatism* **5**, 341–68.

DWIGHT T. (1907) *Variations of the bones of the hand and feet.* Lippincott, Philadelphia.

ENNA C.D., JACOBSON R.R. & RAUSCH R.O. (1971) Bone changes in leprosy. *Radiology* **100**, 295–306.

FAGET G.H. & MAYORAL A. (1944) Bone changes in leprosy: a clinical and roentgenologic study of 505 cases. *Radiology* **42**, 1–13.

FELSON B. (1970) Letter from the Editor. *Seminars in Roentgenology* **4**, 325–6.

FETTERMAN L.E., HARDY R. & LEHRER H. (1967) The clinico-roentgenologic features of ainhum. *American Journal of Roentgenology* **100**, 512–22.

FLETCHER D.E. & ROWLEY K.A. (1952) The radiological features of rheumatoid arthritis. *British Journal of Radiology* **25**, 282–95.

GAMBLE F.O. & YALE I. (1975) *Clinical Foot Roentgenology*, 2nd ed. Robert E. Krieger, New York.

GARDNER E., GRAY D.J. & O'RAHILLY R. (1959) The prenatal development of the skeleton and joints of the human foot. *Journal of Bone and Joint Surgery (Am)* **41A**, 847–76.

GENANT H.K., HECK L.L., LANZI L.H., ROSSMAN K., HORST J.V. & PAYOLAN E. (1973) Primary hyperparathyroidism. *Radiology* **109**, 513–24.

GEOFFROY J., HOEFFEL J.C., POINTEL J.P., DROUIN P., DEBRY G. & MARTIN R. (1979) The feet in diabetes. Roentgenologic observation in 1501 cases. *Diagnostic Imaging* **48**, 286–93.

GERSTER J.C., VISCHER T.L., BENNANI A. & FALLET G.H. (1977) The painful heel. *Annals of the Rheumatic Diseases* **36**, 343–8.

GHEITH S.L. & DIXON A.ST.J. (1973) Tangential X-ray of the forefoot in rheumatoid arthritis. *Annals of the Rheumatic Diseases* **32**, 92–3.

GONDOS B. (1968) Roentgen observations in diabetic osteopathy. *Radiology* **91**, 6–13.

GONDOS B. (1972) The pointed tubular bone. *Radiology* **105**, 541–5.

GORHAM L.W. (1963) Kaposis's sarcoma involving bone. *Archives of Pathology and Laboratory Medicine* **76**, 456–63.

GRALINO B.J., PORTER J.M. & ROSCH J. (1976) Angiography in the diagnosis and therapy of frostbite. *Radiology* **119**, 301–5.

HALL R. (1961) A case of melorheostosis with cutaneous haemangioma and lymphatic vesicles. *Journal of Bone and Joint Surgery (Br)* **43B**, 335–7.

HARRIS J.R. & BRAND P.W. (1966) Patterns of disintegration in the anaesthetic foot. *Journal of Bone and Joint Surgery (Br)* **48B**, 4–16.

HARRIS R.I. & BEATH T. (1948) Aetiology of peroneal spastic flat foot. *Journal of Bone and Joint Surgery (Br)* **30B**, 624–34.

HARRIS R.I. (1965) Retrospect: peroneal spastic flat foot (rigid valgus foot). *Journal of Bone and Joint Surgery (Am)* **47A**, 1657–67.

HLAVAC H.F. (1967) Differences in X-ray findings with varied positioning of the foot. *Journal of the American Podiatry Association* **57**, 465–71.

HOERR N.L., PYLE S.I. & FRANCIS C.C. (1962) *Radiographic Atlas of Skeletal Development of the Foot and Ankle.* Charles C. Thomas, Springfield, Illinois.

HOLLAND C.T. (1928) The accessory bones of the foot. In Fairbank H.A.T. (ed.), *The Robert Jones Birthday Volume.* Oxford University Press, Oxford.

ISHERWOOD I. (1961) A radiological approach to the subtalar joint. *Journal of Bone and Joint Surgery (Br)* **43B**, 566–74.

JACK E.A. (1954) Bone anomalies of the tarsus in relation to 'peroneal spastic flat foot'. *Journal of Bone and Joint Surgery (Br)* **36B**, 530–42.

JACKSON D.M. (1968) Heel pad thickness in obese persons. *Radiology* **90**, 129.

JACOBS P. (1975) In Sutton D. & Grainger R. (eds.), *A Textbook of Radiology*, 2nd ed. Churchill Livingstone, Edinburgh.

JAYAKUMAR S. & COWELL H.R. (1977) *Clinical Orthopaedics* **122**, 77–84.

KATTAN K.R. (1975) Thickening of the heel pad associated with long term Dilantin therapy. *American Journal of Roentgenology* **124**, 52–6.

KELLGREN J.H. & LAWRENCE J.S. (1957) Radiological assessment of rheumatoid arthritis. *Annals of the Rheumatoid Diseases* **16**, 485–93.

KERIN R. (1958) Metastatic tumours of the hand. *Journal of Bone and Joint Surgery (Am)* **40A**, 263–78.

KHO K.M., WRIGHT A.D. & DOYLE F.H. (1970) Heel pad thickness in acromegaly. *British Journal of Radiology* **43**, 119–25.

KINO Y. (1975) Clinical and experimental studies of the congenital constriction band syndrome, with an emphasis on its etiology. *Journal of Bone and Joint Surgery (Am)* **57A**, 636–43.

KIRKUP J.R. (1974) Ankle and tarsal joints in rheumatoid arthritis. *Scandinavian Journal of Rheumatology* **3**, 50–2.

KIRKUP J.R., VIDIGAL E. & JACOBY R.K. (1977) The hallux and rheumatoid arthritis. *Acta Orthopaedica Scandinavica* **48**, 527–44.

KÖHLER A. & ZIMMER E. (1968) In *Borderlands of the normal and early pathologic in skeletal roentgenology*. Grune and Stratton, New York.

KRAFT E., SPYROPOULOS E. & FINBY E. (1975) Neurogenic disorders of the foot in diabetes mellitus. *American Journal of Roentgenology* **124**, 17–24.

LAWS J.W., LILLIE J.G. & SCOTT J.T. (1963) Arteriographic appearances in rheumatoid arthritis and other disorders. *British Journal of Radiology* **36**, 477–93.

LECHAT M.F. (1962) Bone lesions in leprosy. *International Journal of Leprosy* **30**, 125–37.

LUSBY H.L.J. (1959) Naviculocuneiform synostosis. *Journal of Bone and Joint Surgery* **41B**, 150.

MARTEL W., STUCK K.J., DWORIN A.M. & HYLLAND R.G. (1980) Erosive osteoarthritis and psoriatic arthritis. *American Journal of Roentgenology* **134**, 125–35.

MASON R.M., MURRAY R.S., OATES J.K. & YOUNG A.C. (1959) A comparative radiological study of Reiter's disease, rheumatoid arthritis and ankylosing spondylitis. *Journal of Bone and Joint Surgery (Br)* **41B**, 137–48.

MCCARROLL H.R. (1950) Clinical manifestations of congenital neurofibromatosis. *Journal of Bone and Joint Surgery (Am)* **32A**, 601–17.

MESCHAN I. (1970) Radiology of the normal foot. *Seminars in Roentgenology* **4**, 327–40.

MOORE B.H. (1942) Macrodactyly and associated peripheral nerve changes. *Journal of Bone and Joint Surgery* **24**, 617–31.

MORRIS J.M., SAMILSON R.L. & CORLEY C.L. (1963) Melorheostosis. *Journal of Bone and Joint Surgery (Am)* **45A**, 1191–206.

MULVEY R.B. (1964) Peripheral bone metastases. *American Journal of Roentgenology* **91**, 155–60.

MURRAY R.O. (1951) Melorheostosis associated with congenital arteriovenous aneurysms. *Proceedings of the Royal Society of Medicine* **44**, 473–5.

MURRAY R.O. & McCREADY J. (1979) Melorheostosis and the sclerotomes. *Skeletal Radiology* **4**, 57–71.

NETHERLANDS COMMITTEE ON BONE TUMOURS (1966) *Radiological Atlas of Bone Tumours*. Mouton and Co., The Hague.

NORMAN A. (1970) Tumor and tumor-like lesions of the bones of the foot. *Seminars in Roentgenology* **4**, 407–18.

O'RAHILLY R. (1953) A survey of carpal and tarsal anomalies. *Journal of Bone and Joint Surgery (Am)* **35A**, 626–42.

O'RAHILLY R. (1957) Developmental deviations in the carpus and tarsus. *Clinical Orthopaedics* **10**, 9–18.

OUTLAND T. & MURPHY I.D. (1960) The pathomechanics of peroneal spastic flat foot. *Clinical Orthopaedics* **16**, 64–73.

PATERSON D.E. (1961) Bone changes in leprosy. *International Journal of Leprosy* **29**, 393–422.

PATTON J.T. (1976) Differential diagnosis of inflammatory spondylitis. *Skeletal Radiology* **1**, 77–85.

PETERSON C.C. & SILBIGER M.L. (1967) Reiter's syndrome and psoriatic arthropathy. *American Journal of Roentgenology* **101**, 860–71.

PUCKETTE S.E. & SEYMOUR E.Q. (1967) Fallibility of heel pad thickness in the diagnosis of acromegaly. *Radiology* **88**, 982–3.

RAJA R., ADAMALI N. & GRAYBURN J. (1980) Heel pad thickness in Kenyan Africans. *East African medical Journal* **57**, 208–11.

REEDER M.M. (1970) Tropical diseases of the foot. *Seminars in Roentgenology* **4**, 378–90.

RESNICK D. (1976) Roentgen features of the rheumatoid mid and hind foot. *Journal of the Canadian Association of Radiologists* **27**, 99–107.

RESNICK D., NIWAYAMA G. & FEINGOLD M.L. (1977) The sesamoid bones of the hands and feet: participators in arthritis. *Radiology* **123**, 57–62.

RESNICK D., FEINGOLD M.L., CURD J., NIWAYAMA G. & GOERGEN T.D. (1977) Calcaneal abnormalities in articular disorders. *Radiology* **125**, 355–66.

SAUNDERS J.B. DE C. & O'MALLEY C.D. (1950) *Vesalius: The Illustrations from his Works.* World Publishing Company, Cleveland, Ohio.

SEDDON H.J. (1932) Calcaneo-scaphoid coalition. *Proceedings of the Royal Society of Medicine* **26**, 419–24.

SHANDS A.R. & WERTS I.J. (1953) Foot problems in children. *Surgical Clinics of North America* **33**, 1643–66.

SHOLKOFF S.D., GLICKMAN M.G. & STEINBACH H.L. (1970) Roentgenology of Reiter's syndrome. *Radiology* **97**, 497–503.

SKINSNES O.K., SAKURI I. & AQUINO T.I. (1972) Pathogenesis of extremity deformity in leprosy. *International Journal of Leprosy* **40**, 375–88.

SLOMANN H.C. (1926) On the demonstration and analysis of calcaneo-navicular coalition by roentgen examination. *Acta Radiologica* **5**, 304–12.

STAPLE T.W. (1973) Roentenography of the diabetic foot. In Levin M. and O'Neal L. (eds.), *The Diabetic Foot*. C.V. Mosby Company, St Louis.

STEEL M.W., JOHNSON K.A., DEWITZ M.A. & ILSTRUP D.M. (1980) Radiographic measurements of the normal adult foot. *Foot and Ankle* **1**, 151–8.

STEINBACH H.L. & RUSSELL W. (1964) Measurement of the heel pad as an aid to diagnosis of acromegaly. *Radiology* **82**, 418–23.

STOUT A.P. & LATTES R. (1967) *Tumours of the Soft Tissues*, 2nd edn. Armed Forces Institute of Pathology, Washington D.C.

THORNHILL H.L., RICHTER R.W., SHENTON M.L. & JOHNSON C.A. (1973) Neuropathic arthropathy in alcoholics. *Orthopaedic Clinics of North America* **4**, 7–20.

THOULD A.K. & SIMON G. (1966) Assessment of radiological changes in the hands and feet in rheumatoid arthritis. *Annals of the Rheumatic Diseases* **25**, 220–8.

TROLLE D. (1948) *Accessory bones of the human foot.* E. Munksgaard, Copenhagen.

VENNING P. (1960) Variation of the digital skeleton of the foot. *Clinical Orthopaedics* **16**, 26–40.

VIDIGAL E., JACOBY R.K., DIXON A.ST.J., RATLIFF A.H. & KIRKUP J. (1975) The foot in chronic rheumatoid arthritis. *Annals of the Rheumatic Diseases* **34**, 292–7.

WEBSTER F.S. & ROBERTS W.M. (1951) Tarsal anomalies and peroneal flat foot. *Journal of the American medical Association* **146**, 1099–104.

WRIGHT V. (1961) Psoratic arthritis: A comparative radiographic study of rheumatoid arthritis and arthritis associated with psoriasis. *Annals of the Rheumatic Diseases* **20**, 123–32.

WRIGHT V. (1978) Psoriatic Arthritis. In Scott J.T. (ed.) *Copeman's Textbook of the Rheumatic Diseases*, 5th edn. Churchill Livingstone, Edinburgh.

YOUNG A., CORBETT M. & BROOK A. (1980) The clinical assessment of joint inflammatory activity in rheumatoid arthritis related to radiological progression. *Rheumatology and Rehabilitation* **19**, 14–19.

2 RADIOGRAPHY OF THE FOOT

It has been stated that, 'there should be no routine views in orthopaedic radiography; the request should be for a particular projection for the suspected diagnosis' (Lipmann Kessel). Very frequently the radiographic request form only states 'x-ray feet'.

Radiography of the foot can be said to be performed in three age groups—in infants, in adolescents and in adults. The views frequently required for common problems in each age group will be discussed. It is hoped that by having a more detailed knowledge of the views available the orthopaedic surgeon will be able to gain the maximum help from his radiographic department.

THE INFANT (0–8 YEARS)

Anteroposterior and lateral films of both feet should always be taken for comparison. To reduce the radiation dose to infants, it is advisable to take the anteroposterior projection of both feet on the same film. Similarly, the lateral views can be taken on the same film in the prayer position ('saying your prayers with your feet'), both soles being placed against each other with pressure applied on the knees to simulate weight-bearing (see below).

Anteroposterior views are of little help until one year of age. The lateral view may, however, be useful from the third month onwards as the cuboid has appeared by then. If the knee is bent to 90° with a relaxed foot, a bisecting line drawn through the talus passes through the upper third of the cuboid and plantar aspect of the first metatarsal.

Radiographs should demonstrate the bones clearly with the use of a low kilovoltage (penetration). At this early age oblique views do not add any further information, only cause exposure to more radiation. Normal exposures for the forefeet and infants should only be from 40–50 kV at 25 MAS, with non-screen film put through a $3\frac{1}{2}$–5 minute cycle in the automatic processor with the developer temperature at 76°F (24.5°C). The tube–film distance should be 30 inches (76 cm) and all extremities examined with a tube focus of 0.3 or 0.6 mm. A twelve pulse or constant potential unit is useful for minimal exposures to eliminate movement blurring.

Radiographic positioning

The anteroposterior view

Sit the patient on an open-ended box, 18 cm high, with the knees bent and the tibiae inclined 15–30°, as if taking a step forward. This is a natural position without any stress and keeps the radiation well away from the region of the gonads while allowing the x-ray tube to be kept vertical to the film. It is unnecessary to tilt the tube 15° towards the heel at this age, and the vertical tube allows quick positioning if the patient is likely to move (Fig. 12.59).

Weight-bearing can be simulated in the very young by instructing the parent (protected by a lead apron and gloves) to press down on the knees. The tibial tuberosities are positioned facing anteriorly and the feet placed on the film in *their* natural position. It is important that the radiographer does not attempt to place the feet on the film in what *he* considers to be a natural position; the feet should be allowed to lie free. If it is doubtful that the patient will keep still, a bandage across the feet weighed down on either side by sandbags or a bucky band will produce stability with a very short exposure time.

The lateral view

In the very young the prayer position can be used to give lateral views of both feet with a single exposure (Fig. 12.60). Children who might be unsteady standing can

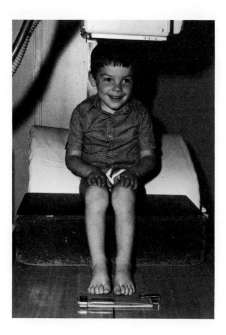

Fig. 12.59 Radiographic positioning: The AP view. The patient is relaxed, the tibiae are sloped back with the tibial tuberosities facing anteriorly. This results in a natural position of the foot on the film.

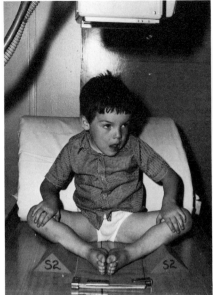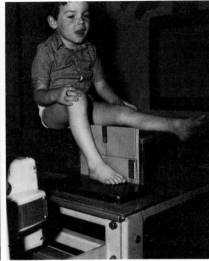

Fig. 12.60 (*Left*) The prayer position for the lateral view of the feet. This position is easily adopted and demonstrates both feet simultaneously.

Fig. 12.61 (*Right*) Lateral view.

be sat on the box with the medial side of the foot in its accustomed position. Pressure can be applied to the knee to simulate weight-bearing (Fig. 12.61).

A lateral radiograph in dorsiflexion may be requested. This can either be taken with the patient standing and the tibia flexed forward towards the foot or with the knee bent and a bandage placed around the forepart of the feet with stress applied in the direction of dorsiflexion. These views demonstrate talar and calcaneal movements.

Metatarsus varus is a common anomaly at this age and the anteroposterior view demonstrates the fan-shaped position of the metatarsals with separation of the heads and the bases close together.

In the case of *club feet*, both anteroposterior and lateral films provide useful information. Sometimes the lateral view shows an apparent flat-topped talus. Some surgeons have in the past considered this to be the result of manipulative overcorrection of the foot, but it is usually due to faulty positioning by the radiographer. The medial malleolus on the side of the varus concavity is rotated forwards, while the lateral malleolus on the convex side is more posterior. The usual lateral radiograph then demonstrates an anteroposterior ankle and a flat-topped talus. To correct this apparent anomaly, the foot has to be further internally rotated until the malleoli are in the same plane, and a true lateral view of the ankle with a round-topped talus will usually be seen. If the film is taken correctly and the true lateral radiograph demonstrates a talus which has a flat top, then this will indeed be due to overcorrection (see Chapter 5, Figs. 5.16, 5.17).

Varus heels can be demonstrated by standing the patient on the film with the knees flexed 15–30° and the tube vertically centred on the heels (Fig. 12.62).

To confirm the diagnosis of *vertical talus* radiographically, a lateral view is taken with pressure applied to the forefoot and the ankle in plantar flexion. If the talus remains vertical and the calcaneum remains at the same angle to the talus, then the vertical talus is genuine. A lateral view with the ankle dorsiflexed will exaggerate the 'rocker bottom' appearance (Fig. 12.63).

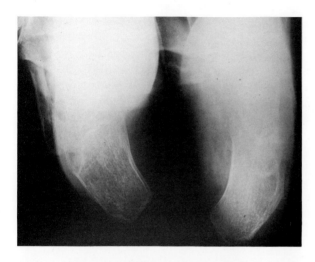

Fig. 12.62 Varus deformity of the heels demonstrated with a vertical beam.

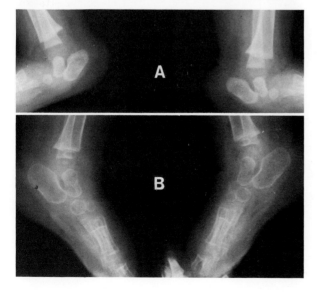

Fig. 12.63 Vertical talus. (A) dorsiflexion, (B) plantar flexion. In (B) the talus is shown to be vertical and its relationship to the calcaneum unaltered.

THE ADOLESCENT (8–18 YEARS)

Anteroposterior views

These can be taken with the patient standing or sitting, though if there is a rigid club foot or flat foot, weight-bearing will make no difference to the resultant radiograph. The situation then is similar to that of the structural curve of the spine in scoliosis. If the patient is bent towards the convexity of the curve it does not straighten.

In the anteroposterior weight-bearing position the film is placed on the floor with the patient standing on it. The tibial tuberosities are positioned facing anteriorly; normally the feet will be parallel to each other. Abnormal feet may be abducted, adducted or supinated etc., but despite this it is essential that the tibial tuberosities are in the correct position and the feet are in the position to which the patient is accustomed (Fig. 12.64). The tube is tilted 15° towards the heels and centred between the two feet at the tarsal region. If the tibiae and fibulae are vertical to the feet the tube is too close to the gonadal region, and it may be difficult to centre with some patients. It is thus preferable to stand the patient so that he can support himself against the radiographic couch with the tibiae sloped back 15°. The 15° angle of the tube towards the heels and the slope of the tibiae give an effective angle of 30° without distortion.

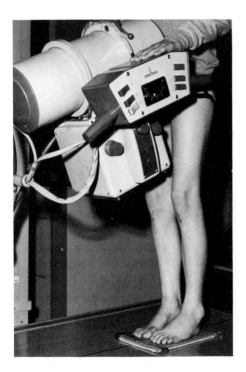

Fig. 12.64 Weight-bearing AP view of the feet. The tube is tilted 15° towards the heels but, in this case, is too near the gonads. Excessive radiation can be avoided by tilting the patient back 15° against the radiographic couch.

It is important to use film giving fine detail. Non-screen film backed by lead ply or lead rubber sheets is used to eliminate scatter and fogging. The film is best processed for five minutes in an automatic machine at a temperature of 76°F (24.5°C). Such a film has a lower contrast level with higher definition, and it is possible to show the phalanges, metatarsals and tarsal bones on one film. With films taken in casettes using fluorescent screens, the contrast range is too high and if the tarsal bones are well demonstrated the forefoot will be blacked out. In the case of 90 second processing of non-screen film (which for practical purposes may be regarded as screen film in an envelope) more radiation is given to the patient to obtain a film of poorer quality.

Radiography of the forefoot (phalanges to metatarsals)

The radiographic request may be for the phalanges to be demonstrated but if the toes are clawed they cannot be shown straight by any variation of the tube angle. In young adolescents it is often possible by lifting the heels to align the phalanges parallel to the film, as some of the patients with claw toes can then correct them (Fig. 12.65).

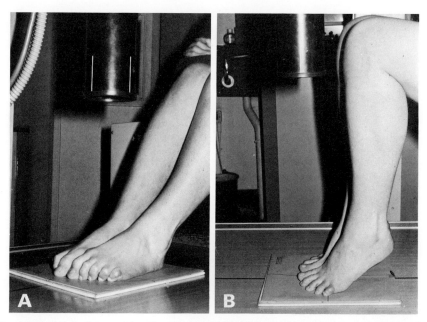

Fig. 12.65 (A) In this position the tibiae are tilted backwards, reducing radiation to the gonads; the feet are firmly on the ground, but the toes remain clawed. (B) In the same patient, with the heels elevated, the toes are now straightened on the film.

The lateral view

A true lateral view superimposes one phalanx upon another and is only useful to show gross malalignment of the phalanges. A better method for a specific phalanx, especially the second, third and fourth, is to place a match or cocktail stick above the adjacent toes, making the particular phalanx more prominent than the others.

The medial oblique view

The routine oblique view is normally taken in the medial oblique position where the medial aspect of the foot rests on the film with the knee bent inwards and steadied against the opposite knee. The foot, with the great toe resting on the film, is angled to 45°. The tube is perpendicular and is centred to the medial edge of the first metatarsophalangeal joint (Fig. 12.66). The film should include the terminal phalanges and the metatarsal bases. Because of the convexity of the dorsum of the foot, this view clearly shows the metatarsal bases and shafts, and also gives a clear view of the tarsus and tarsal joints. This position is important for demonstrating a coalition between the calcaneum and the navicular, in addition to pathology in the calcaneocuboid joint.

The steep medial oblique view

Adolescents may have hallux valgus. The anteroposterior view will demonstrate the varus first metatarsal and the valgus phalanges, and these angles can be

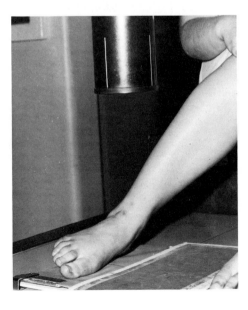

Fig. 12.66   Medial oblique view of the foot.

measured. A true lateral view of the forefoot will have all the metatarsophalangeal joints superimposed one upon the other. The steep oblique view with the foot angled to 75° will give practically a lateral view of the big toe without the other metatarsals being superimposed (Fig. 12.67). The tube is perpendicular and centred 1 inch medially to the first metatarsophalangeal joint.

The lateral oblique view

This is a very useful view to demonstrate any pathology around the first and second toes in the metatarsophalangeal region, as seen in this example of a plantar exostosis (Fig. 12.68). In the lateral oblique view there is no overlapping of the adjacent phalanges. When this position is needed the lateral border of the foot is placed on the film and the medial border raised 45°, the tube is centred to the lateral border of the foot over the fifth toe for the phalanges and over the cuboid for the metatarsals. The pathology is seen more clearly than in the medial oblique view (Fig. 12.69).

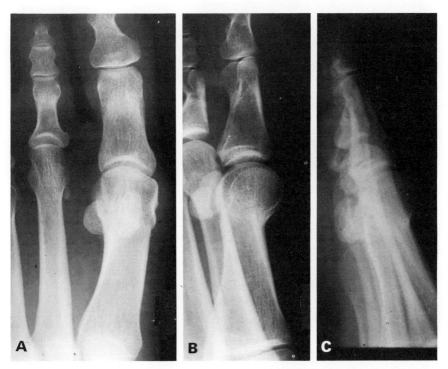

Fig. 12.67 (A) AP view, (B) oblique view, (C) lateral view. Only the steep oblique view clearly demonstrates the joints of the great toe in an almost lateral position.

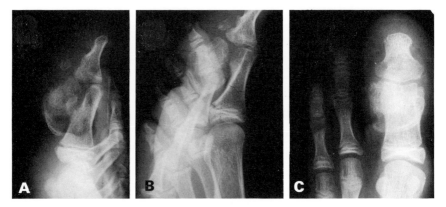

Fig. 12.68 (A) Lateral oblique view. This clearly shows a large dense mass related to the proximal phalanx of the great toe. The lesion was an exostosis arising from the plantar surface of the proximal phalanx of the great toe. (B) and (C) demonstrate the lesion far less clearly.

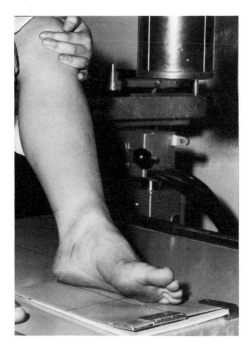

Fig. 12.69 Positioning for the lateral oblique view.

Radiography of the hind-foot

The Harris axial view

Cartilaginous, fibrous or bony fusion of the subtalar joint (talocalcaneal bar) may be demonstrated by this view. The patient stands on the film with the heels on the posterior edge and both feet parallel. The knees are bent forward but will only move about 10° before the heels begin to lift, especially if there is a fusion. The feet must be kept flat on the film; the tube is angled towards the forefeet at 45° and centred between both medial malleoli. In most cases this tube angle is satisfactory but if the joint is not demonstrated clearly two further views with the tube angled at 55° and 35° should be obtained. Radiographically, the main factor is to give enough penetration and exposure (MAS) to illustrate any fusion on the film (Fig. 12.70).

The lateral view

This is useful as it will often show lipping on the superior lateral margin of the head of the talus. A rigid flat foot in a child is usually due to tarsal coalition, and the lateral view in these patients can be taken either standing or non-weight-bearing in the prayer position, whichever happens to be the most convenient. Flexible feet should always have films taken standing, because the apparently normal non-weightbearing lateral view can be abnormal on weight-bearing.

The patient stands on the radiographic couch top, which is usually not difficult for adolescents. The foot is placed on a 1 inch block of wood with the medial border of the foot (which is normally the higher arch) facing the horizontal x-ray

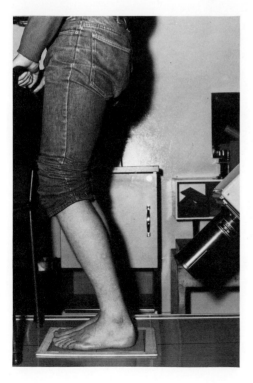

Fig. 12.70 Positioning for Harris's axial view to demonstrate the subtalar joints. Both heels are radiographed simultaneously for comparison.

tube. The film is placed against the lateral border of the foot with the tube centred to the medial longitudinal arch (Fig. 12.71). The patient applies body pressure to the foot being radiographed; the other foot helps maintain stability. With the medial side of the foot facing the x-ray tube, the radiographer can more readily demonstrate pes planus or cavus but, should the clinician prefer the lateral border of the foot nearer the tube, this can be done.

The calcaneal apophysis   The calcaneum is the only tarsal bone that has an apophysis on its posterior aspect. The lateral view will demonstrate the apophysis, which usually runs vertically. Lateral radiographs of both heels can be taken on a single film, with the patient sitting and the feet abducted, to demonstrate the apophyses in younger patients (Fig. 12.72).

The superior plantar view

This is a useful additional radiograph. The patient stands on the film with both heels parallel and the knees slightly bent so that the feet remain flat on the film. The x-ray tube is centred either perpendicularly to the heels or very slightly angled

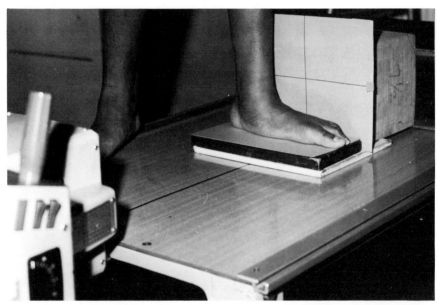

Fig. 12.71 Weight-bearing lateral view of the foot. Placing the lateral aspect of the foot against the film demonstrates the medial aspect of the foot more clearly to the radiographer, enabling him to see pathology, if present. Use of a fine focus does not cause radiographic distortion of the image, as suggested by some authors. A subsequent film of the same patient with the film against the medial aspect of the foot revealed absolutely no difference in the radiographic appearance. This is because we do not move the patient, only the film and the tube.

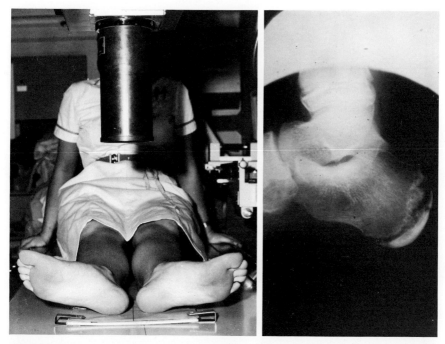

Fig. 12.72 Lateral view of the calcaneal apophysis. The feet are abducted, the heels placed together, and the vertical beam centred between them.

to go through the apophyseal gap, the angulation being varied according to the mobility of the patient (Fig. 12.73).

The routine view for the calcaneum, with the tube angled at 30° towards the heel, does not demonstrate the apophyseal gap, as the apophysis is thrown over the body of the calcaneum. It is nevertheless valuable for other pathology and injuries. The patient sits or lies supine on the radiographic couch with the foot at right-angles to the lower leg. The film is placed under the ankle with its lower border level with the heel pad. The tube is angled 30° towards the base and centred between the two malleoli.

THE ADULT (18 YEARS UPWARDS)

The adult foot is a great challenge to the radiographer as it is a unit with more than 40 whole or part articulations.

Radiography of the forefeet

The appearance of claw toes can be shown on the radiograph. In the anteroposterior position with mobile phalanges, the patient can lift his heels and spread his toes

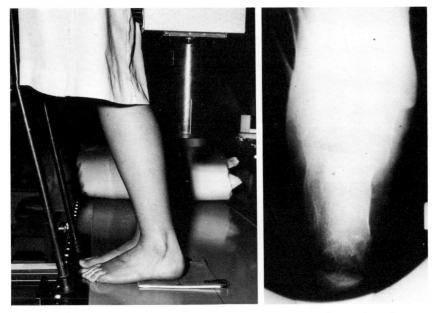

Fig. 12.73   A vertical beam with the knees bent demonstrates the apophyseal gap.

out flat with the radiographer's help (see above), but in older and less mobile patients it is better to place the forefeet on the film and attempt to straighten the toes by padding underneath with cottonwool (Fig. 12.74). The toes should then be parallel to the film. The x-ray tube is centred vertically over the base of the third toe. If both forefeet are to be examined it is best to pad both sets of phalanges. All forefoot films should include the region from the terminal phalanges to the tarso-metatarsal joints.

The second view should be a medial 45° oblique, which can also be taken with the toes separated and straightened as described above.

In the case of a hammer toe, if the phalanges are not protruding enough to them distinctly on the lateral radiograph, a match-stick placed underneath the toe will separate it from the adjacent toes. This may also be useful for demonstrating an injury to a specific toe (Fig. 12.75).

It is frequently difficult for older patients to sit on the x-ray couch, bend their knees and rest their feet plantigrade on a film, as this often induces cramp in the calves. These patients should be sat on the edge of the couch with their feet resting on a chair (Fig. 12.76). Patients after operation who are in wheelchairs can similarly have their films taken without having to be moved if the film is rested on a box. Stretcher patients may remain supine on their trolley while the tube is adjusted to suit the patient, with a box beneath their heels.

To demonstrate bilateral hallux valgus, the feet are placed plantigrade on the film with the tibiae sloping backwards and the weight spread evenly over the feet.

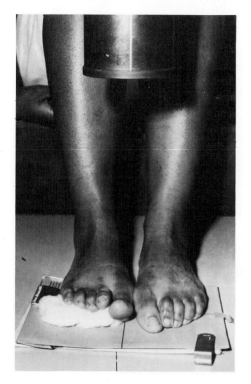

Fig. 12.74 Straightening out of adult claw toes. The left foot demonstrates claw toes, while on the right these have been straightened by placing a pad of cotton wool beneath the toes.

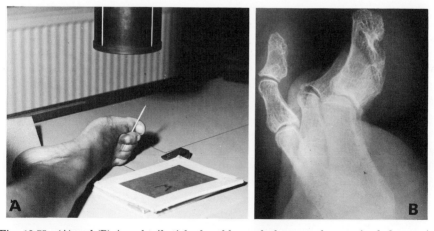

Fig. 12.75 (A) and (B) A cocktail stick placed beneath the toe to be examined elevates it beyond its neighbours for the lateral and oblique views.

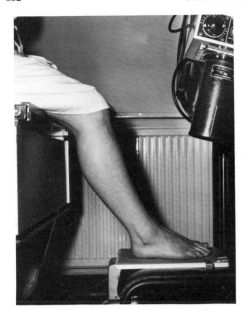

Fig. 12.76 Elderly patients find this position more comfortable for the AP and oblique views.

Simulated weight-bearing can be obtained by asking the patient to press their hands down on their knees. This position can be more effective than standing, for the patient, in an attempt to protect the painful forefoot, may put all the weight on the heels and not on the rest of the foot. The tube is vertical, as for forefoot films, and centred between the metatarsophalangeal joints of the great toes. The metatarsocuneiform joints must be included.

A 45° medial oblique view is not necessary in the demonstration of hallux valgus. It is preferable to take a steeper oblique to give the nearest possible to a lateral view of the first metatarsophalangeal joint without overlapping of the other metatarsals and phalanges. This view may also demonstrate an exostosis in hallux rigidus. After operation a true lateral view may be needed to see the precise position of an arthrodesis of the metatarsophalangeal joint.

The sesamoids

The patient sits on the radiographic couch with both heels resting on the film. Both sets of sesamoids are taken with one exposure. The great toes are placed in contact with each other medially. The line of the heads of the metatarsals should protrude just beyond the heels to throw the sesamoids clear (Fig. 12.77). If the phalanges are dorsiflexed, they can be held clear of the sesamoids with a bandage pulled gently by the patient. Films taken with this technique have the advantage of demonstrating the sesamoids clear of the metatarsal heads, and they are also magnified without loss of detail if a 0.3 or 0.6 mm target focus is used (Fig. 12.78). The heels are slightly lateral to the sesamoids.

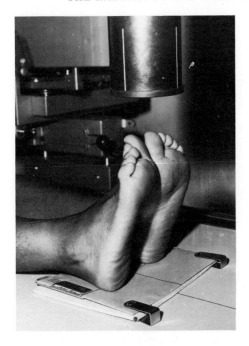

Fig. 12.77 Sesamoid view. The
sesamoids are distal to the heel in
this exposure and the vertical beam
is centred between the great toes, on
the ball of the feet.

An off-lateral view can be taken with the foot positioned as for a normal lateral
view with its lateral border resting on the film, but with the medial border
projecting plantarwards slightly beyond the lateral border. This demonstrates the
medial sesamoid especially well (Fig. 12.79).

Radiograph of the so-called transverse metatarsal arch (the line of the heads of
the metatarsals) is practically the same as for the sesamoids and both sides are
taken simultaneously for comparison. In this situation, the feet must be internally
rotated by about 30° to bring the transverse plane parallel to the film. Flexed toes
are kept out of the way if the patient holds a bandage around both sets of toes and
exerts slight pressure. Young adults can stand tiptoe on a wooden block and the
horizontal tube is centred to both feet with the film set vertically, either behind the
heels or in front of the toes. This should demonstrate whole body weight on the
forefeet (Fig. 12.80).

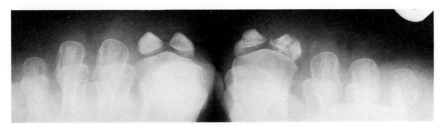

Fig. 12.78 Sesamoid view. Note the osteochondritis of the lateral sesamoid on the right.

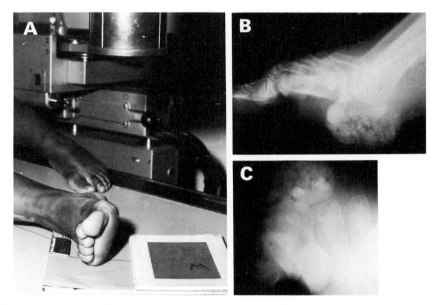

Fig. 12.79   (A) The off-lateral view to show the sesamoid. (B) Radiograph demonstrating the off-lateral view of the sesamoids. These are shown together with a large mass of separate ossicles related to the plantar surface of the metatarso-phalangeal joint of the great toe. At operation this was found to be due to synovial osteochondromatosis. (C) The sesamoid view demonstrates the relationship to the 'transverse arch'.

To demonstrate a *bunionette* or exostosis on the outer aspect of the fifth metatarsal head, an anteroposterior view is obtained. This may show widening of the space between the fourth and fifth metatarsals. The lateral view should be a steep oblique with the lateral border of the foot on the film and the medial border raised 75°. The tube is off-centred laterally from the fifth metatarsophalangeal joint by 1 inch.

If the lateral aspect of the foot is not unduly painful and the patient is mobile, then the lateral dorsal aspect of the foot can be placed on the film and a steepish oblique, centring through the plantar aspect, will give a clear view of the fifth metatarsal region.

Radiography of the tarsal bones

The short dorsal convexity and plantar concavity of the cuneiforms makes them very difficult to visualize clearly. Some overlapping is always seen regardless of the radiographic view obtained. The anteroposterior film, with the tube angled at 15° towards the heel, gives a clear view of the tarsal bones on the inner aspect, the medial cuneiform, the anterior surface of the navicular and its articulations with the talus. The bases of the metatarsals and the tarsal bones on the lateral aspect of the foot are not demonstrated clearly, as the dorsum of the foot slopes convexly

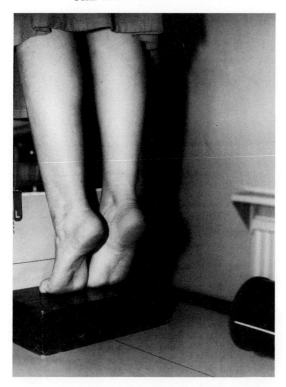

Fig. 12.80 The 'transverse arch' of the metatarsal heads may be demonstrated with the patient standing on tiptoe.

downwards from the medial to the lateral surface. When the patient is positioned for the medial oblique view, the lateral border of the foot is raised 45°. This flattens the dorsal convexity and a far better view of the tarsal bones, joints and metatarsal bases is obtained. It is, in effect, an anteroposterior view of the outer tarsus. This is a very good position for demonstrating a calcaneonavicular bar (Fig. 12.81) and the calcaneocuboid and talonavicular joints.

The lateral oblique view

This is the opposite positioning from the medial oblique view, with the outer border of the foot on the film and the medial aspect raised 45°. It may give a clearer view than the medial oblique view (Fig. 12.82).

The plantar oblique view

The patient lies on the affected side with the dorsal aspect of the foot resting on the film. The opposite leg can be crossed over the foot being examined. The tube is centred to the base of the fifth metatarsal (Fig. 12.83a). If the obliquity of the foot is

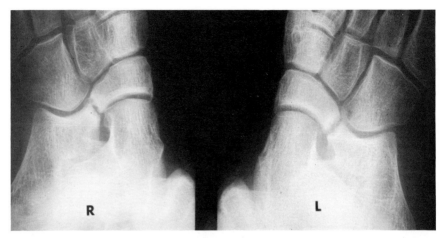

Fig. 12.81 In this adolescent, the presence of bony and cartilaginous union between the calcaneum and navicular is demonstrated with osteoarthritic change between the two bones. The changes are bilateral.

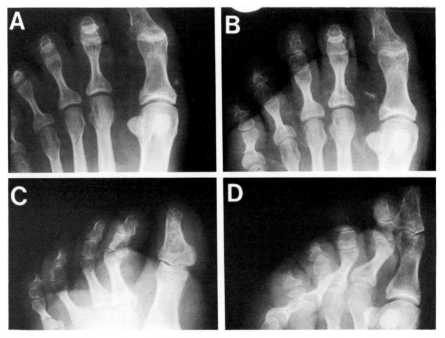

Fig. 12.82 (A) This nursing sister had stubbed her foot on a bed. Claw toes are demonstrated and a fracture of the proximal phalanx of the little toe is seen. (B) With cotton wool under the toes the phalanges are now clearly demonstrated. (C) With the foot in the lateral oblique position, the fracture is much better seen than in (D) with the foot in the medial oblique position. In the latter position, the proximal phalanx is projected oblique over the fourth toe.

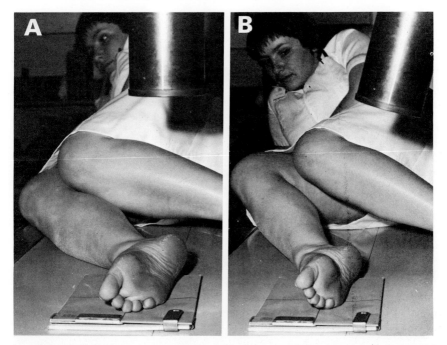

Fig. 12.83   (A) and (B) Plantar oblique view. These are excellent views for the metatarsals and proximal phalanges.

not enough, the tube can be tilted towards the fifth metatarsal at a 10–15° angle medially (Fig. 12.83b).

The 'medial' lateral view

The patient lies on the couch on his right side for his left ankle. The medial malleolus rests on the film with the medial aspect of the knee resting on the couch. The sole of the foot should be at right-angles to the film and the x-ray tube centred to the mid-tarsal region (Fig. 12.84a). If the patient is unable to comfortably rest the medial aspect of the knee on the couch, place an open-ended box over the opposite leg so that the knee of the limb under examination can easily rest on the box (Fig. 12.84b). In mobile adults the prayer position can also be used. The soles of both feet are placed against each other with the film underneath and the knees wide apart. The tube is centred on the mid-tarsal region of both feet.

This view will show the sesamoids laterally, the calcaneum and the longitudinal arch. It is useful for showing both heels on one film and for demonstrating a plantar spur.

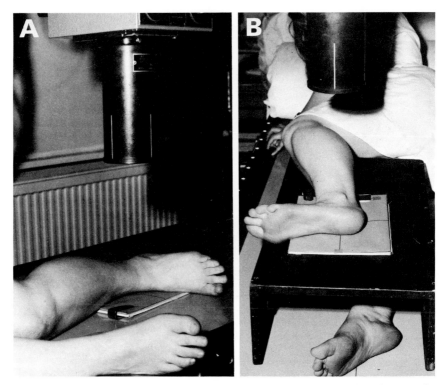

Fig. 12.84 'Medial' lateral view. (A) In our experience, with the knee on the table, a perfect lateral view of the ankle joint and foot is almost inevitably obtained. (B) The obese patient is more easily examined if the foot which is not to be examined is placed beneath a box upon which rests the foot to be examined. At the Royal National Orthopaedic Hospital, these are the standard methods for radiographing the ankle and foot in the lateral position.

The subtalar joint

Initially anteroposterior (dorsiplantar) and lateral views are taken. Bony lipping on the posterior superior surface of the navicular or the anterior superior surface of the talus may be demonstrated together with interruption of the smooth cyma line. A more detailed radiographic examination of the subtalar joint can then be undertaken.

The internal oblique view

In the anteroposterior ankle position the foot is rotated internally 45–50° with its medial aspect resting on a polyfoam block. The tube is angled 20° towards the knee and centred 1 inch below and 1 inch anterior to the lateral malleolus (Fig. 12.85a). This view will demonstrate the talonavicular and calcaneocuboid joints, and is also useful for checking fusion after triple arthrodesis; it often shows the tarsal sinus clearly (Fig. 12.85b).

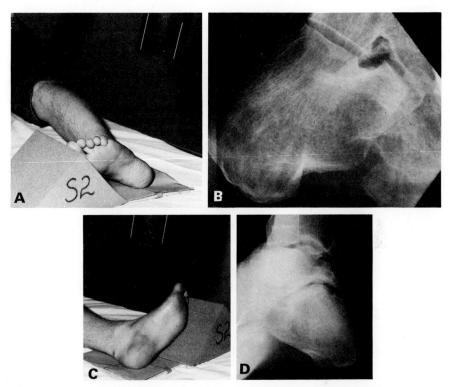

Fig. 12.85 (A) Positioning for the internal oblique view of the subtalar joint. (B) Radiograph using the internal oblique projection. Note the excellent demonstration of the sinus tarsi, as well as the posterior facets of the subtalar joint and, in addition, the talo-navicular joint may also be demonstrated. (C) To demonstrate radiography of the foot in the external oblique position. (D) The radiographic demonstration of the posterior aspect of the subtalar joint using the external oblique method.

The external oblique view

The foot is externally rotated from the anteroposterior ankle position and its lateral aspect rests on a polyfoam pad at a 50° angle. The tube is tilted 20° towards the knee and centred 1 inch below the medial malleolus (Fig. 12.85c). This view demonstrates the posterior aspect of the subtalar joint (Fig. 12.85d). It is particularly useful after triple arthrodesis where fusion of the talocalcaneal joint is well shown.

13

The Principles and Complications of Foot Surgery

L. KLENERMAN

In routine orthopaedic practice problems of the foot are common and usually amount to about 20% of the workload. Inevitably, if one has a general orthopaedic commitment, one will be doing a considerable amount of foot surgery. Although much of the scope of foot surgery is not technically demanding, it does require precision and careful management after operation. Even more important is accurate pre-operative assessment of the patient's symptoms and signs and the correct choice of operation. The guiding principle should be to treat the foot with the same respect as the hand. Patients who have had inadequate and inaccurate operations are very unhappy people.

The complications of foot surgery may be divided into three main groups namely, general, inevitable and preventable.

GENERAL COMPLICATIONS

These may arise from any surgical procedure. An example is deep vein thrombosis, which is rare after foot surgery. Nevertheless, early walking should be encouraged whenever possible.

INEVITABLE COMPLICATIONS

These are features which are always associated with operations on the feet. Swelling is probably the most common, unavoidable sequel. It occurs because of oedema following the use of a tourniquet and the bleeding and trauma of the surgery. It often persists for months, mainly because of the restriction of normal movement by bandages and the dependancy of the foot. Swelling often remains for three months following a simple Keller's operation. The patient is aware of it because even a minor increase in the circumference of the foot makes it impossible to wear a normal shoe. Efforts to reduce swelling must include release of the tourniquet before closure of the wound, so that careful haemostasis can be achieved. Elevation of the foot at the end of the operation and early walking in wooden-soled shoes (Fig. 13.1), which are comfortable, enable the patient to

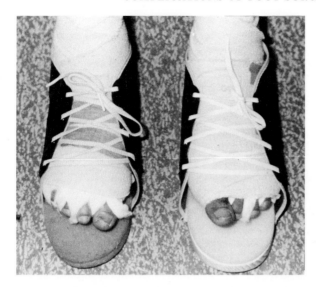

Fig. 13.1 Patient
wearing postoperative
wooden-soled shoe
which is comfortable
and helps early walking.

achieve maximum mobility. Once the wounds are healed, supporting elastic stockings and exercises in elevation may be needed. The prevention of swelling, or reduction to a minimum, is easier than removing it once it has occurred.

Infections should be regarded as almost inevitable and therefore should be foreseen in patients with diabetes or those on immunosuppressive drugs. This applies particularly when one is contemplating the insertion of a silastic implant.

PREVENTABLE COMPLICATIONS

This is the largest and therefore the most important group, and may result from inadequate assessment, failure to be aware of the vascular state of the limb, failure to explain the purpose of the operation and technical failure.

Inadequate assessment

This will result in the wrong choice of operation. The reason for the operation should be clear in one's mind, operate mainly to relieve symptoms and be essentially conservative. Operations are not always needed because the patient has hallux valgus—many middle-aged patients remain symptom-free because they buy broad shoes. Patients with multiple toe deformities may be difficult to assess. Unless the patient's symptoms are discussed in detail, one may easily embark on a series of operations on one or two toes at a time. The diagnosis of forefoot pain can sometimes be difficult. Morton's metatarsalgia due to an underlying neuroma may be overlooked, as the pain in the more severe case is not neatly localized to the cleft between the third and fourth toes, but radiates more widely in the foot and also occurs at night in bed. Although neuromas are often found in feet which have no deformity, they may also occur in association with common deformities such as hallux valgus and hammer toes. Careful palpation of the interdigital clefts and attempts to elicit Mulder's click (see Chapter 7) may help to localize the lesion.

Failure to assess the vascular state

Assessment of the vascular state is vital in the older patient who may need surgery. Failure to do so may result in delayed wound healing, and a sympathectomy or even amputation of a digit may be needed. Sometimes, in the elderly patient, symptoms attributed to hammer toes or bunions may be ischaemic in origin. There should be at least one clearly palpable pulse present (preferably the posterior tibial) and the skin texture and nails should be healthy. In cases of doubt, the pressure index should be measured with a Doppler probe. The ratio of the systolic pressure at the ankle compared with that in the antecubital fossa should normally be approximately one.

If in any doubt, the opinion of a surgeon interested in vascular disorders should be obtained. In rheumatoid arthritis, vasculitis is a contraindication to surgery.

Failure to clearly explain the purpose of the operation

The operation may fail to please the patient simply because the effect of the intended procedure has not been made clear. One has seen several patients who have complained of stiffness of their great toe following a formal arthrodesis of the metatarsophalangeal joint. Careful and prolonged discussion before the operation takes place should avoid this problem. It is not enough to discuss the operation on the day prior to the operation, when the patient is almost on the threshold of the operating theatre. The patient's expectations must be related to surgical reality. It is not possible to restore feet to normal but only to improve them, and patients may not be comfortable wearing fashionable high-heeled shoes with pointed toes.

TECHNICAL FAILURES

These are unfortunately the commonest complications, although they should be the easiest to avoid. In this section the standard procedures in routine practice will be broadly discussed.

Firstly, there is the problem of incisions. The skin on the dorsum of the foot is thin and has very little subcutaneous fat. There is no dense cutaneous vascular plexus to provide abundant quantities of blood for rapid repair of tissues (Pyka & Coventry 1961). Thus, there is little reserve if this skin is subjected to trauma such as excessive retraction at the time of operation. Flaps should always be kept as thick as possible, and care should be taken that instruments used in the depths of the wound are not pressed firmly against the skin. Pyka and Coventry point out that the skin over the belly of the extensor digitorum brevis has the poorest blood supply in the foot. Despite fears to the contrary, incisions on the sole of the foot heal well and have been advocated for many years by Hoffmann (1912), who advocated resection of metatarsal heads through a plantar approach, Gaenslen (1931) in the treatment of osteomyelitis of the heel and Betts (1940) for removal of digital neuromata in Morton's metatarsalgia.

Arthrodesis of the ankle, aside from the need to achieve bony fusion, requires careful positioning of the hindfoot to ensure that the heel is in the neutral position. This will ensure the maximum use of the small amount of movement present in the direction of plantarflexion at the tarsometatarsal function (approximately 10°) (King *et al* 1980). If the heel is in calcaneus the gait is clumsy and uncomfortable for the patient, and if it is in equinus it is difficult to walk barefoot.

Ankle arthroplasty is still a relatively new and untried procedure. Experience so far has shown that it is more likely to be successful in the rheumatoid rather than the osteoarthritic joint (Herberts *et al* 1981).

Triple arthrodesis is an operation less frequently carried out nowadays than in the past, because it is sometimes possible to avoid the need for the procedure by carrying out a calcaneal osteotomy, for instance in the case of peroneal spastic flat feet (Cain & Hyman 1978). In addition, the wide range of pathology for which the procedure has been performed has tended to diminish. The essential of this operation is to leave the patient with a plantigrade foot without a trace of varus, and preferably with a trace of valgus instead (Fig. 13.2). Internal fixation with staples will ensure that the position is maintained and promote fusion. When instability or pain rather than deformity is the problem, extra-articular arthrodesis as suggested by Kilfoyle and Byrne (1976), using dowel-shaped grafts from the iliac crest to block the subtalar, talonavicular and calcaneocuboid joints is effective. Williams and Menelaus (1977) have described the use of a strut of cortical bone from the tibia for the same purpose. Patients with cerebral palsy, spina bifida and poliomyelitis may be suitable for this technique.

Correction of the cavus foot by midtarsal osteotomy and removal of a dorsally based wedge, as described by Cole (1940), is a difficult procedure to carry out accurately. Undercorrection may not satisfy the patient but overcorrection is disastrous, as it will produce a rocker-bottom type of foot (Fig. 13.3). As a simpler but just as effective alternative, the osteotomy described by Japas (1968) is recommended. A V-type osteotomy is produced between the midtarsal and tarsometatarsal joints with its apex proximal and at the highest point of the cavus in the navicular with the limits of the osteotomy extending to the outer and inner borders of the foot through the cuboid and first cuneiform respectively. It does not shorten the foot, as it does not involve the removal of bone and also allows for correction of varus or valgus deformities as well.

Operations for correction of hallux valgus or rigidus are numerous. Keller's procedure, one of the oldest and well-tried, has a relatively small role nowadays. For hallux valgus, osteotomies of the first metatarsal, arthrodeses of the first metatarsophalangeal joint and silastic implants are commonly performed and for

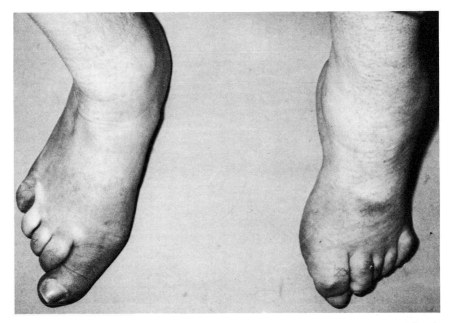

Fig. 13.2   Residual varus deformity of left foot after incomplete correction of old club foot by triple arthrodesis.

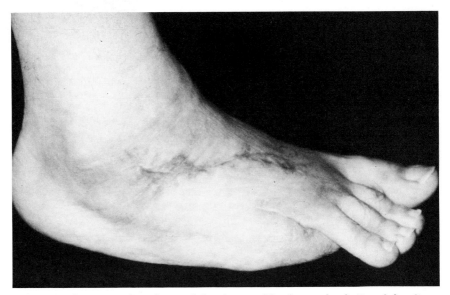

Fig. 13.3   Overcorrection of cavus deformity, resulting in a rocker-bottom deformity.

hallux rigidus the two latter procedures are likewise used by many surgeons. Arthrodesis of the metatarsophalangeal joint of the great toe is a valuable procedure for preservation of the weight-bearing function of the medial ray of the foot. Precise alignment of the toe is vital. The exact position depends on the type of footwear the patient wears. It is less difficult to please men than women, who want to vary the height of heel in different shoes. For most people, 10–15° of dorsiflexion should be sufficient. Excessive dorsiflexion results in a foot where the great toe rubs against the inside of the shoe. In order to check the position at operation, it is important to put the foot at a right angle to the leg in a simulated position of standing before the arthrodesis is made secure.

Silastic prostheses are useful to act as spacers in the preservation of the length and function of the great toe after a modified Keller's type operation. The stud-shaped Swanson prosthesis, which fits into the base of the proximal phalanx, may be associated with a recurrence of deformity in 44% of patients, and is best for hallux rigidus (Sethu et al 1980; Fig. 13.4). For hallux valgus it is preferable to use the flexible hinge implant also designed by Swanson, with one end inserted into the medulla of the proximal phalanx and the other into the metatarsal shaft (Swanson et al 1979). Silastic prostheses should not be used in patients who have a higher potential for sepsis, such as those suffering from diabetes.

Keller's operation still has a small place in the treatment of hallux rigidus and in the elderly with hallux valgus. It does weaken and shorten the great toe, and the patient must be warned of this in advance. However, it does make the foot comfortable. There are some points of technique that should be remembered. Resection of the base of the proximal phalanx should be generous and about one third should be removed; excessive zeal in this part of the operation will produce a very floppy toe. The line of the skin incision should be medial in the region where the dorsal meets the plantar skin, to avoid the tethering of the extensor tendon to the scar that may otherwise occur. Great care should be taken to avoid damage to the flexor hallucis longus, when the base of the proximal phalanx is dissected free.

There are two main complications which are common to the large variety of osteotomies used for the treatment of hallux valgus, delayed or non-union and malalignment of the head of the first metatarsal. Non-union results in aching and swelling after activity. Although it may sometimes be necessary to carry out a sliding bone graft to achieve union, an early operation should be avoided, as spontaneous union may slowly occur (Fig. 13.5 a, b). If the first metatarsal head is angled dorsally, the weight-bearing function of the first ray is shifted laterally and metatarsalgia may be produced.

Overcorrection of hallux valgus, which results in a varus deformity, may occasionally follow McBride's operation (see Chapter 6). From the patient's viewpoint, this is even worse than the original deformity, as it makes the fitting of a comfortable shoe very difficult.

Forefoot arthroplasty for rheumatoid arthritis, using either Fowler's or the Kates–Kessel procedure or a variant, will fail unless there is adequate resection of bone with preservation of the relative lengths of the metatarsals (Fig. 13.6). In

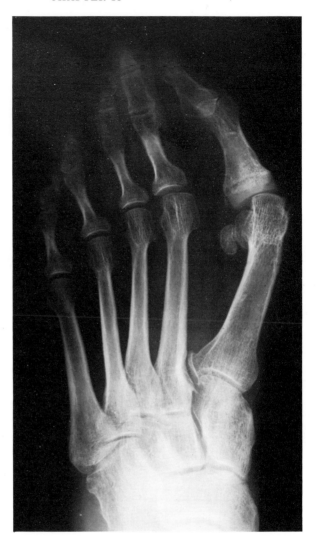

Fig. 13.4 Recurrence
of valgus deformity
despite the use of a
silastic prosthesis.

addition, it is necessary to stabilize the medial ray by means of an arthrodesis of the
metatarsophalangeal joint of the great toe, as otherwise there will be an inevitable
drift back to a valgus position of the lesser toes (Fig. 13.7).

Correction of a hammer toe is one of the most frequently performed operations
on the foot. Fusion of the proximal interphalangeal joint should not be carried out
if dislocation is present at the metatarsophalangeal joint, as otherwise the
straightened toe will point up in the air. Partial proximal phalangectomy is
preferable for the hammer toes with dislocation at the metatarsophalangeal joint,
although waist resection of the proximal phalanx has been suggested, a procedure

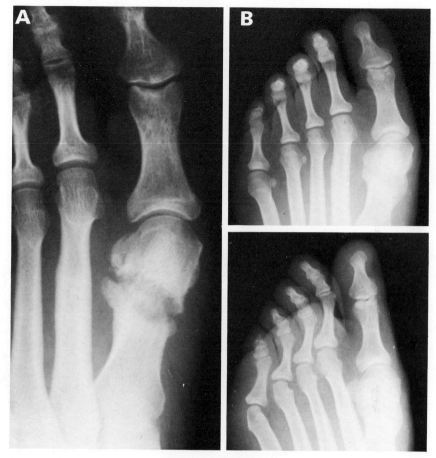

Fig. 13.5 (A) Un-united metatarsal osteotomy for hallux valgus. (B) Nine months later this had spontaneously fused without surgical interference.

of which the author has little experience (McConnell 1975). In this latter procedure a sub-periosteal resection is carried out through a very short incision over the waist of the proximal phalanx, which allows settling of the resection bone ends together within the periosteal tube, resulting in bone union. Routine fusions of the proximal interphalangeal joint with an intramedullary Kirschner wire should include a formal tenotomy of the long extensor tendon and a capsulotomy of the metatarsophalangeal joint, to ensure that the corrected toe lies alongside the other toes.

The principles of surgery of the foot do not differ from those for surgery of the other regions of the body. However, the respect accorded to the hand by orthopaedic surgeons is not also given to the more lowly-placed foot. Provided

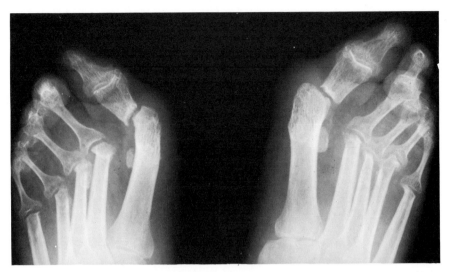

Fig. 13.6   Recurrence of deformity after inadequate resection of bone and failure to stabilize the medial ray of the foot after a filleting procedure for rheumatoid arthritis.

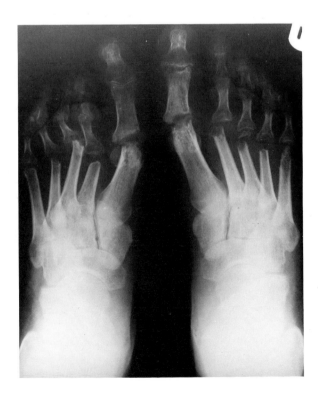

Fig. 13.7   Failure to retain the proportional length of the metatarsals results in localized pressure at the distal end of the long metatarsal.

there has been a careful evaluation of the patient's symptoms and signs, a clear explanation of what operation is planned and how it is expected to improve the situation, and the operation is carried out with a meticulous and precise technique, one should be able to produce a long succession of grateful patients.

REFERENCES

BETTS L.O. (1940) Morton's Metatarsalgia: neuritis of the fourth digital nerve. *Medical Journal of Australia* **1,** 514–15.

CAIN T.J. & HYMAN S. (1978) Peroneal spastic flat foot—its treatment by osteotomy of the os calcis. *Journal of Bone and Joint Surgery* **60B,** 527–9.

COLE W.H. (1940) The treatment of claw foot. *Journal of Bone and Joint Surgery* **22,** 895–908.

GAENSLEN F.J. (1931) Split heel approach of osteomyelitis of os calcis. *Journal of Bone and Joint Surgery* **13,** 759–72.

HERBERTS P., GOLDIE I.F., KOMER L., LARSSON U., LINDBORG G. & ZACHRISSON B.E. (1981) ICLH arthroplasty of the ankle joint. A clinical and radiological follow-up after three years. (In press)

HOFFMAN P. (1919) An operation for severe grades of contracted or claw toes. *American Journal of Orthopaedic Surgery* **9,** 441–9.

JAPAS L.M. (1968) Surgical treatment of pes cavus by tarsal V-osteotomy. *Journal of Bone and Joint Surgery* **59A,** 927–44.

KILFOYLE R.M. & BYRNE D.P.A. (1976) Non-excision triple arthrodesis of the foot. *The Orthopaedic Clinics of North America* **7,** 841–9.

KING H.A., WATKINS T.B. & SAMUELSON K.M. (1980) Analysis of foot position in ankle arthrodesis and its influence on gait. *Foot and Ankle* **1,** 44–9.

McCONNELL B.E. (1975) Hammer toe surgery: waist resection of the proximal phalanx, a more simplified procedure. *Southern medical Journal* **68,** 595–8.

PYKA R.A. & COVENTRY M.B. (1961) Avascular necrosis of the skin after operations on the foot. *Journal of Bone and Joint Surgery* **43A,** 955–60.

SETHU A., D'NETTO D.C. & RAMAKRISHNA B. (1980) Swanson's silastic implants in great toes. *Journal of Bone and Joint Surgery* **62B,** 83–5.

SWANSON A.B., LUMSDEN R.M. & SWANSON G.D. (1979) Silicone implant of the great toe: A review of single and flexible implants. *Clinical Orthopaedics and Related Research* **142,** 30–43.

WILLIAMS P.F. & MENELAUS M.B. (1977) Triple arthrodesis by inlay grafting—a method suitable for the undeformed or valgus foot. *Journal of Bone and Joint Surgery* **59B,** 333–6.

14

Surgical Footwear and Appliances

W.H. TUCK

The relief of many foot deformities depends on the skill of the surgical bootmaker. Over the past years, however, this has become a dying craft, partly because of the lack of training facilities to obtain the high degree of skill that is needed and partly because of the poor pay reward for this type of skill. I think it is well to look back in time to the story of St Crispin and St Crispinian, who were the shoemaker's saints, because a number of the craftsmen who make surgical footwear could well come under this banner. It relates as follows.

Shoemaking may not seem to be a particularly saintly occupation. A cobbler's shop with its continual coming and going, fatiguing smell of leather and clickclacketty tools, may not strike us as quite the sort of place where a saint would choose to live. But on 25th October we celebrate the memory of a pair of saints whose very saintliness inspired them to become shoemakers—St Crispin and St Crispinian. St Crispian and his twin brother, Crispian or Crispinian, were, according to the legend, two young Roman noblemen who lived in the time of the cruel emperor Diocletian. They were converted to the Christian faith and, as at that time Christians were persecuted for their beliefs, they left their native city and all their wealthy connections there and went to live in the country town of Soissons in France.

Here they set up a shoemaker's stall, and started to earn their livelihood by making and mending shoes and sandals. Their trade of course brought them into talk with all sorts of people, and they used every opportunity of telling their customers and neighbours about the new and wonderful religion which they had taken for their own and which had made such an extraordinary difference in their lives. They must have had a very jolly way with them, for it seems that the townsfolk crowded to hear them speak, and they made a great number of converts. Also, in spite of their aristocratic upbringing, they seem to have become experts at their work and famous for the prompt way in which they executed orders, for it used to be jokingly said of the Crispin brothers that their leather was supplied to them by the angels. It hardly seems likely though that they built up a big business, for any customer who was too poor to pay would always be fitted with shoes or sandals for the smallest possible fee, or for nothing at all!

The gallant hardworking lives of the shoemaker Saints came to a tragic end, but the fame which they had earned lived after them, and that they became thoroughly popular saints with the English people is well proved by the famous speech of Henry V before the Battle of Agincourt (October 25th, 1415), in which he reminds the soldiers that they are going to fight on the Feast of 'Crispin Crispian'. The day was long kept as a high holiday by the Shoemaker's Guilds in England and elsewhere—even nowadays you may sometimes hear a shoemaker called a 'Crispin' and shoemaking spoken of as 'St Crispin's Art', in memory of those two shoemaker Saints who became, as a matter of course, the patron saints of shoemakers.

In Camberwell, St Crispin's Workshop was set up by Cambridge University to train disabled people to make surgical footwear, and it was in this particular workshop that I commenced my orthopaedic training. Since that time much has been done to alter the style of making surgical shoes, partly because of the lack of craftsmen and partly because of the extra demand from disabled people, particularly in relation to rheumatoid arthritis.

NEW APPROACH TO ORTHOPAEDIC FOOTWEAR

In 1966 a report in the *International Medical Tribune of Great Britain* on shoes for patients with rheumatoid arthritis described the excellent results obtained with a special type of American polystyrene shoe, the 'space shoe', made by a moulding technique on a positive cast of the patients' foot. A trial was started because the conventional type of surgical shoe supplied to patients with badly deformed feet had often been found unsatisfactory. This confirmed the need for a type of footwear different from the conventional welted shoe.

Since 1968, the Appliance Research Unit of the Institute of Orthopaedics has been making Plastazote shoes for painful feet by the vacuum forming method. The early shoes made by this method were bulky and the method of production was thus changed to the use of one 1/8 inch thick piece of Plastazote for the lining and a layer of plastic material called Yampi for the exterior. This type of footwear has proved to be of value. Because Yampi has the appearance of glacé kid, the shoes are by no means ugly and can be produced in a variety of colours. A special method of fastening has been introduced so that the patient with deformed hands, who finds it impossible to use laces, can very easily manipulate the wide tongue which is fixed over the instep with Velcro fastening. The appearance is not unlike ordinary surgical shoes. The weight is 600 g for a pair of surgical shoes made in glacé kid with microcellular soles, compared with 200 g for a pair of Plastazote/Yampi shoes made on the same lasts with similar soles and heels.

The main advantage of this type of footwear is that, by vacuum forming the uppers, one is assured of a correct fit, as the Plastazote has a memory at 140°C and therefore retains the shape when covered with Yampi. Many of the grossly deformed feet due to rheumatoid arthritis, particularly those with a valgus hindfoot, are more comfortably accommodated in bootees. In some areas it may be difficult to obtain this type of footwear, as a vacuum-forming machine may not be

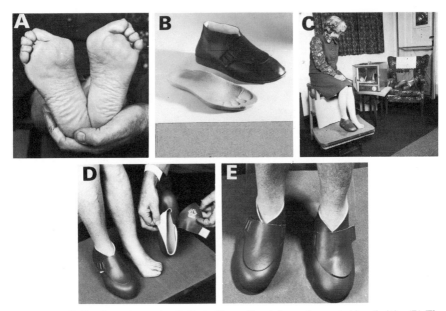

Fig. 14.1 (A) To show the patient's feet. She suffered from rheumatoid arthritis. (B) The moulded insole and moulded bootee. (C) The patient has had her right bootee completed while the left is still in the oven and will soon be ready for moulding. (D) The left heated bootee being applied. (E) The pair of completed shoes which were ready in less than one hour.

available. It has been found that a large number of patients can be fitted with special stock-size Plastazote footwear.

Insoles are made in the customary way and when completed, these are fitted into the patient's stock-size bootee. The bootee is placed in the oven with the insole inside it and heated to 140°C. It is then removed and applied to the patient's foot, and can thus be moulded to accommodate hammer toes or other deformities (Fig. 14.1(A) – (E). A pair of shoes of this type can be made within an hour.

A number of patients that have been referred have had considerable ulceration on the sole of the foot, and provided the Plastazote is moulded with care directly on to the patient's foot, the ulcer will be relieved by this method and some have completely healed. Plastazote has been equally effective for shoes for patients with leprosy, diabetes and all conditions of the insensitive as well as the hypersensitive foot.

MEASUREMENTS, MATERIALS AND METHODS

Measurements, Materials and Methods, a British Standards publication (BS 5943–1980), gives full details of all types of orthopaedic footwear available from the British Standards Institute, 2 Park Street, London W1A 2BS.

It will be of interest and value for orthopaedic surgeons and rheumatologists who frequently prescribe surgical footwear to know some of the details of how measurements are taken and the work which is involved.

The code of practice when measuring a patient for surgical footwear is as follows:

Place the patient sitting with the foot at right angles to the leg on a stool in such a position as is not uncomfortable for the person who is going to do the measuring, i.e. the patient's foot should be at least 18 inches away from the floor, either on a high stool or a platform such as a chiropodist's stool.

Take a profile of the foot with a pencil, starting on the left hand side of the heel and bring it right round the foot along the borders of the foot, keeping the pencil at right angles, making sure that when the toe is reached the pencil is not sloped either in or out. The correct length often depends upon this outline. Mark the arch of the foot by placing the pencil under the arch and bring it forward as far as it will go toward the metatarsal head.

Using a 24-inch bootmaker's tape (this has a metal end), measure three circumferences:

1 At the metatarsals
2 Directly behind the metatarsals
3 In the middle of the instep

Keeping the tape measure at a slight angle, take a fourth measurement around the heel to meet exactly the same place that the instep measurement was taken. If boots are needed, an ankle measurement and also a measurement at the height required for the upper are taken. By this it is meant that, if the boot is for a man and is to be $5\frac{1}{2}$ inches high, mark $5\frac{1}{2}$ inches up and take the measurement round the leg at this point.

Note the age of the patient and the type of foot (whether bony or fat), as measurements will not always show this. Describe (or sketch) the shape of the back of the heel i.e. whether curved or straight, and note any deformities, the height of toes and places of depression. Also give the occupation of adults, because in the case of a farmer or garage worker special uppers must be considered and these do not reflect upon the fitting of the patient. It is as easy to make a pair of surgical boots or shoes with stout leather in the uppers as it is to supply box calf or glacé kid for someone who works in town. The patient usually has a choice of colour of upper and, in the case of ladies, it is as well to give some option as to the style of the shoe required. The leather that is mostly used is glacé kid, box calf, willow calf and grained leathers. The boots are cut in various styles (Fig. 14.2), a whole galosh Balmoral, a joined galosh Balmoral, or there is another style using vamps and quarters (Fig. 14.3). It is permissible to have toe caps, although not always advisable when the toes are painful. In some cases a style known as a Derby can be used (Fig. 14.4). It is as well to examine the feet carefully before finally prescribing. Care must be taken to note if a low opening is necessary, so that the foot can go in easily. This can be done either by prescribing a lace to toe or a lace to toe cap, or the Canadian pattern, i.e. the Derby front is extended to the end of the toes so that there is a flap on either side which tends to give an easier entrance to the flail or deformed foot.

There is a great shortage of bark-tanned leather, which has been the mainstay of the surgical footwear industry for many years. Over the last 15 years a number of tanneries have closed down in England and those remaining cannot maintain the same supply of bellies, shoulders, butts and selected qualities of bends that used to be needed to make very good surgical footwear. Shoulder leather must be used for insoles of a number of these shoes, otherwise the whole balance of the footwear is incorrect.

There is now a very great shortage of labour—the number of youngsters coming into the industry is very small and it is important that those who do come in are taught the new methods of making footwear, which in many cases are easier

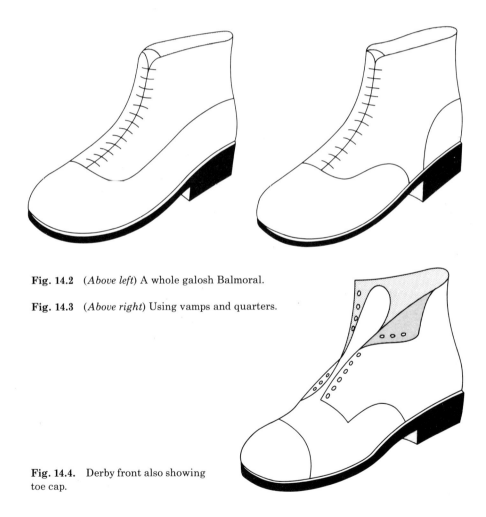

Fig. 14.2   (*Above left*) A whole galosh Balmoral.

Fig. 14.3   (*Above right*) Using vamps and quarters.

Fig. 14.4.   Derby front also showing toe cap.

than the old methods; the process can be streamlined and the footwear often more mass-produced. To a craftsman this perhaps seems a degrading step, but it must be remembered that it is necessary for a first-class skilled man to make the lasts and shape corks. When disguising gross deformities, this is vital.

Another important stage is the cut of the uppers; a great deal of skill is needed in selecting skins and studying designs to meet the requirements of the deformities and to make the surgical footwear as presentable as possible. There has always been the problem of weight. The complaint in the past has invariably been that surgical shoes were too heavy, particularly for the ladies, and this has been because the shoes were welted. This leads again to the question of the materials available for the soles, and particularly for the heels, which are the heaviest part of surgical footwear. Fortunately, there is now a material available which is known as Microcellular. This is made in various thicknesses and densities; some are much harder than others. It is available in black and brown and even in some cases, in shades of brown. It has been my experience that no surgical adaptation is impossible when Microcellular is used in the manufactured footwear.

Sockets can be fitted satisfactorily, heels can be elongated and, where necessary, wedges and metatarsal bars added. By the use of special attachments on finishing machines, the finish of Microcellular can equal that of any fashionable shoe.

To apply this material, it is essential to have a satisfactory press, so that with the use of effective adhesives the Microcellular can be attached to the uppers by pressure. This is labour-saving and produces a much lighter shoe. Also, especially with small children who grow very rapidly, any method which is quick is important. For children who give their shoes excessive wear, Neolite or some of the harder wearing materials can be used in a similar way. I must emphasize that the operator must also have a very good knowledge of adhesives for joining any of the Microcellular plastics to leather or leather uppers. The basic skill of making all surgical footwear using these new materials is exactly the same from the point of view of fitting the last, preparing the stiffeners and toepuffs, preparing the insoles and lasting the uppers, but instead of the welt being sewn in, the upper is braced to the insole and from that point onwards, no further sewing is necessary. If for some reason the patient does need to have leather soles and heels, the footwear can be made lighter by having the main height of the heel made in Microcellular and the top piece which takes the wear made of leather. This has the effect of giving some spring to the heel and also increasing the wear value of the leather because of the springiness of the heel.

In the case of patients using appliances, where it is necessary to fit sockets to the footwear, the seat of the shoe must be strong (i.e. where the socket is fixed). The sockets must be fitted with copper rivets which are placed through the insoles and on to the socket, and the heel very carefully built up over the socket. Where a flat socket is used to take an appliance and there is no joint at the ankle of the appliance, because of a low fracture of the tibia or possibly because of the need to hold the foot at right angles, the plate of the socket must be long and two copper rivets added to the front portion of the socket, otherwise this will pull away from the heel of the shoe.

From the surgeon's point of view, it is difficult for him to know all the new materials which are available when prescribing footwear, and if the orthotist (the orthopaedic technician who attends the clinic) is not fully skilled in the knowledge of surgical bootmaking, this makes the problem more difficult. With the advent of new materials, the Department of Health will no doubt be adding them to their schedule.

There are many gross deformities, for example from rheumatoid arthritis, which do not take kindly to ordinary surgical footwear and Plastazote footwear has been found to be most satisfactory in these cases.

Plastazote

Plastazote is a trade-mark of BXL Plastics Ltd and in 1980 won the Prince Philip Gold Medal Award for 'Plastics in the service of man'.

Plastazote is an expanded cross-linked polyethylene with a closed cell construction which is mouldable and auto-adhesive at 140°C. Plastazote is non-toxic and extremely light with a specific gravity of 0.04 (25 times lighter than water). It is extremely buoyant. The material with closed cell construction is bacteriologically inert and is also unaffected by all common acids, alkalis, solvents and detergents. Although less inflammable than many common materials such as stockinette, lint, etc. Plastazote will melt or burn if exposed to a naked flame.

In dealing with leprosy, my efforts were encouraged by Paul Brand, well known for his surgical expertise in the field, who confirmed the value of Plastazote as a moulding material useful in treating gross deformities of the feet.

During the past 7 years some of the disadvantages of Plastazote have been revealed. The main problem was that Plastazote depressed considerably after wear. The patient would be comfortable for a month and then the material would begin to compress. To counteract this, it was suggested that insoles should always be supplied in duplicate and worn on alternate days. However, with the advent of medium density Plastazote PO 77 (see below), this is no longer a problem.

There are three grades of Plastazote used in connection with footwear. The grade previously most frequently used is PO 53 in white and PO 73 in pink. PO 77 is a white heavier density material now used mainly for insoles, as it withstands compression. HO 62 is a black high-density polythene foam used for elevations instead of cork and where extra support is required.

The machinery required for vacuum-formed shoes is as follows:

1   An oven large enough to take a piece of Plastazote 12 × 16 inches and capable of attaining a temperature of 140°C
2   A vacuum forming machine, with compressor
3   A footwear finishing machine. A smaller type with grinding wheels only may be used

The materials required are:

1   $\frac{1}{8}$ inch thick Plastazote for the upper lining
2   $\frac{1}{2}$–1 inch thick medium Plastazote for the insole and separate support to the base of the foot according to the deformity
3   Material for the uppers in various colours, for the outside covering
4   Velcro for the fastening
5   Adhesives

A plaster cast of the patient's foot is taken, usually by using plaster bandages. When the negative cast is dry it is filled with plaster cream and a positive cast is made. The toe of the cast is extended by approximately $2\frac{1}{2}$ sizes, about $\frac{3}{4}$ inch, to improve the shape of the foot and to give more room for the toes as the patient walks. (If the patient has been wearing surgical shoes, the lasts on which the shoes were made can be used for the vacuum shoes in place of the cast). The cast is cleaned and a medium density insole is moulded, i.e. the insole next to the foot. Where there is a gross deformity as in the case of a valgus hindfoot, 1 inch medium density Plastazote should be used.

Procedure   The cast or last is placed on the vacuum forming machine (Fig. 14.5 A) sole uppermost, and a thin rubber sheet clamped on to the top of the machine (Fig. 14.5 B, C). A piece, not less than $\frac{1}{2}$ inch thick of medium density Plastazote, marked and cut to the shape of the sole with an additional 1 inch all round, is heated in the oven to a temperature of 140°C (Fig. 14.5 D) and placed quickly on the base of the cast or last, the vacuum-forming device switched on and the inner sole mould is made. This is then shaped into position and levelled at the base. Extra Plastazote can be added if the depression is so marked that a level base cannot be achieved with one layer. Having shaped and levelled the base to give the right pitch, an insole of high density Plastazote is then moulded and shaped to the first insole (Fig. 14.5 E). The upper is made by using $\frac{1}{8}$ inch unperforated Plastazote fixed together with solution to a plastic material such as Yampi or Ambla (a vinyl). This is cut to the shape of the upper, remembering that this upper is made in two sections, inside and outside, and each is vacuum-formed each side on the machine (Fig. 14.5 F, G). The upper is joined together at the back and at the toe with an adhesive such as Foss Plast Special 23 8016, which is then secured to the insole by a solution such as Prenofix 825. When this is shaped and securely dry, the base is levelled and the sole is added using Microcellular and, if necessary, a heel is built to balance the foot (Fig. 14.5 H). The front fixing is added and this is usually done by using Velcro so that there is easy access to the foot (Fig. 14.5 I). Obviously this method is much quicker than the conventional method of making footwear. The shoes are about one third the weight, and for people with grossly deformed feet who perhaps do not walk around very much and spend most of their time indoors, will last a considerable time.

In the case of trophic ulcers it is often necessary to mould Plastazote directly on to the foot, and this can then be placed inside the shoe (Fig. 14.1, p. 412). With gross deformities or where there are ulcers or marked metatarsal troubles, it is advisable to mould the Plastazote to the base of the foot. A piece of sponge rubber 2

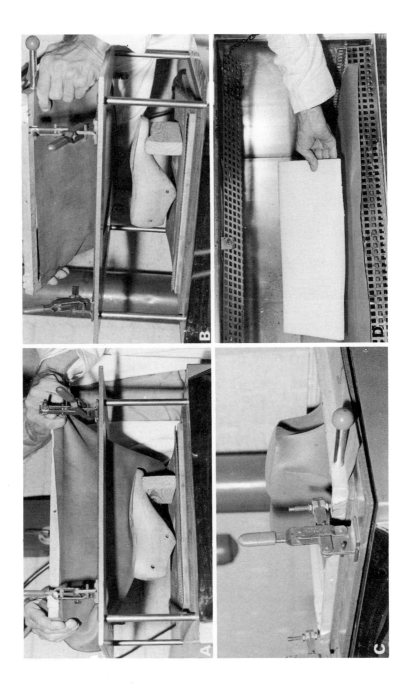

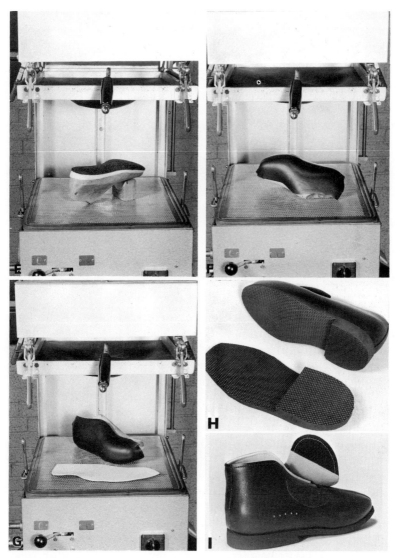

Fig. 14.5 (A) Last placed on vacuum forming machine sole uppermost. (B), (C) Thin rubber sheet is clamped on to the top of the machine. (D) A piece of $\frac{1}{2}$ inch medium density Plastazote to be marked and cut to the shape of the sole. (E) A piece of high density Plastazote moulded and shaped to first insole. (F), (G) The upper is made in two sections. (H) A heel is added. (I) The completed shoe with Velcro front.

inches thick should be used under the Plastazote when moulding. The Plastazote, when heated to 140°C is taken from the oven and placed on top of the sponge rubber. When the patient puts all his weight on to the Plastazote, the sponge rubber depresses and therefore a better moulding of the base of the foot is obtained. This method allows the Plastazote to build up well in the long arch and under the metatarsal arch. The orthotist should mould the edges of the Plastazote very carefully with his fingers into all the deformed positions, particularly in the long arch and on the heel.

It is most important when dealing with valgus ankles to make sure the deformity on the base of the foot is moulded, so that the valgus ankle will be accommodated by the thickness on the inner side—this may be as much as 2 inches to obtain a level base. Very few patients with valgus ankles take kindly to below-knee appliances to the calf and an inside T-strap. The additional weight, together with uneven pressure, causes more discomfort. Microcellular soles and heels have been used on nearly all the footwear made to date. A number of severe cases have been fitted with the wedge type of heel.

It must be understood that orthopaedic footwear, no matter how it is made, requires the skill of craftsmen. If a plaster cast is to be taken a skilled person must do this, otherwise it is very unlikely that a satisfactory shoe will be produced.

Treatment of common foot complaints by shoe alteration

For valgus feet in young children, inside cork wedges or valgus stiffeners can occasionally be added to sensible shoes, but there must not be too much support, which prevents the muscles from working normally. Many shoes supplied today have very little support in the uppers and the valgus stiffener, correctly placed, is very important. This must be made of well-mellowed leather, preferably shoulder leather, skived down to thin edges and shaped to fit into the long arch. This can be fixed by rubber solution and covered with a neat sock.

For children with 'flat feet' (see Chapter 5) and considerable shoe wear, it is sometimes necessary to alter the shoes by adding valgus supports and inside wedges to the heels, but the heels must be floated out on the outer side and this must be done from the seat of the shoe—that is the part of the heel nearest the upper. It is useless to float the heel out on the top piece only, as the whole tends to tread over from the stiffener. After this, observe how the patient walks. It is very seldom necessary to add valgus sole wedges but a short inside wedge of the metatarsal bar type, placed behind the head of the first metatarsal in conjunction with a valgus heel wedge is very important, if there is any weakness in the metatarsal arch. Prolonged heels or fully elongated heels are rarely used today, but in the case of gross deformities it is often necessary to fill in the waist of the shoe to support the whole of this area.

Pes cavus (high arches)

This can be seen in children as well as in adults and if careful alterations are made to shoes, these can be very beneficial. The main object is to take the weight from the high arch toward the heads of the metatarsals and a high arch support extended from the heel forward to the metatarsal heads is the most effective method of giving comfort and distributing weight. One of the main troubles with ordinary footwear for patients with pes cavus is that the metatarsal heads are depressed in the sole and the whole shoe becomes distorted. Sometimes a fairly wide metatarsal bar placed behind the heads of the metatarsals will help. Care must be taken in the purchase of footwear. Patients with high arches have high insteps and any pressure on the instep causes pain. Therefore, careful fitting of shoes before purchase is important, and glacé kid, a soft leather, should be chosen if possible and a thin padding should be added to the tongue.

Hallux valgus (bunions)

Surgery naturally is one of the remedies, but care in obtaining suitable footwear is also very important. Shoes with a straight inner border should be sought and if possible shoes with heels not more than $1\frac{1}{4}$ inches high. Seams on the inner side should be avoided and if conventional surgical footwear is made, the prescription should read as follows: 'One pair surgical shoes, glacé kid, seamless on the inner side, soft lining, valgus supports'. The heels in these cases should be floated out slightly on the outer side. Very often a very slight varus sole wedge is necessary to distribute the weight, because there is always a tendency for the patient to walk on the outer side of the foot. Microcellular soles are advisable in most of these cases because they are springy and light.

Recently the well-known shoe manufacturers, Clarks, have introduced a special brand of shoes (John Locke), specifically to cater for sufferers from bunions and hammer toes. These shoes have a range of fittings well beyond the conventional range and can often be used to avoid the need for specially made footwear.

Hallus rigidus (stiff big toe)

Again this is a very painful condition, and can be treated in various ways with regard to footwear. Firstly, suitable footwear must be obtained with soles as stiff as possible. The alterations that are required to such footwear are as follows: stiffening along the inner border of the sole, preferably with a steel plate or with an Ortholen support, a varus wedge on the outer side of the sole in conjunction with a rocker bar. The rocker bar must be wide enough, possibly 2 inches wide, and more forward than the metatarsal bar (Fig. 14.6). The object of this is to give the foot a natural rocking motion. Because of the pain from the hallux the patient often avoids walking on the inner side of the foot and therefore the varus wedge will bring the foot into balance, knowing the stiffening to the sole or the rocker bar will prevent the pain from recurring. A Plastazote insole is advisable to depress the hallux.

Congenital equinovarus

Infants need splinting and children need special attention to footwear. Surgical

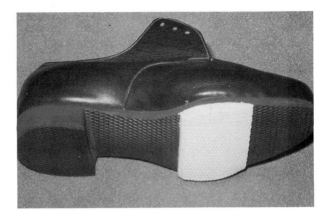

Fig. 14.6 Rocker bar
for hallux valgus.

footwear should be made for severe cases. To enable the foot to go in easily, lacing must be low down and it is important to level the base of the foot with medium density Plastazote. Varus wedges invariably need to be added both to the sole and the heel, and the heel should be floated out on the outer side (Fig. 14.7).

Congenital calcaneovalgus

If the deformity necessitates orthopaedic footwear the prescription may read as follows: surgical boots (and in my opinion, it must be boots) fitted with a special insole to depress the heel and at the same time give valgus and long arch support.

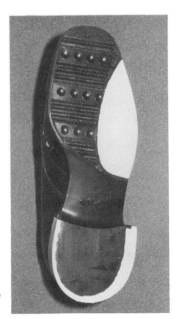

Fig. 14.7. Varus wedge to sole and
heel with the heel 'floated out' on the
outer side.

With this deformity, the back of the upper must be cut straight. The tongue should be wide and padded with a very light piece of Plastazote to avoid pressure on the instep.

Metatarsalgia

This painful condition can be accommodated in various ways but is much dependent upon the type of footwear available. In mild cases a Plastazote insole of medium density should be used, but in more severe cases orthopaedic footwear may have to be made. Sometimes in severe metatarsalgia the support needs very careful fitting and the soles of the shoes should be as stout as possible.

Calcaneal spurs (painful heels)

This is a very painful condition and must be relieved by a support which extends forward from the heel to the base of the metatarsals. The use of Plastazote in these cases is invaluable and the higher densities should be used. Be sure that in moulding the Plastazote for this deformity that the smallest amount of Plastazote remains under the heel but a great deal is left in the long arch to relieve pressure.

Flail feet

As in the case of poliomyelitis, these feet are invariably narrow and need special control. The footwear should be made with lacing low down to the entry of the foot and the tongue should be fairly wide. Any corrective T-straps that are needed will be incorporated in an order for the appliance, but flail feet should have wide tongues which will give stability to the foot and, at the same time, comfort to the patient.

Bony exostosis (bursitis)

The only alteration to surgical footwear in these cases is to place a very small pad of sponge rubber or Plastazote on either side of the exostosis and to remove part of the stiffening. This allows the bony prominence to be housed comfortably and will prevent the shoe from becoming distorted.

Gout

Invariably footwear for this sort of condition means very soft uppers possibly in felt or Plastazote, wide heels and wide soles and wide tongues, with a low opening so that the foot can go in easily without any movement. No wedges or other alterations should be required.

Lobster claw feet (and similar congenital deformities)

Orthopaedic footwear is the only method of dealing with this. Casting of the feet in the correct position is important.

Footwear to accommodate shortening

In dealing with footwear for shortening, that is when there is unequal leg length, cork has been used to accommodate the shortening for many years. For 1 inch shortening only $\frac{1}{2}$ inch raise is necessary to the heel, but for 3 inch shortening it is necessary to raise the heel $2\frac{1}{2}$ inches, the sole $1\frac{1}{2}$ inches and the toe only 1 inch (Fig. 14.8). This enable the foot to rocker forward because cork does not bend very easily and ensures that forward movement of the foot is maintained.

It is now possible to use high density Plastazote for this purpose, which this does not compress, is much more flexible and does not break when the foot bends forward. It is easy to shape and any height can be obtained by fixing layers together with good adhesive. In the cases of elevations to patients' own shoes, due to shortening of one leg or to take the weight off the other leg, this can be done with high density Plastazote instead of cork and it is often unnecessary to cover this with leather as one has to do when using cork.

Instructions to patients who have rheumatoid arthritic feet and who are wearing normal shoes

It is not advisable to wear shoes which:
1 Are welted, such as Tuf shoes
2 Have thin soles
3 Have flexible soles
4 Have plastic heels
Shoes with stout, preferably leather soles are advised, and always to use a full-fitting shoe. The uppers to be preferably suede or glacé kid for painful feet and

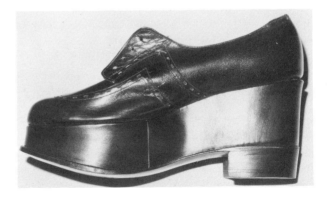

Fig. 14.8 Raise to sole allowing rocker action.

toes, and for patients needing stouter shoes for work, calf leather avoiding toe caps at all times. Keep shoes in good repair. Do not let the heels tread over too far before repairing, this will upset the balance of walking. Remove insoles from shoes at night and if the supports are made of Plastazote, remember that these should be washed regularly.

Footwear problems of the partially amputated foot

When considering the partial amputation of the foot, balance is often very difficult to maintain in walking. This can be even more of a problem when the partially amputated foot has to be housed in a shoe which is inadequate; by this I mean a shoe which is badly balanced. This is quite often the case when dealing with ladies' shoes.

Amputation of the great toe is perhaps a rather rare operation. The balance of the foot is normally dependent on take-off through the great toe itself, and when it is found necessary to amputate this either through trauma or disease, one is left with the problem of the necessity to balance the foot rather than to accommodate the absence of the great toe. Although this has to be done naturally to maintain the shape of the shoe, quite often there is some deformity in the remainder of the foot that needs special attention. The loss of the great toe usually means that the patient will throw his weight on to the outer side of his foot; it is important to maintain the balance necessary to bring the weight through the whole of the metatarsal heads. Usually this can be done by adding an outside wedge to the sole, extended well behind the heads of the metatarsal, to throw the weight well forward on to the great toe area. Care must be taken to see that the weight is evenly distributed. Sometimes a very thin metal plate must be added along the inner border to prevent the shoe from bending, but this should be avoided wherever possible. An amputation block can be made to replace the big toe, preferably of Plastazote, and should be fitted in such a way that when the foot goes forward there is no pressure on the end of the amputation. The block should be fixed on an insole, so that it can easily be removed for adjustments (Fig. 14.9).

In the case of amputation of all the toes, which is more common, it is necessary to fit a full insole with suitable padding to relieve pressure on the metatarsal heads. Often in this type of amputation, one is left with a very high arch similar to that of a cavus foot, and a well moulded cavus low insole with a metatarsal support should be carefully fitted on the same insole to which the toe amputation block is fitted. The old method of doing this was to have a cork in the forefoot to the end of the toes, shaped to match the fellow shoe about one inch from the amputation, then to have sponge rubber facing to the cork carefully fitted, so that when the foot went forward there was no pressure at the end of the amputation.

Plastazote is now the material of choice and it is usually necessary to fit the toe block at least one size, i.e. $\frac{1}{3}$ inch, away from the end of the foot. Again, it must be ensured that the balance is even and it may be necessary to give an adequate rocker to the sole to improve the walking, because with the loss of the forefoot, there is no

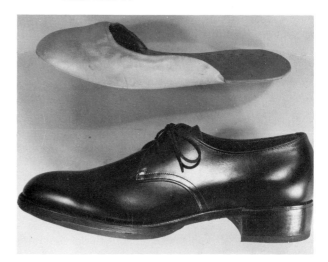

Fig. 14.9 To show toe block on insole and side view of shoe with varus sole wedge for patient who has lost the great toe.

balance of rocking forward. It is therefore necessary to replace this by adding a rocker sole, adding a piece of leather $\frac{1}{4}$ inch thick skived at each end about 2–3 inches wide across the tread of the shoe. Some stiffening must be added to the sole to prevent the front turning up, and for this purpose a steel plate is fixed to the insole of the shoe down the centre of the foot. Spring steel with sufficient flexibility must be used to bring the foot straight. A heavy steel plate should be avoided as this will often break and is much too clumsy. A light sole plate in a high density polythene material (Ortholen) is quite adequate for some patients.

Amputation of toes in cases of leprosy needs special attention; one has to be so very careful in housing the remaining part of the foot because of the loss of sensation and, if possible, to prevent ulceration, as any breakdown of the skin is much more difficult to heal. The method recommended is to use 1 inch Plastazote and to take an impression of the partial foot. The Plastazote is cut to equal the full length of the other foot and it can be rockered up. By using 1 inch Plastazote and careful moulding, a first-class impression is obtained of any part of the foot that is likely to be ulcerated, and the springiness of the material round that area will often encourage healing if there is an ulcer, or certainly prevent an ulcer from developing. An extra piece of Plastazote may be added in the long arch by the fusion method I have described, if required. It must be understood that this type of support cannot be accommodated in ordinary footwear, and surgical footwear made to careful measurements is essential.

In cases of amputation through the midmetarsal (Fig. 14.10) area, one is left with a foot which is difficult from the point of view of walking forward, and it is advisable to mould Plastazote to the remaining portion of the foot and to extend this to the full length of the normal foot (Fig. 14.11).

Almost every partial amputation brings an individual problem and I quote now a case referred to me from another hospital. The surgeon stated: 'Here now is

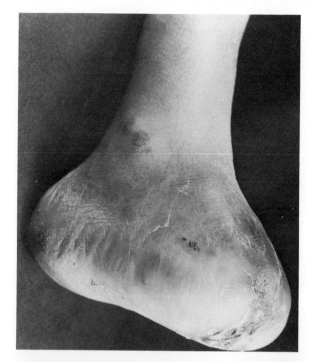

Fig. 14.10 Midmetatarsal amputation of foot.

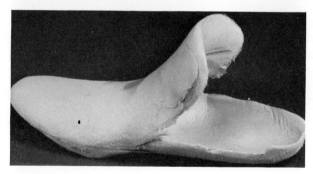

Fig. 14.11 Block on insole to make up the lost length of the foot.

another case presenting a considerable problem in relation to the fitting of a shoe. The patient has a partial amputation of the right foot, the first and second toes and the metarsals have been removed. On the left side the forefoot has been removed and the ankle is really in the equinus position with hardly any movement, although the heel has been flattened to give a good plantar surface at right angles to the line of the tibia, which means that the heel is very prominent'. The surgeon's prescription continued: 'He will need suitable padding to allow him to wear ordinary shoes and I would suggest some form of padding at the back of the left heel above the calcaneum to fill the gap between the back of the Achilles tendon and his shoe. He is keen to wear conventional shoes for cosmetic reasons.'

The surgeon continued: 'This is another challenging case where we seek help using Plastazote or one of these other materials.' When I saw this patient, there was no doubt that he needed a great deal of special attention.

For the left amputation a Plastazote anklet was made to fit in the shoe at the back and a spring plate throughout the sole. The heel of the left shoe was made $3\frac{1}{2}$ inches across, with a float out on both sides. It is advisable in the majority of such cases to make absolutely certain that the heel is wide so that the patient obtains maximum stability. For the right foot, where the great toe had been amputated, including the whole of the metatarsal joint, he required a plastic prosthesis to level the base of the foot. This meant that the whole of the remaining metarsal had to be depressed and the heel of the shoe also required to be floated out on each side and a varus sole wedge added, so that the foot could be evenly balanced. The prosthesis, made in Plastazote, weighed only five ounces, had articulated movement in the toe and fitted into the patient's size $9\frac{1}{2}$ shoes. It is important when fitting this type of appliance to mould the front part so as to grip the front of the foot when the shoe is laced. This holds the foot firm without causing any pressure at the end of the amputation.

Another case is that of Mr A, who has Hansen's disease and has had considerable trouble with his footwear over a number of years. On the left side Mr A has only about half his foot remaining, and on the right side he has lost all his toes and part of the metatarsals. The soles of his feet were in poor condition, having a certain degree of ulceration on the plantar surfaces, and both feet were anaesthetic. He earned his living as an entertainer and was very concerned about the appearance of his footwear. His previous footwear has been made with thick sponge rubber insoles, sponge rubber metatarsal pads, sponge rubber amputation toe blocks plus wedges to accommodate the deformity. With this type of footwear he needed periods of hospitalization and further minor amputations. He had continual discharge from some of the ulcerations. Progress was very slow and unsatisfactory until it was decided to use Plastazote to support his feet. Careful casts were taken of both his feet for surgical footwear and Plastazote was moulded to the base of his feet under pressure to accommodate the ulcerated areas. The result has been that he now has a well-balanced foot; there is no sign of ulceration and the base of his feet are healthy. This has completely altered his outlook on life and he is now able to earn his living as an entertainer without embarrassment.

Most surgical footwear with leather uppers is now made by the direct attachment method (not welted) and patients with partial amputations benefit considerably because footwear made in this way is very much lighter than that made in the welted manner and is also, by being firm but resilient, completely shock-absorbing in walking.

To conclude, having discussed a number of cases using the old method of sponge rubber insoles with pads and toe blocks, there is no doubt that patients with partial amputation of the foot, prone to ulceration and with deformities that result in uneven balance, derive enormous benefit from having Plastazote insoles moulded directly to the base of their feet. This new method has been a major breakthrough in meeting the specialized needs of these particular cases. Another advantage is that Plastazote is completely washable although water-repellent, and can be perforated for ventilation if required. There is one important thing to remember when low density Plastazote supports have been in use for a period of time—it is always necessary to reinforce them by adding $\frac{1}{4}$ inch thick Plastazote under the depressed area. This should be fixed to the original support by a rubber solution—the support itself should not be remoulded. By using medium density Plastazote, however, this may not be necessary.

15

Chiropody

P.J. READ

THE PROFESSION

The official definition of chiropody is circular in nature: 'Chiropody comprises the maintenance of feet in a healthy condition and the treatment of their disabilities by recognized chiropodial methods in which the practitioner has been trained'. Although the treatment of skin lesions is an important part of chiropody treatment, the mere treatment of corns is not the whole or even the majority of chiropody. The up-to-date practitioner is very anxious to avoid the 'cut and come again' image and is concerned to produce a permanent cure wherever this is possible. Again, chiropody is not just the treatment of minor foot disorders; it is equally concerned with the prevention of all foot disorders. The foot, particularly in civilized society, is subjected to considerable strains and stresses of a repetitive nature. These strains and stresses may produce pain or they may produce lesions. Even in an age dominated by the motor-car, very few can escape the forces undergone by the feet in standing or locomotion.

Since 1954 the recognized course of chiropody has been of three academic years. The current entry requirements for most schools are five passes in GCE of which two, including one science subject, must be at 'A' level. Other passes at either 'O' or 'A' level must include English Language and generally another science subject. Equivalent qualifications are accepted. The course of training embraces three important aspects. Firstly, there is the teaching of the practical techniques involved. Secondly, there is the theoretical background of how the foot works and why it does not always work satisfactorily, together with the theoretical basis of mechanical and pharmaceutical treatment. Thirdly, students are taught to recognize and treat conditions which arise from systemic rather than from local causes.

Chiropodists have always received most of their patients direct, without medical reference. The philosophy of the course and its associated examinations has been based on the need for chiropodists to distinguish between systemic disorders affecting the feet and disorders of purely local origin. In addition to the examinations in direct professional subjects, examinations in anatomy and physiology in the second year and medicine and surgery in the final year are conducted by external examiners, who have been approved by the Royal Colleges and who are frequently of consultant or professorial status. In the second year of the course students undertake a course in the administration of local analgesia and take an examination conducted by a consultant anaesthetist approved by the Faculty of Anaesthetists of the Royal College of Surgeons of London. However, in addition to working as individuals, chiropodists are part of the greater medical profession and play a significant role in the medical team in the treatment of diabetics, rheumatoid and osteoarthritics, patients suffering from peripheral neuropathies and many orthopaedic conditions. The community physician is interested in the work of chiropodists in keeping elderly patients mobile.

The Professions Supplementary to Medicine Act 1960 set up the Chiropodists Board, a statutory body having the responsibility for registering qualified chiropodists and regulating their professional education and their professional conduct. The Board consists of a majority of chiropodists elected by the profession, together with medical representatives and a person 'well-versed in educational matters'. To work within the National Health Service a chiropodist has to be registered by the Board. There is however, nothing to prevent any person setting up in private practice as a chiropodist although there are bye-laws in certain areas governing the licensing of premises. Only the titles State Registered Chiropodist, Registered Chiropodist and State Chiropodist are in fact protected. Moves are being made to seek at least restriction on the title 'chiropodist' and to have its use confined to registered chiropodists. Chiropody forms a natural part of medical care and the demand for chiropody at the present time far exceeds the supply. The total numbers of chiropodists registered by the Board stood in 1980 at 5081, while the number of unregistered chiropodists is unknown.

TREATMENT

Chiropody then, is both the treatment of foot conditions and also the methods used to treat certain foot disorders. It covers the whole range of foot disorders, short of those requiring orthopaedic surgery and the whole range of ages from young to old. Perhaps one of the most typical cases a chiropodist treats is a middle-aged patient with plantar callosities and possibly some corns on the toes. These are in fact two separate problems. One is a problem involving the mechanics of the foot and the other relates to the condition of the skin. Some skins are far more prone than others to produce the thickened epidermis which is a feature of so many foot conditions. Nobody has yet discovered why this should be so and treatment tends to lay stress on correcting the faulty mechanics of the foot and palliating the skin condition. Years ago, the plantar callosities over the centre 3 metatarsal heads would have been attributed to a 'fallen metatarsal arch'. In the 1930s it was pointed out that all the metatarsal heads are in contact with the ground, as witnessed by the wet imprint of a foot on a bath mat, as well as by more sophisticated pedographic methods. Morton showed that each of the four outer metatarsals bear equal shares of body in standing and that the first metatarsal bears a double share of the weight (see Chapter 3 for discussion of this aspect).

More recently attention has been focussed on the foot in motion rather than the foot at rest. In brief terms, the heel meets the ground first in what is termed the 'heel strike' and this term occupies 15–20% of the time taken for a single step. In the phase which follows the heel, the lateral border of the foot and the metatarsal heads are all bearing weight. This phase occupies 30–35% of the 'step-time'. This is followed by a very short phase, generally no more than 10% of the step-time, when the metatarsals alone are bearing weight. The weight is then shared between the metatarsals and their respective toes for the remainder of the step, about 30% of the total time. In walking, the centre of gravity is oscillating in the vertical plane so that the pressure exerted by the foot on the ground is not uniform.

It so happens that the metatarsal phase coincides with the phase of maximum pressure. Patients suffering from plantar callosities are frequently found to have toes which do not perform any weight-bearing function. Weight-bearing skin can be determined by an examination of its thickness and texture. Lack of useful function in toes may be due to buckling, to arthritis or to imbalance or inefficiency of the muscles of the foot and leg which act upon the toes. Frequently the toe inefficiency is brought about by footwear, both by shoes and hose, in particular stretch hosiery. The point is made that footwear does not have to do gross damage to the foot in order to produce significant foot conditions.

The treatment of the condition described is firstly to pare away the thickened stratum corneum—in itself a skilled job—and possibly the use of some form of emollient on the skin. Keratolytics are not to be favoured as their action is difficult to control and precision and the smooth removal of the hard skin is necessary if maximum comfort is to be achieved. The mechanical aspect of the problem may be solved by using an orthosis which, for example, provides a platform for the toes to make them do some work, or an orthosis which cushions the metatarsal heads and spreads the load over a larger area of tissue during the metatarsal weight-bearing phase when maximum pressure is being extended on the metatarsal heads. An insole which cushions will also compensate for loss of resiliance in the subcutaneous tissue which is often a feature of middle and old age. These insoles may be made using a variety of materials. Sponge rubber or other closed-cell materials are well-established favourites, but are, at least temporarily, in short supply. Thermoplastic polyurethane foam is another promising material from which effective orthoses may be prepared. Adhesive pads of similar materials may be used, generally as a temporary measure, since it is an obvious advantage if removable and washable orthoses can be provided.

All mechanical treatment of feet is a compromise since we use our feet in two distinctly different ways—one is for locomotion and is related to dynamic weight-bearing; the other way in which we use our feet is standing, which relates to static weight-bearing. Generally the tendency is to cater for dynamic weight-bearing rather than for static weight-bearing although the nature of the patient's job may tilt the balance of the compromise towards static weight-bearing. A shop assistant or a worker at a factory bench provide obvious examples where emphasis would be laid on the static weight-bearing function of the feet in determining the treatment.

Plantar callosities

Plantar callosities result from a diffuse overloading of the plantar metatarsal area. If the pressures are more localized, corns rather than callosities may be the result. The illustration shows a remarkable sandal which is manufactured from very hard wood. This sandal was worn for many years and miles by a Tibetan monk (Fig. 15.1). The imprint of the toes and the metatarsal heads can be seen very clearly. The same small areas of tissues are subjected to stress with every step that is taken. Gait is a repetitive action and repetitive in a remarkably uniform manner. Because of this, slight variations in the relative lengths of the metatarsal bones—the metatarsal formula—may lead to the production of painful corns and other pressure lesions which will be discussed later. There are considerable ranges of metatarsal formula within the normal. A relatively short first metatarsal may produce a pressure lesion over the head of the second metatarsal. The second metatarsal articulates with the first and third cuneiforms as well as with the second cuneiform. The base of the metatarsal is thus held firmly and thus cannot move as freely as the others. Of course, not only may there be skin lesions over the metatarsal head, but the metatarsal itself may be subject to stress fracture or to Freiberg's infraction of the metatarsal head. A comparatively short first metatarsal may lead to a pressure lesion over the fifth metatarsal head because of the manner in which the patient compensates in walking, as the first metatarsal is not able to provide the final push-off area of contact with the ground. While variations in relative lengths of the first metatarsal with its function of providing the take-off point of the foot may produce a variety of patterns of lesions, the relatively short fifth metatarsal is more likely to produce a lesion over the fourth metatarsal head. Slight variations in the

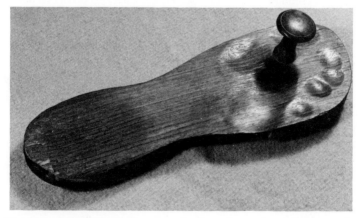

Fig. 15.1 A sandal made from very hard wood worn by a Tibetan monk.

lengths of the centre three metatarsals again may produce trouble because of the repetitive nature of walking. Much more common however, is that a comparatively long second or third metatarsal is associated with a long second or third toe, which gives a digital formula in which these toes are longer than the first or fourth. Short footwear or short hosiery cause the toe or toes to become buckled. Back pressure from the buckled toe presses the associated metatarsal head downwards and it becomes overloaded. The distinction should be noted between the concept of the fallen metatarsal and a metatarsal which is pushed downwards by its associated digit. An important point about buckling of toes is that once the deformity has commenced the musculature of the foot is such that it tends to exacerbate the deformity. Even while there is still mobility in the joints it is difficult for many people to straighten the toes by muscular activity. Toe splints may sometimes help to prevent a toe becoming more buckled or even to straighten a mildly buckled toe. These can be made from a variety of soft materials including silicone rubbers.

Plantar corns

The treatment of plantar corns is again the skilful removal of hyperkeratotic material using a scalpel. The nature of the mechanical problem has then to be analysed as suitable adhesive padding devised. In general, for the sake of hygiene and for aesthetic reasons the adhesive materials should be replaced at the earliest possible moment by orthoses which can be removed when the feet are washed. In the treatment of plantar callosities some general cushioning is often possible, whereas in treating a plantar corn accuracy in positioning a pad or orthosis is essential. For this reason orthoses for plantar corns are often made on a cast of the foot.

There may be several ways of tackling the problem of plantar corns. One may be to spread the weight-bearing load to metatarsals on either side of the overstressed area. Sometimes the weight may be spread backwards along the shaft of the metatarsal or a combination of the two methods may be used. Account must be taken of the degree of mobility of the metatarsal segment involved and of the mobility of the foot in general. A short or inefficient first metatarsal is frequently compensated for by a shaft of fairly firm material placed along the shaft and over the head of the metatarsal. Corns over the heads of the first and fifth metatarsals may call for a pad which transfers the stress to the second, third and fourth metatarsal heads. In the case of rheumatoid arthritis it is likely that the deformity of the metatarsophalangeal joints will give rise to corns which may occur on any combination of metatarsal heads. Often the use of materials of two densities, one appreciably softer than the other with the softer material under the affected heads, will provide comfort for this type of patient.

Digital corns

Buckled toes are themselves likely to be the site of corns from pressure arising from footwear. There is again a number of ways of solving the problem of protecting the tissues from further damage. A fairly recent innovation is a synthetic tubular foam which provides general cushioning and is useful either as a first aid measure, replacing the older corn ring, or in the later stages when the corn is improving (Fig. 15.2). Again, very accurate pads may be required which may be prepared on a plaster cast taken of the toe. The cast is dipped in latex rubber and natural and synthetic foams are incorporated to direct pressure away from the affected joint. Not all digital corns, of course, occur on the joints. The apices of the toes are a common site for painful and intractable corns. In these cases a carefully designed prop may be used to raise the tips of the toes away from the ground. The use of silicone rubber in the manufacture of toe pads is being developed. These are simple to make and do not require casting techniques as they are prepared on the foot.

The question of footwear has been dealt with in another chapter, but it is impossible to talk about chiropody without making mention of it. After all, the shoe is the normal, if not the natural, environment for the foot. The lateral border of the fifth toe is a very common site for a hard corn. This is frequently due to the fact that there is a slightly valgus foot in an inflare shoe; the conflict between the shoe and the foot will centre around the fifth toe (Figs. 15.3, 15.4). In appearance, and even by measurement the shoe is wide enough for the foot. In fact, much of the space is wasted because of the way the foot lies in the shoe.

Interdigital lesions

Corns often occur in the interdigital clefts. These lesions are often referred to as 'soft' corns because on a sweaty foot they may be macerated and present a whitened appearance. Very often, however, interdigital corns are just like other corns in appearance. In some cases they may have a thickened ring on the outside of the lesion where most corns have a central nucleus of extra hard keratinized tissue. Interdigital corns may occur in any cleft but most commonly in the 4–5 cleft. There

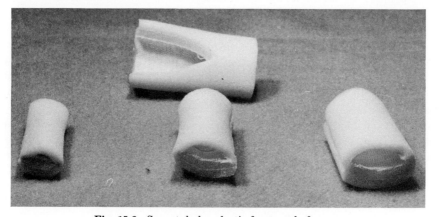

Fig. 15.2 Some tubular plastic foam ready for use.

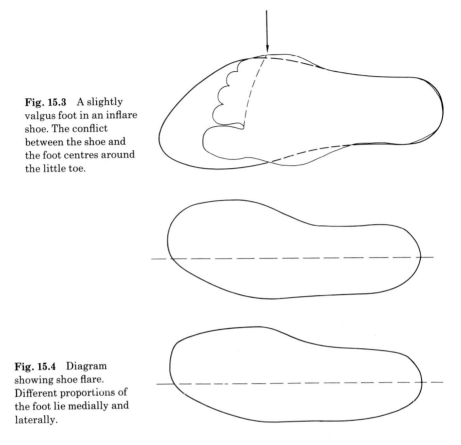

Fig. 15.3 A slightly valgus foot in an inflare shoe. The conflict between the shoe and the foot centres around the little toe.

Fig. 15.4 Diagram showing shoe flare. Different proportions of the foot lie medially and laterally.

are two reasons for this; first, the 4–5 cleft lies more obliquely than the others, and secondly (as is shown in Fig. 15.3) there is often a conflict between the shoe and the foot which centres on the fifth toe.

The sites or occurrence of interdigital corns are determined by the metatarsal and digital formulae. In Fig. 15.5, in the foot on the left the head of the proximal phalanx of the fifth toe impinges on the base of the proximal phalanx of the fourth. In this foot a lesion is likely to occur in the 4–5 cleft. In the foot on the right of the diagram the fifth toe lies snugly but there might be an impingement between the bases of the middle phalanx of the second toe and the distal phalanx of the first toe. The treatment of all these lesions is to remove all the keratinized tissue and to use an astringent medicament such as 25% solution of silver nitrate or the use of a silver nitrate stick. A 2% solution of crystal violet in spirit is often very effective used interdigitally, but it needs to be used with care because staining, which is difficult to remove, can occur on hosiery or on bedding. The treatment of the cause of the condition depends on an analysis of the biomechanics of the forefoot in question. The toes may be held apart using synthetic foam material such as that

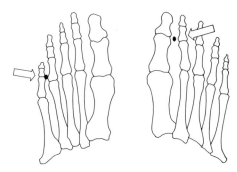

Fig. 15.5 Two common sites for interdigital corns.

shown in Fig. 15.2. In the figure this is shown in its tubular form but it is also available in flat sheets. Alternatively, a device made from silicone rubber may be moulded on to the foot. The condition may be prevented in some cases by altering the alignment of the metatarsal heads using a plantar pad. The alignment of the phalanges need only be changed by as little as 1 mm to avoid the juxtaposition of bony prominences.

Interdigital maceration is frequently seen but does not by any means indicate fungal infections (Athlete's foot) in every case. Probably fewer than 20% of cases give positive results for fungal infections on microscopic examination of scales or on culturing. The problem is often one of lack of evaporation of sweat, which can be solved by attention to hygiene and the use of astringent lotions. Fortunately the use of fungicidal lotions and powder rarely does any harm, so that if they are used unnecessarily there are no ill effects.

Bunions

The bunion ranks next to corn and callus as a cause of foot misery—discomfort is too mild a word. The word bunion is used here to denote a condition of hallux valgus with an overlying bursa or with skin lesions giving rise to pain. Corns and callosities are frequently seen in association with hallux valgus. This definition avoids the need to discuss what degree of angulation must exist between the metatarsal and the digit before one can describe the condition as hallux valgus. The painful bunion/hallux valgus syndrome is not confined to the first metatarso-phalangeal joint. The secondary effects of the hallux valgus on the foot give rise to painful lesions, a common example being a buckled, possibly overriding second toe and a corn on the plantar surface over the second metatarsal head.

The chiropodist has a dual role to play in the treatment of hallux valgus; firstly prevention and secondly the palliative treatment of the bursa or skin lesions. It is generally agreed that the widening of the gap between the first and second metatarsal is an early stage, if not the first stage, in the development of hallux valgus. The first metatarsal swings away from the midline of the foot, and in an established case, slips off the sesamoid bones so that the medial sesamoid articulates with the metatarsal where the lateral sesamoid would normally do so. The deviation of the metatarsal is followed by an increase in the angulation between the metatarsal and the toe, brought about firstly by footwear, including hose, and secondly by the bowstring action of the muscles (see Chapter 6).

While hallux valgus is essentially a disease of civilization, it has been shown to occur amongst barefoot races, although it is rare. This is to say that some feet may produce hallux valgus in the absence of footwear. In contrast, some feet in 'civilized' society will never produce hallux valgus however badly they may have been treated in the matter of choice of footwear. Other feet are at high risk. With experience, those feet which are at risk can be identified by shape, particularly by observation of the metatarsal formula and by observing the general mobility of the foot. The long mobile foot, which is likely to roll over into valgus, is also a prime candidate for hallux valgus. Particular care must be taken during childhood and adolescence in choice of footwear of people who have this type of foot. Choice of socks is as important, if not more, than the choice of shoes.

Treating the lesions associated with hallux valgus may be described as straightforward chiropody. An inflamed bursa may be treated by topical applications and a chronic bursitis may be reduced by the use of rubefacients. Protection of the tissues is essential and the use of modern materials produces cosmetically acceptable appliances. The use of a casting technique, the taking of a cast of the foot and preparing the shield on the cast is the method of choice, since accurately shaped devices are essential. Commercial bunion shields provide only general cushioning, whereas it is generally necessary to remove the pressure from an area of tissue completely. The chiropodial treatment of bunions is essential for the patient awaiting surgery and often surgery can be avoided altogether and the patient kept comfortable and retain an intact foot. Co-operation over footwear is essential but this does not necessitate the wearing of ugly shoes.

The other problems to which the first metatarsal is heir—hallux rigidus and hallux flexus—also produce their effects on foot function and produce their own sets of lesions, as does the 'short' or inefficient first metatarsal of Dudley Morton. Again the pattern may be seen of a defect in foot function causing painful lesions on the feet for which treatment is required. The treatment of the lesions, however, cannot be reduced to an ad hoc level but must be related to an understanding of the functional defect involved and may consist in part of the correction of or compensation for a mechanical deficiency. The pattern is again seen in the valgus or postural valgus foot.

Minor disturbances of gait and foot function

Many foot disorders arise in the forefoot and result from anatomical anomalies such as unusual metatarsal or digital formulae or from buckling of the toes. The result of ill-fitting footwear and the use of 'stretch' socks is buckling of the toes. Buckling may, of course, also arise from rheumatoid or osteoarthritis.

Quite separate from the disorders of the forefoot, foot troubles may occur as the result of anomalies occurring at the subtalar and midtarsal joint. The term 'anomalies' is used here to avoid both the exaggeration of the term 'deformities' and the understatement of the term 'minor'. This group of foot troubles includes valgus foot, inrolling foot or pronated foot. These are cases which do not warrant surgical interference but which may give rise to symptoms or to lesions in the forefoot. A valgus, pronated foot tends to swing outwards from the midline of the body and since all normal shoes have a greater or lesser degree of inflare pressure, lesions may occur in the forefoot as the result of the battle between shoe and foot.

There is much debate as to how far these conditions should be treated, particularly in children. Heel wedges, heel grips and shoe inlays all have their advocates, but particularly in the case of children, it is difficult to assess their value. Any survey of preventative measures as far as feet are concerned is likely to be hampered by the fact that the child is likely to outlive the investigator. The question as to whether asymptomatic feet should be treated in order to prevent hypothetical future foot disorders should always be asked. As Sir Denis Browne once remarked, 'Have you noticed that those who treat normal feet get better results than we do?' The fact of the matter is that there is in the foot a wide range of normality.

Whether or not corrective shoes or orthoses are prescribed the chiropodist has a role in advising on footwear and in foot health education. The chief faults in footwear are that they may be either fitted too short or, in the case of children, have been outgrown. Nearly as important as shoe length is the way the shoe is fastened to the foot. As a general rule, a shoe should have a fastening at least two thirds up the instep. The fastening does not need to be a lace—it may be a thin strap. The foot must be held back in the shoe and must not be allowed to slip forward so that the forefoot is wedged into the V-shaped front. Much is always made of the fact that a high-heeled shoe throws body weight forward on to the metatarsals; the foot slipping forwards down the inclined plane is equally damaging. Hosiery must not be overlooked, particularly stretch socks and tights. It is axiomatic that if the foot stretches the sock then the sock compresses the foot. This will all too often lead to buckling of the toes. Unfortunately, particularly in children but also to a degree in adults, the buckling process does not hurt. Pain comes a long time after the toes have become buckled when secondary skin lesions have been produced. In the case of both tights for adults and most importantly in tight-like garments for babies, the foot length of the garment must be adequate or more than adequate when related to the rest of the garment, since the garments tend to be selected for their general size, rather than for foot size.

In the older age groups chiropodists will often be able to make simple modifications to ordinary shoes or will prescribe alterations to be made by a local cobbler. These alterations may take the form of soft leather inserts over pressure points or, in many cases, of simply stretching the shoe. Shoe stretching needs to be done accurately and can be very effective. Leather shoes tend to be readily stretchable and maintain their stretch; some synthetics have a 'memory' and tend to regain their former shape. It is often important for patients' morale that they should be able to wear as near normal footwear as possible. If a chiropodist can keep a patient in 'normal' footwear, a good job is being done for the patient.

Foot strain

Not all foot troubles which a chiropodist may be called upon to treat manifest themselves as skin lesions. A strained foot is defined as one where the soft tissues of the foot are unable to stand up to the stresses to which they are subjected. The feet may ache, but quite often the pain is severe and the condition is described as acute. Frequently, if not always, a condition of hyperhidrosis accompanies foot strain. The strain may arise because the foot is being over-used or it may be the result of some comparatively minor structural or functional defect. Foot strain often centres round the joints of the foot, particularly the subtalar joint complex where inversion and eversion of the foot takes place. One tends in these days not to talk too much about the arches of the foot, even the longitudinal arch, but one looks rather at how the foot is related to the leg and how it meets the ground. Sometimes an inrolling foot is a strained foot but the two conditions are not synonymous. The plantar calcaneonavicular ('spring') ligament is often affected and is the site of pain and is tender on palpation. This is what frequently leads to a diagnosis of fallen arch or pain associated with the longitudinal arch of the foot. It may be that the appliance which is used to rest the strained foot may look very much like an 'arch support' but its function in reality is to limit the range of movement at the subtalar joint rather than to give any support to the arch. The treatment for a strained foot is rest and the identification and correction of the cause. The ideal is a short period of bed rest; even a weekend may be sufficient. It is not always easy for a patient to change a job involving standing for a sedentary occupation. However, often the use of shoe modifications can provide just sufficient help to produce comfort. During the Second World War a very simple device proved very effective in factories where a lot of standing was involved. The workers were given a platform on which to stand, the centre of the platform being raised 2–3 inches and sloping downwards toward the outside. This was sufficient to alter the angle at which the feet met the ground and to throw weight towards the outer border of the foot, lessening the stresses on the more susceptible inner border.

The condition of foot strain arises more commonly from static weight-bearing than from walking or running. In army days and in more recent times in association with sponsored walks, chiropodists were and are called upon to treat skin lesions, mostly blisters, rather than pain from deep structures. It is static or nearly static weight-bearing which appears to produce trouble. Foot strain is not to be confused with a syndrome which has been labelled for want of a better term, the 'barking dog syndrome'. To the uninitiated, if a Cockney says 'my dogs are barking', he means 'his feet are killing him'. The 'barking dog syndrome' consists of hot, tender and sweaty feet combined with the sensation that one's footwear has suddenly become too small. It is generally brought about by a visit to a zoo, museum or gallery or by a shopping expedition or by travel home in the rush hour by Tube. It is to be noted that the feet are hot and tender—this denotes pain arising from the skin rather than from deeper structures which cause an aching or dull pain. The condition probably has little to do with the feet but is rather a circulatory problem. Venous drainage from the feet is dependent on the action of leg muscles and the barking dog syndrome occurs when people have either been meandering or standing still. The feet are, in fact, slightly oedematous which again relates to a temporarily inefficient venous drainage. The treatment is to wash the feet, change the socks and stockings and rest for a period with the legs elevated above heart level.

Systemic manifestations

Systemic diseases affect the feet in various ways which call for chiropodial treatment or treatment which chiropodists are particularly well qualified to give. For example, a motor neuropathy may produce a defect in gait which leads to foot lesions or, as in the aftermath of poliomyelitis, from a distorted foot which does not call for surgical intervention. The skin of the feet is not excluded from dermatological conditions—a case of exfoliative dermatitis affecting the feet can be a chiropodist's nightmare. In some systemic diseases the feet are particularly affected and chiropody can play a highly significant role in the management of such cases.

Rheumatoid arthritis produces its own typical lesions on the feet. Firstly there is distortion, often gross, of the small joints of the foot, in particular the metatarsophalangeal and interphalangeal joints. Secondly the periarticular tissues produce a typical lesion resulting in thickening of the epidermis in the region of the joints. Not only is there gross deformity of the forefoot but problems occur in the plantar metatarsal area as well. Surgeons will sometimes amputate the toes, but even after toe amputation there may still be lesions over the metatarsal heads which require a moccasin type of appliance to keep the patient comfortable. Many patients with rheumatoid arthritis can be kept in a reasonable degree of comfort by a combination of the treatment of skin lesions, padding and attention to footwear. Surgical shoes are not always practical and often they are not acceptable. With the use of vacuum-forming apparatus it is possible to make very light comfortable footwear from thermoplastic materials quite cheaply. If it is at all possible to adapt standard footwear by the use of balloon patches, made by cutting a hole in the shoe and covering with a piece of matching leather, this is to be preferred (Chapter 14).

Patients suffering from diabetes have special problems with their feet (Chapter 9). Indeed, the diabetic department of a hospital generally demands priority of the chiropody services available. The skin of diabetics appears to be particularly prone to produce corns and callosities and in particular, diabetics tend to get an accumulation of skin debris in the nail sulci which gives rise to discomfort. Because of this, they are particularly prone to indulge in home chiropody. In the case of diabetics merely keeping the patient comfortable is not in itself sufficient. Chiropody has a much more positive role to play. Features of diabetes which particularly affect the feet are firstly the microangiopathy which affects the local resistance of the tissues, and secondly the peripheral neuropathy which diminishes, or even eliminates pain sensation. These pathological features frequently lead to ulceration over pressure points in the foot. The treatment of these ulcers is quite straightforward; the ulcer must be kept clean and all pressure removed from the area. This is straightforward but it is not easy. Many diabetics are allergic to, or cannot tolerate adhesive dressings and the problem is to devise accurate replaceable dressings. Once the ulcer has healed more permanent protective devices may be provided. Weekly, even daily, treatment may be necessary, treatment often being slow and tedious. Because diabetics frequently suffer from arteriosclerosis, ulceration is more prone to occur during the winter months. It is also significant that not infrequently the manifestations of diabetes in the feet are the first symptoms which suggest the disease. A history of intermittent claudication (ischaemic pain on exercise), of night cramps or of burning sensations of the feet in bed may well be given to the chiropodist. Suspicions may also be roused by lesions which do not heal as readily as they should. The chiropodist is a captive audience in a white coat and may hear things from a patient who is loath to 'waste' their family doctor's time with what they feel may be trivia. It is not for the chiropodist to establish a diagnosis of diabetes, nor would he wish to alarm the patient unnecessarily. He may therefore couch his referral in general and very cautious terms rather than as a specific expression of his suspicions. Due attention should be paid to such guarded referrals.

A number of more dramatic cases of anaesthetic feet are now being seen in this country—the after-effects of leprosy. These cases are normally in the hands of specialists, but they do have special foot problems with which trained chiropodists are particularly well able to cope. In countries where leprosy is endemic, special measures are taken to protect the feet and much attention is paid to foot health education. In this country leprosy cases are rare and the chiropodist has an important counselling function in addition to carrying out protective treatment.

Many general diseases affect the feet, especially those which involve the circulatory or nervous systems. Tabetic ulcerations or ulcers associated with arteriosclerosis are not uncommon. Occasionally focal infections may occur in the feet and quite often the results of systemic infection may give rise to foot pain rather than to specific lesions. Problems arise from the fact that people live longer; after all feet are extremities and are the first parts to suffer from ageing arteries and deficiency in nerve supply. Many chiropodists think wryly of the truth of the expression 'dying from the feet upwards'. The fact is that one of the social results of a longer life span is an increased demand for chiropody.

NAILS

The foot has its fair share of skin disorders (see Chapter 7). It has perhaps three specialities of its own; fungal infection (Athlete's foot), plantar warts and the effects of hyperidrosis (excessive sweating). All of these are more annoying than dangerous, although the adverse psychological effect of foot ailments should not be underestimated, particularly the effects of hyperidrosis. Much advertising pressure is placed upon the public who are brainwashed to fear that they smell offensive to their neighbours. Sweaty feet are often the result of foot strain, but the control of sweating on the palms of the hands and soles of the feet is emotional rather than thermal. One's hands sweat with nervousness or with emotional tension, be it love or an important interview. Feet sweat in the same way and worry or emotional tension wondering whether one's feet smell creates a vicious circle of cause and effect.

Nails are an important skin appendage and toe nails give rise to a good deal of trouble, mostly of a minor nature. Nails are, of course, subject to fungal infestations and diseases such as psoriasis and eczamatous conditions. Nail shape may be affected by respiratory, cardiac or alimentary disease (clubbing of the nails); and by certain anaemias (spoon-shaped nails), and defects in nutritional supply may produce gross distortion of the nails (onychogryphosis).

However, most nail troubles arise from mechanical causes. The nail plates of the toes may be distorted by external pressures and once distorted they tend to remain so. There are also two important anatomical features of the nails which are all too often overlooked. If the thumb is pressed against a hard surface it will be seen that the blood is forced out of the nail bed. This is because the nail plate is intimately attached to the nail bed, which in turn has a strong fibrous attachment to the underlying phalanx. Thus the soft tissues are pressed up around the nail plate which is, as it were, pulled into the soft tissues. This sets the stage for corns and callous in the nail groove. The second feature of the anatomy of the nail is that the nail sulci are formed of desquamating epithelium. Normally skin squames are shed into the air to form household dust. In the nail sulci they collect to form impacted debris (often referred to by patients as 'chalk'), which causes discomfort, even pain in an area well known for its rich sensory nerve supply.

Patients often attempt to relieve pain by 'poking' down the sides of the nails. If this is done with some cotton wool on an orange stick little harm results, particularly if the wool has been soaked with hydrogen peroxide solution which will soften the impacted debris. If a sharp instrument is used, or if the patient attempts to cut down the side of the nail, onychocryptosis may result (Fig. 15.6). A point of nomenclature is that chiropodists refer to an ingrowing toe nail only when the nail plate has actually pierced the flesh. Nail plates which are exaggeratedly curved are not referred to as ingrown but as involuted or sometimes convoluted. Generally an ingrowing toe nail is caused by cutting down the side of the nail and leaving a splinter of nail which pierces the nail sulcus as the nail grows forward.

Onychocryptosis may often be treated conservatively; as little of the nail is removed as possible. A thin sliver of nail plate is removed from the side of the nail making sure that the sliver includes the offending splinter of nail. If the nail is tender and the procedure would cause pain an injection of 3% Carbocaine without adrenalin may be used as a local analgesic. An average dose would be 2.5–3.0 ml.

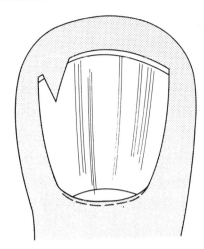

Fig. 15.6 Injudicious cutting of the
nail down the sulcus to relieve pain
from accumulated debris. A splinter
of nail remains and this leads on to a
true ingrowing toe nail.

Often this operation can be carried out without the use of local analgesia. The nail
sulcus is then packed with gauze or some synthetic material or with a soft leather
and the nail kept under observation. It may be necessary to harden the tissues of
the sulcus using a solution of ferric chloride BPC or a 10–25% solution of silver
nitrate. The sulcus is repacked as often as necessary during the period of nail
growth and is, needless to say, kept free from debris. This procedure produces
satisfactory results in a high proportion of cases.

There are, however, a number of cases where this simple procedure is not
sufficient. This may occur where there is some nail deformity which may appear to
be quite minor but which in practice gives rise to recurrent episodes of
onychocryptosis. In some nails this deformity may be in the form of excessive
curvature of the nail plate and be confined to one side of the nail. In these cases
partial avulsion of the nail is indicated and, very occasionally, total avulsion.
Partial nail avulsion may also be carried out where excessive curvature is giving
rise to recurrent pain due to accumulated debris or thickening of the epidermis of
the sulcus, even though there is no actual penetration of the flesh by the nail plate.

The technique used is as follows. The toe is anaesthetized using a plain
solution of 3% Carbocaine or similar analgesic. Generally two injections are
given, one on either side of the base of the digit. If satisfactory analgesia is not
achieved in 3–4 minutes a third injection may be given across the plantar surface of
the toe. The eponychium, that is the 'quick' of the nail, is raised at the base of the
nail near to the nail matrix in the area of the nail plate to be removed. A blunt
instrument resembling a small, stiff metal spatula is used as a retractor for this
purpose. After the eponychium has been loosened a special nipper having one
cutting blade which acts as a shallow anvil is then inserted under the free edge of
the nail on the side of the nail to be removed and is forced towards the base of the
nail. A single cut is made by closing the nippers and the effect is to loosen a section

of nail, 2–5 mm wide, depending on the degree of curvature, from the nail bed and also freeing the nail from the main nail plate. At this stage the nail is not entirely separated at the base and separation is completed using a nail chisel. The cut with the chisel must be carried completely to the base of the nail and the section of nail must be removed from the nail bed and especially from the nail matrix. The portion of nail to be removed is gripped with a pair of locking forceps which are used to twist the section out; this is best done towards the midline of the nail.

The next part of the procedure is perhaps the most important. The removal of nails surgically has in the past been bedevilled by the regrowth of nail or parts of the nail. Removal of the nail section is not in itself sufficient—the nail matrix from which the section of nail grew must be destroyed. Complete destruction of the matrix is essential; unless this is thoroughly carried out the nail will regrow and the procedure will have been valueless. One method used to destroy the nail matrix is 'phenolization', that is using liquefied phenol (80% strength) applied on a swab for 3–5 minutes. The action of the phenol is stopped by washing thoroughly with industrial methylated spirit or surgical spirit in which phenol is highly soluble. This method has the advantage of utilizing both the caustic and haemostatic effect of phenol. An alternative method is to use negative galvanism. The negative electrode of the galvanic apparatus is placed on the tissue to be destroyed and the positive electrode is strapped to the patient's calf over a saline pack. The dose varies—6 mA for 7 minutes is an average dose. Again it is essential that complete destruction of the nail matrix is achieved.

The toe is dressed using a light packing of Bactigras or similar product and a thick non-adherent sterile dressing is applied and fixed in position using tubular gauze. The procedure is undertaken on an out-patient basis and the patient may return home immediately after completion. It is, however, undesirable that full activity is resumed until it is comfortable to do so—usually after 12–24 hours. The dressing is renewed 48 hours after the operation and redressing is carried out again after one week and thereafter as required. The final result is a nail plate of acceptable shape which is slightly narrower than the original. Healing is normally complete in six weeks. The patient may wear a sandal or a shoe from which the toe cap has been removed for a short period, but normal footwear can be worn fairly soon after the operation provided that the footwear gives adequate room for the dressing. This technique is simple, highly effective and interferes minimally with the patient's normal activities.

Modifications of the basic technique to include excision of part of the tissue of the sulcus as well as the nail plate may be indicated in certain cases. Clinical judgment and selection of technique is based on the degree and nature of the curvature of the nail plate and the depth of the nail sulcus, which may vary considerably.

Patients often ask how nails should be cut. Generally it is better to recommend a rounded nail following the line of the hyponychium—the recess of skin underlying the free edge of the nail plate—rather than the older 'cut straight across' convention. There is no evidence that a 'V' cut in the centre of the nail does any good. The most important point, especially about the great toe nail, is that it should not be cut too short, however hard this may be on the hosiery. The nail should be left sufficiently long that it rests on the pulp on the distal end of the toe so that it is supported against the downward pull of the phalanx in walking (Fig. 15.7).

The natural curvature of the nail is an important factor which may cause

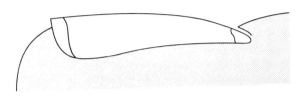

Fig. 15.7 The nail plate should be left sufficiently long for the free edge to rest on the pulp of the toe (top).

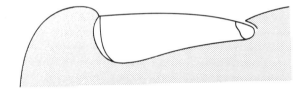

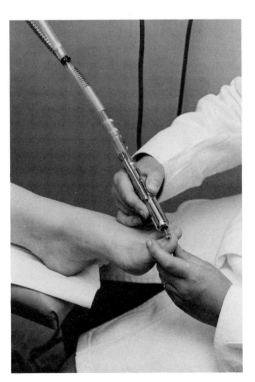

Fig. 15.8 A nail drill used for gryphotic nails.

trouble in the nail sulcus. This curvature may be increased by trauma or by external pressure on the nail resulting in distortion of the nail matrix. There are techniques for reducing the curvature of the nail. If necessary the nail plate is thinned and the sides of the nails are packed. Amadou is often used as a pack because it has astringent properties and also stays soft when impregnated with moisture. A more modern technique is to use a wire brace which, when worn over a period, will considerably reduce curvature of a nail plate.

Gryphotic nails, that is nails which thicken and distort, are common in the feet. They are difficult to cure but they are easy to reduce although the procedure gives scope for considerable skill. Cutting through thickened toe nails is not for the inexperienced (Fig. 15.8). Onychogryphosis caused by simple trauma is not common. Generally there is an underlying systemic cause (including old age), which calls for considerable care and expertise in treatment. Such nails do not grow quickly and it is generally not necessary to thin them more frequently than twice a year.

Some of the aspects of a chiropodist's work have been discussed and some of the methods of treatment described. By their nature, the use to which they are put, the environment in which they are used, feet give rise to a complex of problems the resolution of which calls for a knowledge of foot function, attention to detail and ingenuity and imagination in the use of material and the devising of methods of protective and corrective treatment.

Index

A

Accessory bones 21–2, 360–4
  in pes planovalgus 58
Achilles tendon *see* Tendon-Achilles
'Achillobursitis', radiology 326
Adaptation of the foot 1–2
Adductor hallucis imbalance in hallux
    valgus 86–7
Adventitious bursa 145
Age, effects on disease 164
Ainhum 369
Ambla in surgical footwear 417
Amputation
  Burgess 190, 191
  in diabetes 182, 187
Faraboeuf 189, 190
  partial footwear 425–9
  and the ruined foot 204
Anatomy
  evolutional, comparative 2
    bone changes 3–4
    functional 2–6
    lever systems 4–5
    locomotor muscles 3, 4–5
    shape of joint surface 5
  functional 19–30
    bone structure 19–22
    gait cycle 25–6
    joints 22–4
    pulses 26–7
    skin 27–8
    toes 24–5
Aneurysmal bone cyst, radiology 358–9
Ankle joint 22–4
  axes of movement 22–4
  ball and socket 24
Ankylosing spondylitis, radiology 325,
  329
  juvenile 334

Anterior foot strain 140
Aponeurosis, plantar 7
  windlass action 7
Arches of the foot 19
Arches
  footwear 420
  longitudinal, collapse 44
  in pes cavus 71–2
  in pes planovalgus 420
  weight-bearing 19–21
Arterial disease, diabetes 181–2
Arteriography in diabetes 184
Arthritis 165–72
  juvenile chronic 77, 132
  seronegative 170, 172
  see also Rheumatoid arthritis
Arthrodesis
  in calcaneum fractures 242
  complications 403,404
  in congenital talipes equinovarus
    70
  first metatarsophalangeal joint, hallux
    valgus 107
    combined with arthroplasty 112
  in hallux rigidus 122–4
    complications 122
    methods 123–4
  in hammer toe 148
  in pes cavus 73
  in pes planovalgus 59
  radiography 399
Arthroplasty
  complications 405
  in hallux rigidus 124
    Keller's 107–10, 114, 115, 124
    Mayo's 110–11
    Mayo's combined with
      osteotomy 111
Athlete's foot 442–3
Athletics and natural selection 2–3
Atopic eczema 158

B

Balmoral galosh   413
Basal osteotomy in hallux valgus   100–3
  combined with arthroplasty   111
Beak fractures, calcaneum   210, 215, 216
Bean-shaped foot in clubfoot   66
Big feet, causes   367–8
Biphalangism   313–16
Blair operations, modified, avascular
      necrosis, talar
      fracture-dislocation   271
Bone(s)
  changes and function   3–4
  evolutionary changes   3–4
  structure   19–22
    accessory bones   21–2
    weight-bearing   19–21
  tumours, radiology   352–60
  types   354
Bony exostosis (bursitis) and
      footwear   423
Boot
  Denis Browne   67, 68
  Derby front   414
  Galosh Balmoral   413
Bunion
  and footwear   421
    in hallux valgus   92
  see also Hallux valgus
Bunionette   115–16, 165
  radiography   394
Burgess operation in diabetic
    amputation   190, 191
Bursa
  adventitious   145
  around heel   129
    peritendinitis   129
    'winter heel'   129
  intermetatarsophalangeal   140
Bursitis
  footwear   423
  hypertrophic   141
  rheumatoid   141–2

C

Calcaneonavicular bar,
    radiography   395, 396
Calcaneum apophysitis   76
Calcaneum, fractures   205–43
  anatomy   205

  anterior end   218–20
    anterosuperior   218–19
    comminuted   220
  beak   210, 215
  central   220–31
    additional lines   226–31
    comminuted   231
    displaced primary   221, 225, 226,
      234–43
    management   234–43
    secondary   222–31
    seesaw   224, 229, 230, 240
    sustentaculum tali   221, 224, 225
    trapdoor   222, 227, 228, 240
    undisplaced primary   220, 222, 223,
      232, 235
  in children   231–2, 233
  classification   205, 210, 213
  incidence   210, 214
  management   234–43
    closed reduction   237, 238, 240
    conservative   236, 240
    disability, residual, sources   234
    early mobilization   237, 238
    end result, factors influencing   235
    late operative procedures   242–3
    manipulation   237, 238
    open reduction   237, 238, 241
    plaster cast   237
    recovery time   239
    traction   237, 238
  posterior end (tuberosity)   210–18
    posteromedial process   216
    posterior primary   216–18
    posterosuperior avulsion   210, 215
    vertical   217, 219
  ossification, radiology   313
  Paget's disease   131–2
  radiography   388–9
  radiology   205, 206–10
  rheumatoid arthritis   323–9
  spurs, footwear   423
  stress   232–4
  trabecular pattern   8
Callosities, plantar   152–3
  chiropody   433, 434
  in claw toes   148
  treatment   136
Cerebral palsy   193–5
Chevron osteotomy, hallux valgus   106
Chiropody   175–6, 430–47
  training   430–1
  treatment   431–47

Chiropody, treatment (cont.)
    bunions 437–8
    corns, plantar 431, 432, 434
    digital corns 434–5
    foot dysfunction 438–40
    foot strain 440–1
    gait dysfunction 438
    insoles 432
    interdigital lesions 435–7
    metatarsal heads 431–2
    nails 442–7
    plantar callosities 432, 433–4
    systemic manifestations 441–2
Christmas disease 173
Claw feet, footwear 424
Claw toes 148–50
  in diabetes 178–80
    treatment 186
  in paraplegia 201
  radiography 389, 391, 396
Clubfoot *see* Congenital talipes
    equinovarus
Congenital hypotonia 58
Congenital metatarsus adductus and
    varus 61–3
  differential diagnosis 61
  fixed adductovarus and valgus 63
  treatment 61–3
Congenital pes cavus
  see Pes cavus
Congenital talipes calcaneovalgus 71
  associated conditions 71
  differentiation 59
  footwear 422–3
  manipuation 71
Congenital talipes equinovarus 63–70
  anatomy 63–4
  associated conditions 64
  conservative treatment 66–7
  differential diagnosis 59, 61
  footwear 67, 68, 421
  incidence 64
  manipulation 65–6
  midfoot horizontal breach
      (bean-shape) 66
  neurological associations 64–5
  in paraplegia 201
  radiographic assessment 66, 69, 380
  rocker-bottomed foot 59, 66
  splintage 65–6
  surgical treatment 68–70
    complications 404
  treatment 65–70

uncorrected 66, 68
Congenital vertical talus 59–61
  associated disorders 55
  differential diagnosis 59
  features 55–7
  incidence 59
  treatment 61
Contact eczema 158
Contractures
  aponeurosis 138
  Volkmann's ischaemic
      contracture 139
Corns 153
  digital, chiropody 434–5
  plantar, chiropody 434
Crush fractures, midtarsus 280
Cuneiform fracture, radiology 352
Cuneometatarsal joint in hallux
    valgus 91–2
Curretage, plantar wart 152, 153
Cushing's disease 175
Cyst
  aneurysmal bone, radiology 358–9
  bone, simple, radiology 359
  epidermoid 145
  rheumatoid 145–6
  sole 144–5

D

Dactolysis spontanea, foot in 369
Davies–Colley arthroplasty in hallux
    rigidus 124
Denis Browne hobble boots and bar 67,
    68
Dermatitis, peridigital 158
Dermatophytes 155
Dermatosis, juvenile plantar 158
Diabetes 176, 177–92
  aetiology 177–83
  amputation 182, 187
  amyotrophy 181
  arterial disease 181–2
  arteriography 184
  chiropody 441
  combined lesions 182
  Doppler scanning 184
  footwear 186
  infection 188–90
    ischaemic 189
    neuropathic 189–91
  load distribution 46

Diabetes (cont.)
  neuropathy   177–81
  radiography   183–4
  radiology   346–50
    atheromatous calcification   349
    osteopathy   347
    peripheral neuropathy   347
    pointed tubular bone   343, 348
  sepsis   177
  treatment   185–91
    conservative   186–7
    operative   188–91
    prophylactic   185–6
Dislocations
  interphalangeal joints   297–8
  metatarsophalangeal joints, great
      toe   296
  talus   262–4
  see also Talus and peritalar injuries
Distal osteotomy in hallux valgus   103
Doppler scanning in diabetes   184
Dupuytren's contracture (plantar
      fibromatosis)   138

                E

Eczema   157–8
Ehlers–Danlos syndrome   58
Ellis osteotomy, hallux valgus   101
Enchondroma, radiology   355
Endocrine problems   175
Endogenous eczema   157
Epidermoid cyst   145
Equinovarus deformities,   see Congenital
      talipes equinovarus
Erosions in rheumatoid arthritis,
      radiology   319
  calcaneum   323–9
Eversion   23
Evolution   1–18
  adaptation   1–2
  comparative anatomy   2–6
  fossil record   9–16
  functional correlation   6–9
  natural selection   1–2
Ewing's tumour, radiology   356–7
Examination of the foot   50–4
  ankle   53
  circulation   52
  gait   50
  heel   51
  joints   52, 53

  midtarsal joint   53
  movements   53–4
  normal newborn   50
  in recumbency   51
  subtalar joint   52
Exostectomy in hallux valgus   112
Exostosis, bones   423
  osteocartilaginous, radiology   354
  subungual   150

                F

Faraboeuf amputation   189, 190
Fasciitis, plantar   137
Fibromatosis, plantar   138
Flail feet, footwear   423
Flat foot,   see Pes planovalgus, peroneal
      spastic flat foot
Flexion-extension movements   24
Foot
  examination   50–4
  function   19–30
  in children   55–82
  mechanics   31–49
    methods of study   32–6
Footwear
  contact eczema   158
  in diabetes   186–7
  fittings   175–6
  in hallux valgus   87–8, 95
  in pes cavus   73
  in pes planovalgus   57, 58, 67, 69
  surgical   410–29
    alterations   420, 421
    history   410–11
    leather   414
    Microcellular   415, 417, 421
    in partly amputated foot   425–9
    Plastazote shoes   410–20, 422–30
      see also Plastazote shoes
    in unequal leg length   424
    Yampi   411, 417
Force distribution measurement   34–6
Force plates   33
  modification   35
Fossil records   9–16
  bipedalism   11
  chronology   10–11
  hominid sites   11–13
  measurements   13
  photoelastic stress   13

Fracture-dislocations
  midtarsal joint   274
    navicular   280
  talus   257–62
    see also Talus and peritalar injuries
Fractures   203–304
  calcaneum   205–43
    see also Calcaneum, fractures
  complications   204
  diagnosis   203
  joints   204
  metatarsal   292–6
  midtarsus   272–82
    see also Midtarsal injuries
  sesamoids   150–1
  severe trauma   204
  shape of foot   204
  skin   203
  stress   140–1
    midtarsus   281–2
  talus and peritalar   243–72
    see also Talus and peritalar injuries
  tarsometatarsal region   283–92
Fungal infections   442–3

G

Gait
  cycle   25–6
  kinematics   32
Giant-cell tumour, radiology   356–7
Girdlestone's operation, hallux
    valgus   112
Glomus tumour   150
Gout
  footwear   423
  and pseudogout   172
Gryphotic nails   446, 447

H

Haddar, hominid specimens   11–15
Haemophilia   173
Hallux rigidus   116–24
  aetiology   116–19
  arthrodesis   122–4
  arthroplasty   124
  callosity   136
  childhood   78
  clinical features   119
  familial pattern   118

foot shape   117
metatarsus elevatus   117
osteochondritis dissecans of first
    metatarsal head   116
osteotomy   121–2
pathology   119
radiography   118, 120–1
trauma   116–17
treatment   121–4
  conservative   121
  surgery   121–4
Hallux valgus   83–115
  aetiology   84–9
  bunion   92
  clinical features   94–8
  congenital   88
  conservative treatment   98
  cosmetic complaints   95
  definition   83
  epidemiology   85
  first cuneometatarsal joint   91–2
  first metatarsophalangeal joint   89–91
  foot pronation   87
  footwear   95, 421
    rocker-bar   422
  hallux rotation   93
  hereditary factors   84
  lateral toes   93
  in leprosy   344
  load distribution   44–6
  metatarsals   91–2
  metatarsus primus varus   84–6
  muscle imbalance   86–7, 92–3
  osteotomy, recurrence rate   85
  pain   94–5
  pathology   84–94
  physical signs   95–6
  radiography   384, 390
  rheumatoid arthritis   88–9, 165–6
    radiology   321
  sex incidence   84
  shod/unshod people   87–8
  stiffness   95
  surgery   98–115
    adolescent patients   113
    arthrodesis   107
    arthroplasty   107–11, 100
    combined operations   111–12
    complications   403, 405, 407
    exostosis excision   112
    intermetatarsal suture   112–13
    lateral toe operations   113
    older patients   114–15

Hallux valgus, surgery (cont.)
  osteotomy procedures   100–7
  over-correction   405
  policy   113–14
  recurrence   406
  salvage procedures   115
  silastic replacement   113
  soft tissue procedures   98–100
  young adults   114
symptoms   94
and toe amputation   89
treatment   98–115
X-rays   96–8
  classification   97
Hammer toes   146–8
  radiography   390
  surgical complications   406
Heel
  bumps, winter heel   129, 130
  in foot examination   51
  osteomyelitis   131
  pad thickness, health and
      disease   364–6
    in acromegaly   364–5
    racial differences   365–6
    trauma   77
  Paget's disease   131, 132
  pain, childhood   77
  painful, bursae   129
  peritendinitis   129
  pistol-grip   199
  spurs, rheumatoid arthritis,
      radiology   324–9
  tuberculosis   131
Hemiplegia   193, 198–9
  treatment   198–9
Hindfoot, pain, childhood   77
Hohmann's osteotomy, hallux
    valgus   103, 104
Hook foot   61
Hyperhidrosis   135, 158, 443
Hyperlaxity syndromes   173–4
Hypertrophy, nail   153
Hypostatic eczema   157
Hypotonia, congenital   58

I

Incisions, surgical   402–3
Inflammatory skin diseases   156–9
Ingrowing toe nail   154, 155
Insoles, metatarsal   186, 187

Intermetatarsal suture in hallux
    valgus   112
Intermittent claudication, in
    diabetes   182, 186
Inversion   23
Ischaemia, diabetic   182, 187, 188, 189

J

Joplin's sling procedure in hallux
    valgus   98, 99
Juvenile rheumatoid arthritis (chronic
    polyarthritis)   77, 132, 172
  radiology   333

K

Kaposi sarcoma   161–2, 371–4
Keller's arthroplasty
  in hallux rigidus   124
  in hallux valgus   107–10, 114, 115, 124
    combined with arthrodesis   112
    combined with osteotomy   111
    complications   400, 403, 405
Keratolysis, pitted   158–9
Kinematics of gait   32
Kinetics, foot   33
Kinetograph   35
Kohler's disease   77–8
Koobi Fora, fossils   15
  KNM-ER 3733, 406 and 1470   15

L

Laetoli, hominid specimens   11
Lambrinudi's operation for claw toes   148
Lapidus osteotomy, hallux valgus   101,
    104
Leprosy   199–200
  bony change, radiology   343–6
    lateral ray destruction   353
    pointed tubular bone   343–6
  chiropody   442
  lepromatous   200
  tuberculoid   200
Load distribution   40, 41, 43
  in diseased foot   44–7
Locomotion, and functional changes   3,
    4–5
'Lucy'   11, 15–16

M

McBride's conservative operation hallux
valgus 98, 99, 114
combine with arthroplasty 111
Macrodystrophia lipomatosa, and
overgrowth of foot bones 367–8
Madura foot 370–1
Mallet toes 147
see also Hammer toes
Marfan's syndrome 58
Mechanics, foot 31–49
methods of study 32–6
Melanoma, malignant 159
amelanotic 160
subungual 161
Melorheostosis 367, 368
Metastatic tumours, radiology 359
Metatarsal accessory bones 361–2
Metatarsalgia
childhood 78
footwear 423
Morton's 142–4
postoperative, after Keller's
procedure 115
Metatarsals in hallus valgus 91–2
Metatarsophalangeal joint
in hallus valgus 89–91
Reiter's syndrome 332
Metatarsus
adductus and varus, *see* Congenital
metatarsus adductus and varus
elevatus 117
fractures 292–6
direct trauma 294
fifth metatarsal, 293, 294–6
indirect trauma 294
neck with gross displacement 292,
295
stress 296
primus varus and hallux valgus 84–6
radiography 380
Microcellular in surgical footwear 415
Mid- and hindfoot rheumatoid arthritis,
radiology 322
Midtarsal joint, examination 53
Midtarsus injuries 272–82
classification 274
dislocations
incidence 275
isolated 281
lateral 275, 276, 277, 278
medial 275, 276, 277, 278

swivel 275–8
fracture-dislocation 274
navicular 280
fractures, crush 280
navicular tuberosity 278
navicular 278–9
incidence 275
results of treatment 282, 283
sprains 272–3
incidence 275
Mitchell's osteotomy in hallux
valgus 99, 100, 104, 105–6, 115
non-union 115
Morquio's disease 237
Morton's metatarsalgia 142–4, 401–2
Moulded baby syndrome 71
Movements
ankle 22–4
examination 53–4
Mulder's click 142
Muscle imbalance in hallux valgus 86–7,
92–3
Myelomeningocele 195–6

N

Nails
big toe, shedding 154
chiropody 442–7
cutting 445–7
dystrophies 153–6
fungal infections 443
gryphotic 446, 447
ingrowing 154
onychogryptosis 443–5
overcurvature 155
senile 155
Natural selection, foot 1–2
Navicular
disintegration, radiology 351
fracture 278–9
tuberosity, fracture dislocation 280
fracture 278–9
Neurofibromatosis, and overgrowth of
great toes 366–7
Neurological disorders affecting
foot 193–202
'Neuroma' 143
Neuropathies 174
arthropathy and pointed tubular
bone 342

Neuropathies (cont.)
  diabetic   177–81
    autonomic   181
    chronic (sensory)   178–9
    classification   178
    motor   181
    single nerve lesions   181
    subacute   180–1, 186
Neutron diffraction studies   9

O

Oblique osteotomy of metatarsal shaft, in
    hallux valgus   103
Olduvai hominid 8 (OH8)   12, 13–15
Oligohydramnios   71
Onychogryphosis   153, 443
Os intermetatarsium and hallux
    valgus   88
Ossification
  radiology   313
  of tendo-Achilles   130
Osteoarthrosis (osteoarthritis)   132,
    173
  talus   272
  subtalar joint   273
Osteoblastoma, benign   354
Osteocartilaginous exostosis,
    radiology   354
Osteochondritis dissecans of first
    metatarsal head   116
Osteochondritis, navicular   77–8
Osteochondrodystrophy   337
Osteogenesis imperfecta   58
Osteogenic sarcoma, radiology   356
Osteoid osteoma, radiology   353–4,
    355
Osteomyelitis
  heel   131
  talus   77
Osteoporosis, radiology   317–18
Osteotomy
  complications   403
    un-united   407
  in hallux valgus   100–7
    combined with arthroplasty
      111–12
  in pes cavus   73
  of the proximal phalanx in hallux
    rigidus   121–2
  wedge, in pes planovalgus   58, 59
Overcurvature, toe nails   155

P

Paget's disease, heel   131, 132
Pain, foot   129–63
  ankle   131
  childhood   76–9
    forefoot   78–9
    heel pad   77
    hindfoot   76
    juvenile chronic arthritis   77
    midtarsal region   77–8
  in hallux valgus   94–5
  heel   129–30, 131
  persistent, calcaneum fractures   242
  skin   151–62
  sole   134–45
  subtalar joint   132
  systemic disorders   164–76
  tendo-Achilles   130, 132–4
  toes   146–51
Paraplegia, traumatic   200–1
Peabody osteotomy, hallux valgus   103,
    104, 106
Peridigital dermatitis of children
    158
Peripheral neuropathy
  diabetic foot   347
  plantar muscle atrophy   139
Peritalar joint injuries   see Talar and
    peritalar joint injuries
Peritendinitis   129
Peritalar joint injuries   *see* Talar and
    peritalar joint injuries
Peritendinitis   129
Peroneal spastic flat foot   335–9
Pes arcuatus   72–3
Pes cavus   71–3, 174
  family history   71
  footwear   420
  surgical complications   403, 404
    overcorrection   404
Pes planovalgus   55–9
  accessory ossicle   54
  associated conditions   58
  categories   58
  definition   55
  differential diagnosis   59
  exercises   55
  family history   58
  footwear   420
    adjustments   57, 58
  infection   58
  peroneal spastic   337–8
    causes   337
    incidence   337
    see also Tarsal coalition

Pes planovalgus (cont.)
  positions 55–7
  in rheumatoid arthritis 321, 322
  treatment 58–9
  triple arthrodesis 59
  true 57–8
Phalanges, fractures 296–8
  metatarsophalangeal joints 296
    dislocation 296
Pistol-grip heel 199
Plantar
  callosities, chiropody 433, 434
  fascia 137–9
    contracture 138
    deep structures 138–9
    fasciitis 137
    fibromatosis 138
plantar warts 151–2
Plastazote shoes 410–20, 422–9
  characteristics 416
  in leprosy 412, 416, 426–9
  measurements, materials and
      methods 412–20
  in partly amputated foot 425–9
  procedure 417–20
  insoles 421, 423
  in rheumatoid arthritis 412, 416
  in specific disorders 421–30
  in ulceration 412, 417, 428–9
Pointed tubular bone 342–6, 349–50
  conditions causing 342
  diabetes 343, 347, 348, 349–50
  in leprosy 343–6
  and neuropathic arthropathy 342,
      349
  Raynaud's phenomenon 346
  rheumatoid arthritis 346
Poliomyelitis, anterior 199
Pompholyx, recurrent summer
      157
Pressure sores
  in diabetes 186, 188
  in paraplegia 200
Pressure transducers 34
Pronation 23
  in hallux valgus 87
Psoriasis
  and arthritis, radiology 329–31,
      333
    in children 335
  feet 156–7
  nails 156
Pulses, foot 26–7

R

Radiography 378–99
  adolescent (8 –18 years) 382–3
    forefoot 383–6
    hindfoot 386–9
  adult 389–99
    forefoot 389
    sesamoids 392–4
    subtalar joint 398–9
    tarsal bones 394–7
  infant (0–8 years) 378–82
    anteroposterior view 378, 379
    lateral view 378, 379–81
Radiology 305–78
  accessory bones 360–4
  children 333
  development, foot 313–16
  diabetes 346–50
    neuropathic destruction of
        tarsus 350–2
  normal foot 305–15
    anteroposterior
        measurements 314–15
    lateral measurements 309–10
    structures 305–12
  pointed tubular bone 342–6
  psoriasis and arthritis 325, 329–31
  Reiter's syndrome 325, 327, 329, 331–3
  rheumatoid arthritis 316–29
  tumours 352–60
Ray, lateral, destruction 352
  leprosy 353
Raynaud's phenomenon, pointed tubular
      bone 346
Reiter's syndrome 172
  radiology 325, 327, 329, 331–3
Rheumatoid arthritis 132, 165–72, 175
  advanced 169–70
  chiropody 441
  early 165
  footprint 167
  footwear 412, 416, 424–5
  and hallux valgus 88–9
  juvenile chronic (Still's disease) 132, 172
  later 165–9
  load distribution 46–7
  nodules 168
  Plastazote shoes 412, 416
  radiology 316–29
    abnormalities of aligment 320
    calcaneum 323–9
    erosions 319, 323–9

Rheumatoid arthritis, radiology (cont.)
    hallux valgus   321
    mid- and hindfoot   321
    osteoporosis   317–18
    secondary osteoarthritis   319
    soft tissues   317
    spurs   324
Rheumatoid bursitis   141–2
Rheumatoid cyst   145–6
Robert Jones
    operation for claw toes   148
    tendon transfer   73
Rocker-bar for hallux valgus   422
Rocker-bottomed foot, talipes
    equinovarus   59, 66

S

Sarcoma, Kaposi   371–4
Senile nail   155
Sepsis   177
Sesamoids
    causing pain   150–1
    fractures   151, 298–9
    in hallux valgus   90
    at metatarsal heads   361, 362–4
    radiography   392, 393
Sever's disease   76
Shoes   see Footwear
Silastic prostheses   403, 405
    of metatarsophalangeal joint, great
      toe   113
Silver's procedure, hallux valgus   100
Skew foot   61
Skin of foot, diseases   151–62
Soft tissue
    changes in rheumatoid arthritis   317
    injury   204
Sole, disorders   134–45
    anterior foot strain   140
    callosities   135–6
    chronic hypertrophic bursitis   141
    cystic swellings   144–5
    middle of the tread   139
    Morton's metatarsalgia   142–4
    plantar fascia   137–9
    rheumatoid bursitis   141
    stress fractures   140–1
    structure   139–140
    subcutaneous tissues   136–7
Spastic diplegia   195
Spina bifida occulta   196–8
    clinical presentation   197–8

    treatment   198
Spinal dysraphism   195–8
    clinical presentation   197–8
    treatment   198
Sprain, midtarsus   272–3
Spurs, heel (calcaneal)
    footwear   423
    in rheumatoid arthritis,
      radiology   324–9
Standing, foot in   40–4
    arches   43, 44
    distribution of body weight   40, 41, 43
    toes   42
Stamm combined procedure in hallux
    valgus   111
Steindler's procedure
    in aponeurosis contracture   138
    in clubfoot   73
Still's disease   see Juvenile rheumatoid
    arthritis
Streeter's bands   369
Stress fractures   140–1
    calcaneum   232–4
    metatarsals   296
    midtarsus   281–2
Subtalar joint
    arthrodesis   242
    disability, and calcaneum fractures,
      management   234, 235
    dislocations   245
    examination   52, 53
    pain, causes   132
    radiography   399
    rheumatoid arthritis radiology   322
Subungual exostosis   150
Supination   23
Surgery, complications   400–9
    failure to assess vascular state   402
    failure to clearly explain purpose of
      operation   402
    inadequate assessment   401
    incisions   402
    inevitable   400–1
    infections   401
    preventable   401–2
    swelling   400
    technical failures   402–9
Sweat glands, hyperhidrosis   135
Systemic disorders, painful foot   164–76
    examination   164–5
    history   164–5
    treatment   175–6
    see also specific diseases
Systemic sclerosis   172

T

Talipes
  calcaneovalgus 55, 56
  equinovarus, congenital *see*
    Congenital talipes equinovarus
Talus
  avascular necrosis, incidence 282
    results of treatment 271
  blood supply 264–8
    extra-osseous 264–8
    intra-osseous 268
  congenital vertical *see* Congenital
    vertical talus
  dislocations 262–4
    classification 244
    incidence 245
    peritalar 262–4
    results of treatment 265
    transcervical 258–60
  fracture–dislocations 257–62
    classification 244
    incidence 245
    results of treatment 265
    transcervical 258–60, 271
      management 260–2
    transcervical peritalar dislocation of
      tarsus 257, 260, 271
  fractures 243–57
    avulsion 243, 245, 246
    experimental 257
    management 260–2
  neuropathic destruction,
    radiology 351
  and peritalar injuries 243–72
    classification 244
    compound 269
  incidence 245
  inadequate reduction, redisplacement
    mal-union and delayed union 269
  infection 269
  osteoarthritis 272
  potential problems and
    treatment 268–72
    results of treatment 265
  skin 268–9
  processes 243–57
    head 247–8, 250
    lateral 243, 246, 247, 248, 249
    lateral/medial incidence 252
    osteochondral 249–53, 254
    posterior 243–6, 247
    transcervical 253–7, 271

transcorporeal 246, 251, 271
Tarsometatarsal
  injuries 283–92
    classification 284
    clinical picture 288
    dislocation 285, 286
      irreducible 291–2
    experimental work 285–8
    fracture-dislocation 287
    sprains 292
    treatment 288–9
    results 289
  joints, rheumatoid arthritis
    radiology 322
Tarsus
  accessory bones 361–2
  bones, radiography 394
  coalition 73–4
    acquired 337, 338
    axial view 338, 339
    calconeonavicular 335, 337
    congenital 337, 338
    diagrammatic representation 336
    double tube tilt 339
    incidence 337
    peroneal spastic flat foot 337–9
    primary signs 340–1
    secondary signs 341–2
    surgery 74
    talocalcaneal 335, 337
  joints 23–4
  neuropathic destruction,
    radiology 350–2
  transcervical peritalar
    dislocation 257–8
  tarsal tunnel syndrome 130
Tendo-Achilles
  and hallux valgus 88
  lengthening in cerebral palsy 194–5
    in hemiplegia 198–9
  ossification 130
  rheumatoid arthritis, radiology 323–7
    achillobursitis 326
  rupture 132–4
    complete 132–4
    partial 134
  xanthoma 130
Tendovaginitis, tibialis posterior 131
Tinea unguium 155
Toe(s) 146–51
  amputations, footwear 425
  anatomy 24–5
  function 25

Toe(s), anatomy (cont.)
   lengths, variations   24
  biphalangism   313–16
  claw   148–50
  curly congenital   74–6
   treatment   75–6
  examination   53
  fractures   292
   and metatarsal joints   292–6
   and phalanges   296–8
  hammer   146–8
   metatarsophalangeal dislocation
    296
  overlapping, congenital   74–6
   treatment   75–6
  in standing   42
  in walking   4
  see also Hallux rigidus, Hallux valgus
Transverse metatarsal arch
   radiography   393
Trethowan osteotomy, hallux valgus   101
Tropical feet   369–74
Tuberculosis, heel   131
Tumours
  bone, radiology   352–60
  classification of   354
  skin   159–62

V

Valgus deformities   59–61
Varus deformities   61–3
  heels radiography   381
  in hemiplegia   194
Volkmann's ischaemic contracture   139

W

Walking, foot in   36–40
  axial rotations   37, 38
  cycle   25–6, 37
  forces and joint movements   39–40
  gravity   36–7
  heel strike   34, 39
  pronation   37–8
  steps per minute   36
  toes   40
  torques   37, 39
Warts, plantar   151–2, 442–3
  differential diagnosis   152
  treatment   152
Wedge osteotomy in pes planovalgus   58,
  59
Weight-bearing   19–22
Werner's syndrome   172
Wilson's cone arthrodesis in hallux
  rigidus   123
Wilson's oblique osteotomy in hallux
  valgus   103, 114
Winter heel   130

Y

Yampi plastic in surgical footwear   411,
  417